Optimizing Health Monitoring Systems With Wireless Technology

Nilmini Wickramasinghe
Swinburne University of Technology, Australia & Epworth HealthCare, Australia

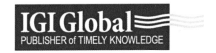

A volume in the Advances in Medical Technologies and Clinical Practice (AMTCP) Book Series

Published in the United States of America by
    IGI Global
    Medical Information Science Reference (an imprint of IGI Global)
    701 E. Chocolate Avenue
    Hershey PA, USA 17033
    Tel: 717-533-8845
    Fax: 717-533-8661
    E-mail: cust@igi-global.com
    Web site: http://www.igi-global.com

Library of Congress Cataloging-in-Publication Data

Names: Wickramasinghe, Nilmini, editor
Title: Optimizing health monitoring systems with wireless technology /
  Nilmini Wickramasinghe, editor.
Description: Hershey, PA : Medical Information Science Reference, [2019]
Identifiers: LCCN 2018010761I ISBN 9781522560678 (hardcover) I ISBN
  9781522560685 (ebook)
Subjects: I MESH: Monitoring, Physiologic I Wireless Technology I Wearable
  Electronic Devices I Telemedicine--methods I Cloud Computing
Classification: LCC R855.3 I NLM WB 142 I DDC 610.285--dc23 LC record available at https://lccn.loc.gov/2018010761

This book is published in the IGI Global book series Advances in Medical Technologies and Clinical Practice (AMTCP) (ISSN: 2327-9354; eISSN: 2327-9370)

British Cataloguing in Publication Data
A Cataloguing in Publication record for this book is available from the British Library.

For electronic access to this publication, please contact: eresources@igi-global.com.

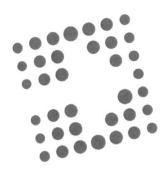

Advances in Medical Technologies and Clinical Practice (AMTCP) Book Series

Srikanta Patnaik
SOA University, India
Priti Das
S.C.B. Medical College, India

ISSN:2327-9354
EISSN:2327-9370

MISSION

Medical technological innovation continues to provide avenues of research for faster and safer diagnosis and treatments for patients. Practitioners must stay up to date with these latest advancements to provide the best care for nursing and clinical practices.

The **Advances in Medical Technologies and Clinical Practice (AMTCP) Book Series** brings together the most recent research on the latest technology used in areas of nursing informatics, clinical technology, biomedicine, diagnostic technologies, and more. Researchers, students, and practitioners in this field will benefit from this fundamental coverage on the use of technology in clinical practices.

COVERAGE

- Neural Engineering
- Nursing Informatics
- Medical Informatics
- Nutrition
- Patient-Centered Care
- Telemedicine
- Clinical High-Performance Computing
- Biomedical Applications
- Diagnostic Technologies
- Clinical Data Mining

IGI Global is currently accepting manuscripts for publication within this series. To submit a proposal for a volume in this series, please contact our Acquisition Editors at Acquisitions@igi-global.com or visit: http://www.igi-global.com/publish/.

Titles in this Series

For a list of additional titles in this series, please visit:
http://www.igi-global.com/book-series/advances-medical-technologies-clinical-practice/73682

Deep Learning Applications in Medical Imaging
Sanjay Saxena (International Institute of Information Technology, India) and Sudip Paul (North-Eastern Hill Universit, India)
Medical Information Science Reference • © 2021 • 274pp • H/C (ISBN: 9781799850717) • US $245.00

Design and Quality Considerations for Developing Mobile Apps for Medication Management Emerging Research and Opportunities
Kevin Yap (La Trobe University, Australia) Eskinder Eshetu Ali (Addis Ababa University, Ethiopia) and Lita Chew (National University of Singapore, Singapore)
Medical Information Science Reference • © 2021 • 256pp • H/C (ISBN: 9781799838326) • US $225.00

Expert Approaches to Health IT Tools in Clinical Practice
Ramgopal Kashyap (Amity University, Raipur, India)
Medical Information Science Reference • © 2021 • 300pp • H/C (ISBN: 9781799840510) • US $245.00

Opportunities and Challenges in Digital Healthcare Innovation
Kamaljeet Sandhu (University of New England, Australia)
Medical Information Science Reference • © 2020 • 261pp • H/C (ISBN: 9781799832744) • US $285.00

Mathematical Models of Infectious Diseases and Social Issues
Nita H. Shah (Department of Mathematics, Gujarat University, Ahmedabad, India) and Mandeep Mittal (Department of Mathematics, Amity Institute of Applied Sciences, Amity University, Noida, India)
Medical Information Science Reference • © 2020 • 316pp • H/C (ISBN: 9781799837411) • US $245.00

Nano-Strategies for Combatting Antimicrobial Resistance and Cancer
Muthupandian Saravanan (Mekelle University, Ethiopia) Venkatraman Gopinath (University of Malaya, Malaysia) and Karthik Deekonda (Monash University, Sunway Campus, India)
Medical Information Science Reference • © 2020 • 300pp • H/C (ISBN: 9781799850496) • US $285.00

Exploring the Role of ICTs in Healthy Aging
David Mendes (Universidade de Évora, Portugal) César Fonseca (Universidade de Évora, Portugal) Manuel José Lopes (Universidade de Évora, Portugal) José García-Alonso (Universidad de Extremadura, Spain) and Juan Manuel Murillo (Universidad de Extremadura, Spain)
Medical Information Science Reference • © 2020 • 292pp • H/C (ISBN: 9781799819370) • US $285.00

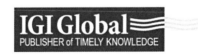

701 East Chocolate Avenue, Hershey, PA 17033, USA
Tel: 717-533-8845 x100 • Fax: 717-533-8661
E-Mail: cust@igi-global.com • www.igi-global.com

This book is dedicated to Goody, Aunty Damayanthi, and MM.

Editorial Advisory Board

Table of Contents

Detailed Table of Contents

Chapter 1
Nilmini Wickramasinghe, Swinburne University, Australia & Epworth HealthCare, Australia
Juergen Seitz, Baden-Wuerttemberg Cooperative State University, Germany

The novel coronavirus (SARS-CoV-2) first identified in Wuhan, China in late December 2019 was identified as a pandemic by the World Health Organization (WHO) in March 2020 and has caused tremendous disruption to economies around the world and significant loss of life and serious illness. The current outbreak which has been thought to have originated in an animal wet market in late 2019, being transferred from the horse shoe bat to the pangolin, is well adapted to human cell receptors. This enables it to easily infect people with an R0 of approximately 2.2 causing a respiratory illness (COVID-19) which can develop into pneumonia in moderate to severe cases. Older adults and people with underlying medical conditions are at higher risk. The following outlines a responsible digital health solution.

Chapter 2
Chinazunwa Uwaoma, Claremont Graduate University, USA
Clement C. Aladi, Claremont Graduate University, USA

The early months in 2020 saw a rapid increase in the adoption of mHealth and telehealth across the globe. The obvious reason being the sudden outbreak of coronavirus infectious disease (COVID-19), which sent the entire world scrambling for solutions to contain and mitigate the spread. Ordinarily, telehealth and mHealth are considered optional in most traditional healthcare systems even in developed countries, but today, these technologies have become the most sought-after tools required to augment the overwhelmed healthcare systems orchestrated by COVID-19. Mobile technology in particular has continued to play important roles in the monitoring, surveillance, and the assessment of the outbreak in so many ways. This chapter offers a window into different ways mHealth and telemedicine are used to provide healthcare services and disease management, as well as the challenges in the implementation of these technologies as the world braces for the devastating effects of COVID-19.

Chapter 3
Kodieswari A., Bannari Amman Institute of Technology, India

Cancer disease is the second largest disease in the world with high death mortality. Cancer is an abnormal growth of a normal cell. There are more than 100 types of cancer like blood cancer, brain cancer, small intestine cancer, lung cancer, liver cancer, etc. The type of cancer can be classified by the type of cell which is initially affected. When cancer grows it does not show any symptom. The symptom will appear when the cancer cell grows in mass and the symptom of cancer depends on the type of cancer. The cause of cancers is environmental pollutants, food habits, inherited genetics, tobacco, stress, etc., but in practice, it is not possible to prove the cause of cancer since various cancers do not have specific fingerprints. After the heart attack, cancer is a second killer disease in India. The death mortality is high in cancer because in most of the cases it is identified at the final stage which causes more death. According to ICMR, among 1.27 billion Indian populations, the incidence of cancer is 70-90 per 100,000 populations and 70% of cancer is identified in the last stage accounting for high morality. There are many types of treatment to treat cancer and they are surgery, radiation therapy, chemotherapy, targeted therapy, hormone therapy, stem cell transplant, etc. All cancer treatments will have side effects and the treatments will help only if the cancer cells are identified at the early stage. So time factor is important in diagnosing of cancer cells; hence, early detection of cancer will reduce the mortality rate. This chapter proposed the early detection of cancer cells using image processing techniques by the structure of circulating tumor cell. Early detection of cancer cells is very difficult because the concentration of cancer cells are extremely small and about one million malignant cell is encountered per billion of healthy cells. The circulating tumor cells, CTC, are shed into the bloodstream as a tumor grows, and it is believed these cells initiate the spread of cancer. CTC are rare, existing as only a few per one billion blood cells, and a highly efficient technology like chip-based biosensor platforms is required to capture the CTC, which in turn helps to detect cancer cell at an early stage before spreading. In proposed method, the circulating tumor cell has used a marker to detect cancer at early stage.

Chapter 4
Nalika Ulapane, Swinburne University of Technology, Australia
Nilmini Wickramasinghe, Swinburne University of Technology, Australia & Epworth
HealthCare, Australia

The use of mobile solutions for clinical decision support is still a rather nascent area within digital health. Shedding light on this important application of mobile technology, this chapter presents the initial findings of a scoping review. The review's primary objective is to identify the state of the art of mobile solution based clinical decision support systems and the persisting critical issues. The authors contribute by classifying identified critical issues into two matrices. Firstly, the issues are classified according to a matrix the authors developed, to be indicative of the stage (or timing) at which the issues occur along the timeline of mobile solution development. This classification includes the three classes: issues persisting at the (1) stage of developing mobile solutions, (2) stage of evaluating developed solutions, and (3) stage of adoption of developed solutions. Secondly, the authors present a classification of the same issues according to a standard socio-technical matrix containing the three classes: (1) technological, (2) process, and (3) people issues.

The prevalence of diabetes type 2 among the population and the increasing rate of new diagnoses as well as other co-morbidities make it imperative that we develop a richer understanding of type 2 diabetes. An Australian survey of diabetes type 2 people for different co-morbidities was carried out to obtain information about the possible connections of the co-morbidities with type 2 diabetes. The analysis is done with the logit model and Pearson's chi-square and the results indicate that gender, age of the patients, and the duration of the diabetes type 2 diagnosis play a significant role in the exposure of individuals to different comorbidities. The influence of the duration of diagnosis and age of the patients is limited in comparison to the gender, which has females at a very high risk of developing the studied co-morbidities compared to males. The findings can improve diabetes type 2 management to boost high quality, proactive, and cost-effective caregiving for the patients.

Chapter 6

Diabetes is one of the most significant global health emergencies affecting populations in the 21st century, where one out of 15 adults has type II diabetes. Impaired glucose tolerance contributes to more than half of all causes of diabetes. Further, depression has adverse economic and health outcomes. The condition also contributes to poor outcomes in screening efforts among type II diabetes patients. E-health intervention is one of the means for reducing depression. There is, therefore, a need to investigate whether the strategy effectively reduces depression among patients with type II diabetes. The research examined the e-health interventions, which include personal health records (PHRs), diabetes mobile apps, patient portals, information repositories, telehealth, and electronic health records (EHRs). The research findings indicated that e-health would significantly help in reducing depression among people with type II diabetes.

Type II diabetes is a rapidly growing non-communicable chronic disease that is causing significant concern to healthcare systems around the world. As there is no foreseeable cure, the most effective solution is to focus on strategies to control blood glucose levels by regular monitoring of diet, exercise, and when necessary, medication management. In today's environment, to do so effectively necessitates the need for a personalised self-management technology solution which can help patients take control of their diabetes. This chapter presents initial data from a research in progress study focused on designing a personalised diabetic application. The authors proffer a design science research methodology (DSRM) approach to design, develop, and ultimately, evaluate a patient-centric diabetes platform. This application is not only a smart patient empowering solution which serves to guide patients and assist their care team with regard to diet, exercise, medication and their respective impacts on blood sugar levels but is also designed to be culturally sensitive.

Chapter 8

Saranya Vasanthamani, Sri Krishna College of Engineering and Technology, India
S. Shankar, Hindusthan College of Engineering and Technology, India

The wireless body area network (WBAN) consists of wearable or implantable sensor nodes, which is a technology that enables pervasive observing and delivery of health-related information and services. The network capability of body devices and integration with wireless infrastructure can result in pervasive environment deliver the information about the patients to health care service providers. WBAN has a major part in e-health observing system. Due to sensitivity and critical of the data carried and handled by WBAN, reliability becomes a critical issues. WBAN loads a high degree of reliability as it openly affects the quality of patient observing. A main requirement is that the health care professionals receive the monitored data correctly. Thus reliability can be measured to achieve reliable network are fault tolerance, QoS, and security. As WBAN is a special type of WSN. The objective is to achieve a reliable network with minimum delay and maximum throughput while considering power consumption by reducing unnecessary communication.

Chapter 9

Reima Suomi, University of Turku, Finland
Eila Lindfors, University of Turku, Finland
Brita Marianne Somerkoski, University of Turku, Finland

Cardiovascular diseases are a leading death cause in the world. Cardiac arrest is one of the most usual, and very quickly fatal, especially in out-of-hospital environments. Defibrillation, aside with cardiopulmonary resuscitation, is an effective means to restart blood circulation and heart operation, even though even these forms of treatment can help just in sadly few situations. Defibrillation was invented and first demonstrated already year 1899, but first in the 2000s portable defibrillators with good automatic functions started to penetrate daily environments of people, especially in urban settings. Nowadays the starting point is that every citizen with normal human functionality should be able to use automated defibrillators. The chapter discusses how modern information and communication technology, especially mobiles services, internet, and location services based on them, could help citizens in the first crucial step in implementing their safety competence in emergency situations by using automatic defibrillators if they could only find them.

Chapter 10

Rima Gibbings, UIC, USA
Nilmini Wickramasinghe, Swinburne University, Australia & Epworth HealthCare, Australia

Care delivery services have been traditionally dependent on direct encounters between providers and patients. With the increase in the number of aging population and the added demand for most expensive and advanced care delivery services, healthcare organizations are investing in care services that are more effective and less costly. Use of technology in healthcare systems has been a significant driver for care improvement initiatives used for controlling cost and extending care delivery services that enhance healthcare accessibility. Implementing technology in healthcare demands proper alignment between newly developed tools and care delivery system needs. In this chapter, the authors discuss the role of technology in healthcare and the value of mHealth in diverse clinical settings.

Chapter 11

Martinson Q. Ofori, Dakota State University, USA
Omar F. El-Gayar, Dakota State University, USA

Access to the internet and the proliferation of mobile phones has resulted in a rising trend of mobile apps developed for disease self-management. This use of mobile health technology (mHealth) is viewed as an effective way to induce health behavior change. The authors conducted an evidence review of articles published in PubMed/Medline, Web of Science, and ACM Digital Library between January 2015 and January 2020 that developed and evaluated mHealth apps informed by behavior change theory. A total of 31 studies reviewed developed apps to encourage physical activity, dietary changes, diabetes, Alzheimer's disease, and others. The prevalent way of applying behavior theory to apps was through behavior change techniques (BCT) applied in 45% of the selected studies. Over 54% of the selected studies reported positive outcomes in inducing health behavior change. The results indicate that the use of behavior change theory to inform application design will result in statistically significant effects in improving health outcomes of a condition.

Chapter 12

Samaneh Madanian, Auckland University of Technology, New Zealand
Reem Abubakr Abbas, Auckland University of Technology, New Zealand
Tony Norris, Auckland University of Technology, New Zealand
Dave Parry, Auckland University of Technology, New Zealand

The increasing penetration of smartphones and their ability to host mobile technologies have shown valuable outcomes in disaster management; albeit, their application in disaster medicine remains limited. In this chapter, the authors explore the role of mobile technologies for clinical applications and communication and information exchange during disasters. The chapter synthesizes the literature on disaster healthcare and mobile technologies before, during, and after disasters discusses technological and operational aspects. They conclude by discussing limitations in the field and prospects for the future.

Chapter 13

Anitha Mary, Karunya University, India
Jegan R., Karunya Institute of Technology and Sciences, India
Suganthi Evangeline, Karunya Institute of Technology and Sciences, India

In today's world, people are most concerned about their health and safe living especially bed ridden people needing extensive care and assistance. A strict routine has to be followed by the patients after operation. Wearable sensors play an important role in monitoring physiological signals for the patient at home. With wireless technology, these physiological parameters can be monitored continuously. Also, the medical staffs and doctors are given immediate warning and causality services can be provided as early as possible. This chapter addresses the importance of wireless technology in healthcare sector.

Chapter 14

    Oleg Victorovich Sytnik, A. Ya. Usikov Institute for Radiophysics and Electronics of the
        National Academy of Science of Ukraine, Ukraine

The problem of detecting and identifying the heat transfer processes in living tissues using a noninvasive ultrasound technique is discussed. An optimal method, which is optimal in terms of maximum of likelihood, is proposed to detect the temperature variations within internal layers of the living tissue. The properties of signals returned from different tissues are examined. The ultrasound velocity for different temperatures and the salt composition of a specimen under study is estimated. Results of the algorithm simulation are given.

Chapter 15

    Eeva Kettunen, University of Jyvaskyla, Finland
    Markus Makkonen, University of Jyvaskyla, Finland
    Tuomas Kari, University of Jyvaskyla, Finland
    Will Critchley, University of Jyvaskyla, Finland

Life-long physical activity patterns are established during teenage years, so promoting physical activity is important. Sport and wellness technology has potential for promoting physical activity. Yet, research concerning its use among teenage populations is sparse. This intervention study investigated whether using a sport and wellness technology application could affect teenagers' physical activity intention, its antecedents, and the effects of these antecedents on intention. The study uses the theory of planned behavior (TPB) combined with self-efficacy as a theoretical model. The results showed no statistically significant difference between the intervention and control group in terms of the means and variances of the four constructs (attitude, subjective norm, self-efficacy, and intention) in the theoretical model. However, there was a statistically significant difference in the effect of self-efficacy on intention in the intervention group. Using sport and wellness technology in physical activity interventions among teenagers has potential and further research is warranted.

Chapter 16

    Nilmini Wickramasinghe, Swinburne University, Australia & Epworth HealthCare, Australia
    Vijay Geholt, Vilanova University, USA
    Elliot Sloane, Vilanova University, USA
    Philip James Smart, Austin Health, Australia
    Jonathan L. Schaffer, Cleveland Clinic, USA

Healthcare delivery is facing multiple orthogonal challenges around escalating costs and providing quality care, especially in OECD countries. This research examines the opportunity to leverage Health 4.0 technology and techniques to address the post-operative discharge phase of the patient journey. In so doing it serves to proffer a technology enabled model that supports not only a quality care experience post discharge but also prudent management to minimize costly unplanned readmissions and thereby subscribe to a value-based care paradigm. The chosen context is stoma patients but the solution can be easily generalized to other contexts. Next steps include the conducting of clinical trials to establish proof of concept, validity, and usability.

The current management to prevent Protein Energy Malnutrition (PEM) is examined and the use of technological tools such as Electronic Health Records (EHR) systems and mobile solutions are employed to prevent the development of PEM and its complications. Implementation of technological solutions in healthcare is a critical factor in achieving better health outcomes as documented in some parts of the world. Sub-Saharan Africa is behind on the adoption of electronic health records and other health information technology solutions due to several challenges such as lack of funding and infrastructure required to implement its use. Recent studies show that Sub-Saharan Africa is slowly gravitating towards adoption of health information technology particularly EHR systems and mobile solutions because of the need to find solutions to its healthcare crisis. Development of a PEM prevention system using these tools to enhance the current management will improve patient health outcomes and decrease the mortality rate of PEM.

Elderly population in the Asian countries is increasing at a very fast rate. Lack of healthcare resources and infrastructure in many countries makes the task of provding proper healthcare difficult. Internet of things (IoT) in healthcare can address the problem effectively. Patient care is possible at home using IoT devices. IoT devices are used to collect different types of data. Various algorithms may be used to analyse data. IoT devices are connected to the internet and all the data of the patients with various health reports are available online and hence security issues arise. IoT sensors, IoT communication technologies, IoT gadgets, components of IoT, IoT layers, cloud and fog computing, benefits of IoT, IoT-based algorithms, IoT security issues, and IoT challenges are discussed in the chapter. Nowadays global epidemic COVID19 has demolished the economy and health services of all the countries worldwide. Usefulness of IoT in COVID19-related issues is explained here.

Foreword

It is indeed a pleasure to write a foreword for this book. The topics addressed are extraordinarily relevant given the issues we face locally and globally in an era of increased challenges and rapid change. Healthcare is an especially complex domain that is important to all of us and will continue to be at the forefront of societal challenges. Wellness is multi-faceted and requires attention to a wide range of issues. Tensions and tradeoffs abound in the consideration and creation of robust systems.

Wireless technology use in conjunction with health monitoring systems is widely recognized as a key component of solution strategies for a myriad of contemporary problems. People, processes and technology all work together and are intertwined in the creation of robust systems that transcend time and enable rapid adaptation to change. Technology continues to evolve to meet changing needs and opportunities.

The socio-technical focus taken in this book enables consideration of a wide range of social as well as technical aspects of systems aimed at becoming used and useful and able to adapt to changing circumstances. I well remember conversations with Eric Trist and Enid Mumford that long ago influenced my own thinking and broadened my horizons of consideration at a crucial time in my personal development.

COVID-19 is not the first pandemic the world has grappled with nor will it likely be the last. Further, a wide range of chronic and other diseases will present continuing healthcare and wellness challenges. The need for health systems making good use of wireless technology will only increase and presents opportunities for application that we are only beginning to appreciate.

The chapter authors represent a broad range of backgrounds and perspectives which adds to the value and credibility of the book in promoting broad-based readership and impact. The insights based on peer-reviewed research provide a level of credibility and robustness rarely witnessed in a book. At the same time, the book encourages forward thinking to influence policy that can effectively and efficiently deal with the future.

Douglas R. Vogel
City University of Hong Kong, China

Preface

Never before has healthcare and wellness of people been more important. The defining moment of 2020 without a doubt has been the COVID-19 pandemic. With the impacts of the virus affecting countries all over the world, top of all agendas has been navigating the health and wellbeing of individuals, families, communities and citizens. A key enabler during this dark hour has been without a doubt digital health solutions. In particular, mobile and wireless solutions have served as a beacon of hope, like a light house shining a bright light to help navigate to a safer better future.

Even before COVID-19, healthcare delivery in all OECD countries was facing tremendous challenges around escalating cost of care, an aging population and longer life expectancy which from a healthcare delivery perspective translates to even more complex and expensive healthcare interventions and the rapid rise of chronic conditions which in turn adds a further burden to a troubled healthcare system. Now with COVID-19 and looking to a post COVID-19 environment, these challenges are even more heightened. But as the COVID-19 pandemic has highlighted with our digital health technologies and most especially mobile and wireless initiatives, it is possible to deliver superior quality care, provide targeted preventative strategies, almost ubiquitous access efficiently, effectively and high value.

However, to do this on an ongoing basis we need to reexamine current practices, processes and people issues so that at all times we can leverage the best results from our digital health solutions. There are many lessons to be learnt form COVID-19 but one thing that is clear post COVID-19 we need a new dawn for healthcare delivery and wellness support that is enabled, supported and leveraged by the latest innovations and developments in digital health.

Optimizing Health Monitoring Systems With Wireless Technologies is a definitive volume that serves to shine light on the possibilities for mobile and wireless solutions to support and enable superior healthcare and heightened wellness strategies in a post COVID-19 healthcare world. This volume provides insights from research conducted in various countries that delves into critical issues around effecting better processes, addressing key people issues and maximizing advances in technology solutions. This socio-technical focus that is integral to the books structure and all the 18 chapters therein and serves to ensure that in all initiatives a patient/people perspective is kept front and centre to ensure optimizing of health monitoring systems and sustained use which will ensure realization of their full benefits and value.

Specifically, the 18 chapters are as follows;

Chapter 1
How can Digital Health be best leveraged to provide optimal support during pandemics like the COVID-19 crisis? by Wickramasinghe and Seitz, presents how we can leverage digital health solutions to assist the delivery of care in pandemics like COVID-19.

Chapter 2

Mobile Technology Support for the Assessment and Management of COVID-19 Outbreak: Benefits and Challenges by Uwaoma and Aladi, also focusses on the COVID-19 pandemic and the key enabling role for mobile technology support.

Chapter 3

Early detection of cancer using Smartphone by Bannari discusses the opportunities for digital health solutions to assist with earlier and precise detection of cancer, a growing and troubling chronic condition that is impacting all countries throughout the world.

Chapter 4

Critical Issues in Mobile Solution based Clinical Decision Support Systems—A Scoping Review by Ulapane and Wickramasinghe begins to unpack critical issues for clinicians around decision making in real time and how digital health solutions can support superior decision making

Chapter 5

Comorbidities and Diabetes Type 2: A Gender-Driven Probabilistic Estimate of Patient's Risk Factor by Ossai et al focusses on another key and problematic chronic condition for the 21st Century; namely, that of diabetes and suggests strategies enabled by digital health solutions that will enable better risk mitigation for patients with diabetes.

Chapter 6

Depression Reduction For Patients With Type II Diabetes Via E-Health Interventions by Wong looks at the impact of diabetes and how e-health can assist in diminishing depression, a noted impact with longer term diabetes patients.

Chapter 7

Developing personalised diabetic platform using a Design Science Research Methodology by Joachim et al focusses on how to incorporate design science research methodology, user-centred design principles and co-creation to develop superior technology solutions that are more patient centric in nature.

Chapter 8

Lifetime Enhancement and Reliability in Wireless Body Area Network by Vasanthamani and Hindusthan looks at the possibilities for the design and development of wireless body area networks and their applicability for numerous health and wellness contexts.

Chapter 9

Location Information Services Of Automated External Defibrillators (AEDs): Location Information Services Of Automated External Defibrillators (AEDs) by Suomi et al discusses the benefits of having automated external defibrillators at the ready to assist as and when required in situ.

Chapter 10

MHealth and Care Coordination by Gibbings and Wickramasinghe identifies the critical role of holistic care coordination enabled through mobile solutions to provide superior care delivery.

Chapter 11

Mobile Applications for Behavioral Change: A Systematic Literature Review by Ofori and El-Gayar presents critical issues around the importance of ensuring appropriate and sustained behavior change vis mobile applications.

Chapter 12

Mobile Technologies in Disaster Healthcare: Technology and Operational Aspects by Madanian et al. provides critical insights into how mobile technologies can play vital enabling roles to deliver healthcare in emergency and disaster scenarios.

Chapter 13

Modern Health Care with Wearable Sensors and Wireless Technology by, Karunya et al. presents several opportunities for utilizing wearable and sensor solutions for assisting with health monitoring and care delivery.

Chapter 14

Non-invasive Active Acousto-Thermometer by Sytnik describes developments in non-invasive temperature assessments for various contexts.

Chapter 15

Sport and Wellness Technology to Promote Physical Activity of Teenagers: An Intervention Study by Kettunen et al. examines how technology can be used to promote sport and wellness activities especially for younger groups in the population.

Chapter 16

Using Health 4.0 to enable Post Operative Wellness Monitoring: the case of colorectal surgery by Wickramasinghe et al looks at the opportunities to support enhanced recovery after surgery through post operative wellness management enabled by developments in health 4.0.

Chapter 17

Protein Energy Malnutrition in Children -Prevention System by Onaleye identifies an opportunity for incorporating mobile solutions to assist vulnerable groups in the community so that a better health state can be realized.

Chapter 18

Health Care-Internet of Things and Its Components: Technologies, Benefits, Algorithms, Security and Challenges by Tyagi discusses key aspects around the Internet of Things and what aspects are significant for delivering superior healthcare and wellness initiatives.

Taken together, this miscellany of chapters covers the breadth of possibilities for digital health and in particular mobile and wireless solutions to assist, enable and support the delivery of superior healthcare care and wellness initiatives. As we enter the post COVID-19 world, healthcare and wellness have become more important than ever while we try to build back better. It becomes imperative that we focus on digital health solutions to enable us to effectively, efficiently and successfully cut the Gordian knot of providing access to all, high quality and optimal value care that is patient centred and personalized. While no book can be a comprehensive and definitive presentation of all that is required to succeed, this handbook goes a long way to meeting a key and current need to inform and advise scholars, researchers, practitioners, clinicians and allied health workers, regulators and policy makers, individuals and the community at large on the critical aspects around wireless and mobile technologies to deliver superior healthcare and wellness initiatives. Moreover, this handbook highlights critical issues around responsible design, development and deployment of digital health solutions; a critical success factor especially in today's dynamic and complex healthcare environment. It is my hope that all readers will find this a useful resource to guide them in the journey to ensure we have superior healthcare and wellness initiatives for all in a post COVID-19 world.

Nilmini Wickramasinghe
Swinburne University of Technology, Australia & Epworth HealthCare, Australia

Acknowledgment

This book would not be possible without the efforts of many people. First and foremost, a big thank you to all the authors who have contributed to this volume as well as the reviewers who gave their time to provide detailed and specific comments which have helped to enhance all the chapters within this compilation. I am also grateful to my institutions; Swinburne University of Technology and Epworth HealthCare, for affording me the time to work on pulling this volume together. I wish to express thanks to my colleagues around the world for time set apart for discussions of critical ideas and issues and their support and suggestions which have collectively made this work a quality work. In addition, and as always, thank you to my family. Lastly, I am particularly grateful to Jan and the team at IGI for their assistance and efforts in progressing this book project to publication. Especially during this COVID-19 time, we have all been under tremendous pressure and yet it has been possible to complete this project as planned and without delays which would not have been the case without everyone's support and efforts – thank you!

Chapter 1

How Can Digital Health Be Best Leveraged to Provide Optimal Support During Pandemics Like the COVID–19 Crisis?

Nilmini Wickramasinghe

ⓘ https://orcid.org/0000-0002-1314-8843

Swinburne University, Australia & Epworth HealthCare, Australia

Juergen Seitz

Baden-Wuerttemberg Cooperative State University, Germany

ABSTRACT

The novel coronavirus (SARS-CoV-2) first identified in Wuhan, China in late December 2019 was identified as a pandemic by the World Health Organization (WHO) in March 2020 and has caused tremendous disruption to economies around the world and significant loss of life and serious illness. The current outbreak which has been thought to have originated in an animal wet market in late 2019, being transferred from the horse shoe bat to the pangolin, is well adapted to human cell receptors. This enables it to easily infect people with an R0 of approximately 2.2 causing a respiratory illness (COVID-19) which can develop into pneumonia in moderate to severe cases. Older adults and people with underlying medical conditions are at higher risk. The following outlines a responsible digital health solution.

INTRODUCTION

In the first three months of 2020, we have witnessed country after country enforcing lock downs of various degrees of severity in an attempt to flatten the curve and reduce the spread of COVID-19; a severe respiratory illness that has been deemed a pandemic by the WHO in March 2020 and has led to the death of thousands of people and the serious illness of many more. Current medications appear to have little impact in controlling and/or curing this disease and while we wait for the identification and

DOI: 10.4018/978-1-5225-6067-8.ch001

deployment of an appropriate vaccine, it is useful to identify suitable measures that can be taken to contain and slow down the spread of this deadly virus. We contend that digital health can offer us several solutions that can provide timely and facilitate the rapid containment and development of prevention strategies. The following serves to identify critical factors that must be considered in the design and development of such digital health solutions to enable maximum benefit and minis potentially negative unintended consequences.

BACKGROUND

Digital health, a relatively new and developing domain which lies at the confluence of medicine, computer science and business management is characterized by key sub-streams as follows (Wickramasinghe, 2019): 1) analytics, 2) augmented and virtual reality (AR/VR), 3) 3D printing, 4) sensors and 5) mobile and wireless solutions. Clearly, there are opportunities for all these areas to assist in the containment and prevention of COVID-19. For example: i) analytic techniques can be harnessed and applied to the multi-spectral data currently being generated around the world to develop surveillance networks or prediction models, ii) AR/VR solutions can be developed to support people from a distance and replace much face-to-face health interactions around many issues such as mental health and more especially anxiety or depression mood states, iii) 3D-printing can be harnessed to rapidly produce more equipment such as masks and ventilators and sensors can assist in particular older or disabled members of a community to manage more effectively while iv) telemedicine is effective to provide at a distance necessary and required healthcare advice and support. However, one area that has been seen to be particularly powerful during the initial months of the COVID-19 pandemic is the rapid development of mobile solutions and/or apps.

Mobile Apps

Currently, there are over 300,000 mobile apps both android and iOS available to support diet and exercise needs (Jimenez et al., 2019). This, in itself, highlights the appeal of such apps to the general population and the fact that there is a relatively low learning curve today for large sections of the community to adopt and use such apps. Moreover, such solutions provide anywhere, anytime support and advice which is particularly beneficial. However, it is important to note that while there are several thousands of apps available that focus on what can loosely be identified as wellness or prevention aspects, when it comes to healthcare or medical focus the uptake of such apps typically rapidly falls away. The major reason for this is around the high requirements in many (in particular) western countries for specific data privacy and security features (Trepte, et al., 2017). We acknowledge that security and privacy concerns are necessary and important but we question the impact such a focus has in terms of reducing the rapid development and deployment of appropriate solutions because of what might be considered "over regulation" around security and privacy. Hence, the research question guiding this inquiry is *How can we rapidly design, develop and deploy suitable digital health solutions for emergency and disaster situations?*

Fit Viability

From theory, it is possible to try to unpack the potential poor sustained use of mobile solutions in terms of poor fit. Proffer the fit-viability morel as a suitable analysis lens which combines the dimensions of fit viability and Task technology fit. Tjan (2001) proposed fit viability dimensions for evaluating Internet initiative projects. Liang and Wei (2004), incorporated these two dimensions with Task Technology Fit (TTF) theory, to develop the fit-viability model to study m-commerce applications. In this context, viability measures the readiness for the technology adoption and implementation, and fit measures capabilities of the systems to optimally perform the required tasks.

Task-Technology Fit

The theoretical basis of the fit construct is derived from the Task-Technology Fit model which according to Goodhue (1995; 1998) argues that a fit between task characteristics and system features needs to be high for the better performance and success. Research (Madapusi 2008; Soh et al. 2000) has indicated that if a system is more aligned with the requirements of the users then there is a greater likelihood of the system having sustained use; ie if the features offered by the system fit with the task requirements the users will be more inclined to continually use it.

Viability

Viability, in contrast, refers to the degree of impact of environment and other external or macro factors on the adoption and implementation decision for a system (Liang et al., 2007). These factors can include political and social, economic, environmental as well as infrastructure/technology factors. At the organizational level literature has proposed many factors at the strategic and tactical levels (Umble et al., 2003). These factors include leadership, management style, polices, information sharing, training and learning, technical staff, and user behaviour. Thus, in the context of mobile apps for addressing critical aspects around COVID-19, a fit viability assessment strongly suggests that it is essential that these solutions address key tasks be it who was in contact with whom to assist with disease containment and spread and that in doing so the technological aspects do not lead to other problems e.g. unintended consequences around privacy and security of personal / private information.

Case Vignettes

By March 2020, several countries had already started to develop and deploy mobile apps to assist with curbing and tracking the spread of COVID-19 as well as sharing important information.

Tracing apps from China (BBC, 2020) (Mehta, 2020), India (The Hindu, 2020) and South Korea (Ministry of Health and Welfare of South Korea, 2020) (Central Disaster and Safety Countermeasures Headquarters, CDSCHQ, 2020) are not acceptable in Western countries because they ask for personal data and observe the geographical location where the holder of the mobile device is. In Singapore the government knows, who the owner of a mobile device is. If somebody is in quarantine, he or she is asked from time to time to send photos from the environment to make sure that he or she is at home. (Ungku, 2020) (Government of Singapore, 2020) Similar features has the Taiwanese app. (Shan, 2020) (Chang, 2020) (Sander & Lemcke, 2020) In India and South Korea, even the neighborhood will be informed if somebody is infected. (The Hindu, 2020) (Ministry of Health and Welfare of South Korea, 2020) (Central Disaster and Safety Countermeasures Headquarters, CDSCHQ, 2020) The Australian government has come out with an app. The key features of this app include: (Australian Government, Department of Health, 2020)

- stay up to date with the official information and advice
- important health advice to help stop the spread and stay healthy
- get a quick snapshot of the current official status within Australia
- check your symptoms if you are concerned about yourself or someone else
- find relevant contact information
- access updated information from the Australian Government
- receive push notifications of urgent information and updates

There has been concern raised in some corners throughout Australia that especially given the rapid launch of this app how secure and private is the information and what is the potential for collected data to be misused or mishandled (The Guardian, 2020). Moreover, many question whether the public should blindly trust the government and how can we be confident that apps like these do address necessary security and privacy aspects.

Returning briefly to fit-viability, what these case vignettes highlight is that the fit with respect to all these app solutions appears, at face value at least, to be quite high; however, the question around the viability of these solutions is at best vague and difficult to assess at this time.

Method

To answer the posed research question, we adopt a mixed method approach. In particular, we perform a hermeneutic analysis of extant literature (Allen, 1995), including grey literature and media releases around the world and apply OODA thinking and Boyds OODA loop to rapidly synthesize these various multispectral data inputs and make sense in or der to then extract pertinent information and germane knowledge that can be used to develop a sound practice for rapidly designing, developing and deploying suitable digital health solutions in this context (Wickramasinghe and vin Lubitz, 2007).

The OODA Loop

What is "critical thinking"? What is "prudent decision making"? Both terms are typically connected to successful outcome sand sound leadership (ibid). Making a prudent decision without prior analysis of the essential characteristics of the event that requires making such decision is, obviously, a foolhardy approach to problem solving. It thus appears that critical thinking and decision making consist of two sub-elements each:

- Critical thinking – summary and analysis
- Prudent decision making - selection of action and implementation of action

The process of critical thinking and decision making has been analyzed and subsequently formalized by the late Col. John Boyd, USAF (ibid) who presented the results in the form of the famous "Boyd Briefing" given to countless politicians, military officers, and businessmen. Boyd's major achievement was the observation that essentially any form of human activity can be broken into four main subcomponents interacting with each other in a sequential, loop-like manner – the OODA Loop (Figure 1).

As can be seen in Figure 1, the Loop is based on a cycle of four critical and interrelated stages: Observation followed by Orientation, then by Decision, and finally Action. The cycle revolves both in

Figure 1. The OODA Loop by John Boyd
(adapted from Wickramasinghe and von Lubitz, 2007)

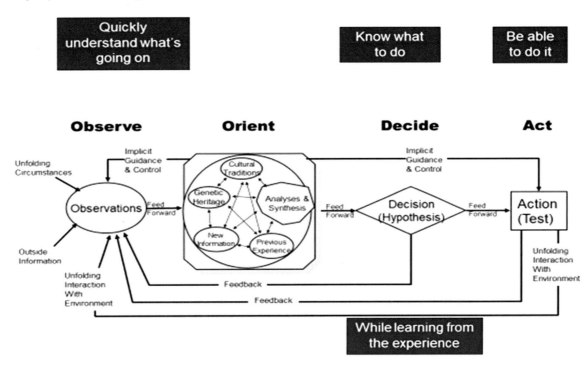

Defense and the National Interest, http://www.d-n-i.net, 2006

time and in space (ibid). Observation and Orientation stages of the Loop are its critical aspects at which the plurality of implicit and explicit inputs determines the sequential Decision- and Action steps (ibid). The outcome of the latter affects, in turn, the character of the next initiation point (Observation) in the forward progression of the rolling loop (Figure 1) The Orientation stage specifies the characteristics and the nature of the "center of thrust" (Boyd used the German expression "Schwerpunkt") at which the most significant activity is to concentrate and which, in turn, determines the specifics of the sequential stages (Determination and Decision – i.e., the definition of action to be taken, and Action – its specific execution)(ibid). However, the progression of the Loop is not linear – a commonly made error in the interpretation of its progression. It does not merely roll along the time axis - the stages within the Loop are simultaneous, delicately intertwined, and balanced (ibid). Action does not interrupt Observation, or Decision does not halt Orientation (ibid). The domain of the Loop is thus multidimensional, and embraces all constituents of the environment within which the Loop revolves. Time is only one of those elements.

Implementation of Boyd's OODA Loop-based training rapidly develops the art of critical thinking and decision-making. Importantly, it also provides the ideal solution to the dilemma of training these skills in a manner consistent with their practical use within a constantly changing environment of multiple situational inputs that are, in turn, characterized by their own temporal and physical instability.

The dynamic nature of the OODA paradigm makes it a pre-eminently suitable readiness development tool in the context of the frequently fluid business operations. However, the commonly employed pattern of training prevents such implementation. As already mentioned, today's "training" is based predominantly on didactic lectures or seminars that quite effectively eliminate the very active nature Observation and Orientation stages by predetermining their characteristics – in fact there is not much to observe or to orient, and everything is offered by the instructor. As a result, both stages are entirely static and the course of the sequential steps (Determination/Decision and Action) is enforced a priori. The result is a rigid, algorithmic training structure whose implementation produces be at best inconclusive and, at worst, entirely misleading lessons.

Suggested Infrastructure

As data privacy and security is an intangible good of high value data should be stored decentral on the mobile device only, which collects the data (GDPR, 2020). Similar to the PEPP-PT approach (PEPP-PT e. V. i. Gr., 2020) we do not store GPS data. GPS can be deactivated. GPS data in combination with timestamps allow building a detailed profile of the mobile device user. We also log only meetings. Mobile devices connect to each other using Bluetooth and/or other short distance transmission technologies. That means, they have to be activated. The mobile device broadcasts an ID. PEPP-PT: 'broadcasts over a short distance a temporarily valid authenticated and anonymous identifier (ID) that cannot be connected to a user'. The challenge is the generation of a globally unique ID that is independent of everything (GPS, time, device,…). Without a central institution, this is not possible. Coincidentally, always a number can be generated independently multiple times. Neither timestamp, nor GPS position allow uniqueness. Many people meet other people at the same time. The GPS position is not exactly enough and at different times, different people can meet at the same place. Only in combination with the device number uniqueness is possible. So, a mobile device generates ID integrating the device ID. However, this generated ID is never broadcasted or exchanged with anybody else. This ID is only stored in the storage of the mobile device. Broadcasted will be only a hash value of the ID. The ID is hashed by a cryptographic (collision resistant) hash algorithm, e. g., SHA-3. (Bertoni, et al., 2020) (NIST, 2012) Using a cryptographic hash algorithm means that it needs a lot of computing power and much time to find out the device ID. Only the mobile device owner can check an ID like checking digital signatures. (Menezes, van Oorschot, & Vanstone, 2001) (Menezes & Smart, 2004) (Schneier, 1995)

A person, who has an infection with a specified disease, has to report this according to German Infection Protection Law. In the law is defined which data have to be reported depending on the disease. In defined cases, the infected person has also to report which person has been met in a defined period. It is often hard to remember, which person were met in a period. Often people don't know who they met, especially in the case of spontaneous meetings like in a grocery store or a super market. People that are not known personally. That means that the list is usually not complete and health departments can only inform a subset of people. Especially in the case of a disease like COVID-19 with a longer incubation time this is critical. At the beginning, health departments have published places, e. g., ski resorts in Austria or Italy were probably many people were infected, and asked people to make appointments to get checked. This was not really effective, because most people don't know each other.

If an infection is confirmed and the person has to report to the health department additionally lists of received hashed IDs and broadcasted hashed IDs can be transferred to the health department without telling anything about the people that have been met. The health department stores these data in the data set of the infected person, but only the hashed IDs and the information, if it is a broadcasted or received ID of the infected person, will be published.

Figure 2. Groups of people and information channels

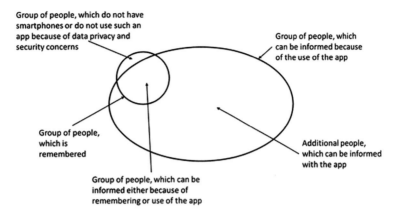

Everybody can download these data and the app checks if there was a contact with an infected person. If the downloaded hashed IDs contains hash values of broadcasted IDs in the list of received IDs and/or contains collected hash IDs in the list of broadcasted IDs of infected people this means that there was a contact with an infected person. An alert tells the mobile device owner what to do. Because of the risk of an infection, the mobile device owner should be motivated to talk to a doctor. It does not mean that an infection happened. If there is no match between the IDs stored on the own mobile device

Figure 3. Process of publication of hashed IDs in case of an infection

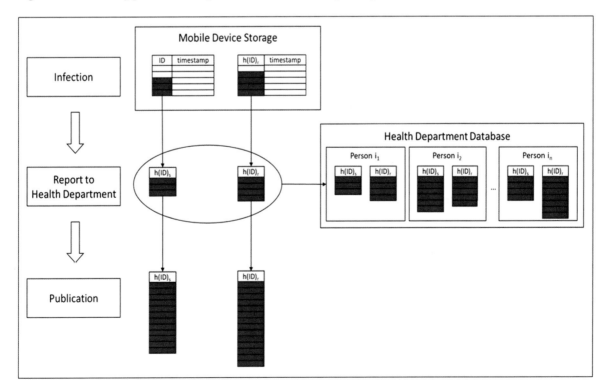

and the published data this is no guarantee that there is no infection, but the probability that there is no infection is much higher. It is also possible that there are several matches or a match only with one list. If there is a match only with one list the reason could be a very short meeting during that, there was not enough time that both parties send and receive an ID. If there are several matches, these matches are not necessarily from one other person. It could be a longer meeting with one person, but also a meeting with more people is possible. It does not matter.

Figure 4. Self-check of meetings with infected people

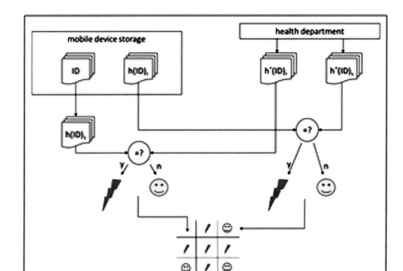

The app follows high data privacy standards. If there is an infection detected, the infected person gives only the own personal data to the health department. The app delivers only numbers, but not names of people, who were met in the last days. These numbers does not allow identifying other people. Other people can check if they have met an infected person. In their own interest, they call a doctor to check, if they are infected. If they are infected, they also have to report to the health department. From these numbers the health department can build chains who was in contact with whom. However, they can built these chains only with people, who have been diagnosed with the infection. From the pattern of infections, the health department is able to analyze later, if there were meetings that were very infectious. However, it is not known when and where this meeting took place.

DISCUSSION

The current pandemic of COVID-19 has served to illustrate the need for public health to be prepared and ready to support at large scale critical prevention and deployment of advice in such contexts so that correct, pertinent information and germane knowledge can be rapidly deployed. To do this effectively and efficiently mobile apps are essential. By briefly examining some of the mobile apps deployed in various countries it was possible to identify that these apps have been designed around key tasks connected with disease containment and spread and/or information provision to the population. The area that appears to be less well addressed has been around the viability of these solutions. In particular, we identified concerns around privacy and security. To address this element in an expeditious fashion we incorporated the principles of OODA thinking and design and developed a model to facilitate a better rapid development for data and information security and privacy. We contend that the model outlined above provides a robust yet agile rubric to design, develop and deploy suitable apps to address any/all emergency and disaster scenarios. In addition, by drawing upon task technology fit theory, we highlight the critical success criteria of strong fit to the specific task as a necessary condition for success.

An important aspect of public health and the interactions of people with their government during this pandemic period has been that of trust. For a population to embrace solutions and follow directives they must have a high level of trust with the government advice and protocols. This means that the mobile solutions designed and deployed to assist and ameliorate critical aspects around COVID-19 need to be designed in a responsible fashion.

Thus, this study also has a significant contribution to highlighting an important area with regards to IS research for healthcare contexts and that is its role in outlining an IS study that is focused on enabling a "better world" (Wickramasinghe, 2019). Given the impact of the COVID 19 pandemic and the number of people globally and the impact there is broad recognition that not only is COVID -19 a serious global health concern, but we need a solution for us to better manage social distancing and likely impacts and many countries are developing apps.

This initial research serves to highlight how we can do this rapidly to ensure the design, development and deployment of mobile apps for emergency and disaster scenarios such as COVID-19. We have answered the posed research question by proffering a model to address the rapid design and development of a suitable security/privacy infrastructure for the mobile apps that are being developed. In addition, we have suggested that it is necessary for such solutions to have a high fit with the specific tasks for which they are designed as well as having a high level of viability, in this way successful, rapid and sustained uptake of such mobile solutions is more likely to ensue. These are currently dynamic and challenging times for healthcare; however we are confident that digital health and health 4.0 hold some of the keys to successfully navigating this time as long as central to all solutions is a responsible approach to its design, development and deployment.

REFERENCES

Allen, D. (1995). Hermeneutics: Philosophical traditions and nursing practice research. *Nursing Science Quarterly*, *8*(4), 174–182. doi:10.1177/089431849500800408 PMID:8684726

Australian Government, Department of Health. (2020, March 31). *Coronavirus Australia app*. Retrieved May 17, 2020, from https://www.health.gov.au/resources/apps-and-tools/coronavirus-australia-app

BBC. (2020, February 11). *China launches coronavirus 'close contact detector' app*. Retrieved May 17, 2020, from https://www.bbc.com/news/technology-51439401

Bertoni, G., Daemen, J., Hoffert, S., Peeters, M., Van Assche, G., & Van Keer, R. (2020). Retrieved May 17, 2020, from Team Keccak: https://keccak.team/keccak_specs_summary.html

Cascella, M., Rajnik, M., Cuomo, A., Dulebohn, S. C., & Di Napoli, R. (2020, April 6). Features, Evaluation and Treatment Coronavirus (COVID-19). *StatPearls*. Treasure Island, FL: StatPearls Publishing. Retrieved May 17, 2020, from https://www.ncbi.nlm.nih.gov/books/NBK554776/

Centers for Desease Control and Prevention. (2020, May 13). *Symptoms of Coronavirus*. Retrieved May 17, 2020, from https://www.cdc.gov/coronavirus/2019-ncov/symptoms-testing/symptoms.html

Central Disaster and Safety Countermeasures Headquarters (CDSCHQ). (2020, April 1). *Guide on the Installation of 'Self-quarantine Safety Protection App'*. Retrieved May 17, 2020, from http://ncov.mohw.go.kr/upload/ncov/file/202004/1585732793827_20200401181953.pdf

Chang, H. (2020, March 26). *Taiwan's Epidemic Prevention Technology: An Inside Look*. Retrieved May 17, 2020, from https://english.cw.com.tw/article/article.action?id=2682

GDPR. (2020). *What is GDPR, the EU's new data protection law?* Retrieved May 17, 2020, from https://gdpr.eu/what-is-gdpr/

Goodhue, D. (1995). Understanding user evaluations of information systems. *Management Science*, *41*(12), 1827–1844. doi:10.1287/mnsc.41.12.1827

Goodhue, D. (1998). Development and measurement validity of a task-technology fit instrument for user evaluations of information systems. *Decision Sciences*, *29*(1), 105–138. doi:10.1111/j.1540-5915.1998.tb01346.x

Government of Singapore. (2020, April 29). *SafeEntry*. Retrieved May 17, 2020, from https://safeentry.gov.sg/

Jimenez, G., Lum, E., & Car, J. (2019). Examining Diabetes Management Apps Recommended From a Google Search: Content Analysis. *JMIR mHealth and uHealth*, *7*(1), e11848. doi:10.2196/11848 PMID:30303485

Johns Hopkins University. (2020). *Coronavirus Resource Center*. Retrieved from https://coronavirus.jhu.edu/map.html

Liang, T.-P., Huang, C.-W., Yeh, Y.-H., & Lin, B. (2007). Adoption of mobile technology in business: A fit-viability model. *Industrial Management & Data Systems*, *107*(8), 1154–1169. doi:10.1108/02635570710822796

Liang, T. P., & Wei, C. P. (2004). Introduction to the special issue: A framework for mobile commerce applications. *International Journal of Electronic Commerce*, *8*(3), 7–17. doi:10.1080/10864415.2004.11044303

Madapusi, A. (2008). *Post-Implementation Evaluation of Enterprise Resource Planning (ERP) Systems* (Doctoral Dissertation). University of North Texas.

Mehta, I. (2020, March 3). *China's coronavirus detection app is reportedly sharing citizen data with police*. Retrieved May 17, 2020, from https://thenextweb.com/china/2020/03/03/chinas-covid-19-app-reportedly-color-codes-people-and-shares-data-with-cops/

Menezes, A., & Smart, N. (2004). Security of signature schemes in a multi-user setting. *Designs, Codes and Cryptography, 33*(3), 261–274. doi:10.1023/B:DESI.0000036250.18062.3f

Menezes, A. J., van Oorschot, P. C., & Vanstone, S. A. (2001). *Handbook of Applied Cryptography* (5th ed.). CRC Press.

Ministry of Health and Welfare of South Korea. (2020). *Self-Check*. Apple App Store. Retrieved May 17, 2020, from https://apps.apple.com/us/app/self-diagnosis/id1501467779

NIST. (2012, October 2). *NIST Selects Winner of Secure Hash Algorithm (SHA-3) Competition*. Retrieved May 17, 2020, from https://www.nist.gov/news-events/news/2012/10/nist-selects-winner-secure-hash-algorithm-sha-3-competition

PEPP-PT e. V. i. Gr. (2020). *Pan-European Privacy-Preserving Proximity Tracing*. Retrieved May 17, 2020, from https://www.pepp-pt.org

Sander, M., & Lemcke, A. (2020, April 19). Radius erlaubt: wie Taiwans Handy-Überwachung funktioniert. *Neue Zürcher Zeitung*. Retrieved May 17, 2020, from https://www.nzz.ch/technologie/wie-taiwans-handy-ueberwachung-funktioniert-ld.1551839

Schneier, B. (1995). *Applied Cryptography: Protocols, Algorithms and Source Code in C* (2nd ed.). John Wiley & Sons.

Shan, S. (2020, March 25). Virus Outbreak: CHT working alone on tracking system: agency. *Taipei Times*, 3. Retrieved May 17, 2020, from https://www.taipeitimes.com/News/taiwan/archives/2020/03/25/2003733339

Soh, C., Kien, S. S., & Tay-Yap, J. (2000). Cultural fi t and misfi t: Is ERP a universal solution? *Communications of the ACM, 43*(4), 47–51. doi:10.1145/332051.332070

The Guardian. (2020). *Coronavirus app: will Australians trust a government with a history of tech fails and data breaches?* Available at: https://www.theguardian.com/australia-news/2020/apr/26/coronavirus-app-will-australians-trust-a-government-with-a-history-of-tech-fails-and-data-breaches

The Hindu. (2020, May 8). Watch | How does the Aarogya Setu app work? *The Hindu*. Retrieved May 17, 2020, from https://www.thehindu.com/news/national/how-does-the-aarogya-setu-appwork/

Tjan, A. (2001). Finally, a way to put your internet portfolio in order. *Harvard Business Review, 79*(2), 76–85. PMID:11213700

Trepte, S., Reinecke, L., Ellison, N. B., Quiring, O., Yao, M. Z., & Ziegele, M. (2017, January-March). A Cross-Cultural Perspective on the Privacy Calculus. *Social Media + Society*, 1-13. doi:10.1177/2056305116688035

Umble, E., Haft, R., & Umble, M. (2003). Enterprise Resource Planning: Implementation Procedures and Critical Success Factors. *European Journal of Operational Research, 146*(2), 241-257.

Ungku, F. (2020, March 20). Singapore launches contact tracing mobile app to track coronavirus infections. *Technology News*. Retrieved May 17, 2020, from https://www.reuters.com/article/us-health-coronavirus-singapore-technolo-idUSKBN2171ZQ

Wickramasinghe, N. (2019). *Handbook of Research on Optimizing Healthcare Management Techniques*. IGI.

Wickramasinghe, N., & von Lubitz, D. (2007). *Knowledge-Based Enterprise: Theories and Fundamentals*. IGI Global. doi:10.4018/978-1-59904-237-4

World Health Organization. (2020, March 26). *Virus origin / Reducing animal-human transmission of emerging pathogens*. Retrieved May 17, 2020, from https://www.who.int/health-topics/coronavirus/who-recommendations-to-reduce-risk-of-transmission-of-emerging-pathogens-from-animals-to-humans-in-live-animal-markets

World Health Organization. (2020, March 11). *WHO Director-General's opening remarks at the media briefing on COVID-19 - 11 March 2020*. Retrieved May 17, 2020, from https://www.who.int/dg/speeches/detail/who-director-general-s-opening-remarks-at-the-media-briefing-on-covid-19---11-march-2020

Chapter 2
Mobile Technology Support for the Assessment and Management of COVID–19 Outbreak:
Benefits and Challenges

Chinazunwa Uwaoma
Claremont Graduate University, USA

Clement C. Aladi
Claremont Graduate University, USA

ABSTRACT

The early months in 2020 saw a rapid increase in the adoption of mHealth and telehealth across the globe. The obvious reason being the sudden outbreak of coronavirus infectious disease (COVID-19), which sent the entire world scrambling for solutions to contain and mitigate the spread. Ordinarily, telehealth and mHealth are considered optional in most traditional healthcare systems even in developed countries, but today, these technologies have become the most sought-after tools required to augment the overwhelmed healthcare systems orchestrated by COVID-19. Mobile technology in particular has continued to play important roles in the monitoring, surveillance, and the assessment of the outbreak in so many ways. This chapter offers a window into different ways mHealth and telemedicine are used to provide healthcare services and disease management, as well as the challenges in the implementation of these technologies as the world braces for the devastating effects of COVID-19.

DOI: 10.4018/978-1-5225-6067-8.ch002

INTRODUCTION

The influence of mobile technology on the assessment and management of COVID-19 crisis has been seen in the areas of disease detection and diagnosis, monitoring the trend of the infection, as well as reducing the impact on healthcare systems. Various online databases have been developed in the USA, China, UK, Australia, Israel, and many other countries for tracing the spread and providing live updates of the disease in real-time. There is also live tracking of exposed localities in Korea, and virtual clinics in China, as well as public information dissemination via WhatsApp and other mobile apps in Singapore (Ting et al., 2020; Buchan, 2020).

Different use cases from all over the world have provided context for how mobile health strategy has supported healthcare and citizen needs during the pandemic. For instance, it is reported in China that mobile technology "increased the efficiency in diagnosis and treatment of patients through 5G-enabled telemedicine" (ITUNews, 2020b). In South Korea, mobile devices were used in early contact tracing which essentially helped in flattening the curve of the disease infection in the country. Also, "free smartphone apps" warned people with text alerts about at-risk locations, based on local cases of the infection that has been identified (ITUNews, 2020a). According to a UN report on COVID-19 response, "location data from mobile phones, credit-card transaction records and CCTV footage are used to trace and test people who might have recently come into contact with an infected person" (UN Department of Global Communications, 2020). There are also myriads of apps with detailed map that indicate exact travel locations or movement of persons that are infected, and to encourage those that have been exposed to infected individuals to go for test or possibly self-quarantine.

Adoption of mobile technology in mitigating the impact of COVID-19 have been extended to healthcare services in the form of mHealth and telehealth. The current structure of the health sector is based on the model of in-person interaction between patients and their caregivers. However, such model of primary care that requires office visit by a patient, is no longer feasible in the face of the current global pandemic; and therefore, has resulted in the urgent transformation of the health sector. The guidelines issued by federal and state governments in tackling the pandemic have helped health care professionals to leverage the various telehealth and mHealth services to provide care for their patients. Through virtual care, physicians have been able to see more patients than before, thus overcoming traditional barriers that have slowed down the penetration of digital technologies in healthcare (Keesara et al., 2020).

Apart from transforming healthcare delivery which has seen a sudden uptake of digital technologies, there is the need to consider strategies that can bring about needed revolutionary expansion of mHealth and telemedicine to address other challenges of the healthcare system, especially security (Keesara et al., 2020). Scalability is also another issue that needs to be considered, particularly longitudinal data-capturing to determine within-person variation of the disease and possible treatments.

The objective of this study is to examine how mobile technology has been instrumental in combating the COVID-19 outbreak. First, the chapter explores existing mobile solutions that have been used in recent times, and presents taxonomy and benefits of mobile solutions that have been developed so far towards this end. It then highlights the setbacks in wider adoption of the mobile applications; and finally, the authors recommend strategies that could enhance the existing solutions.

BACKGROUND

In the past decade, quite a number of mobile phone applications have been developed to monitor and manage certain health conditions. Whereas some are based on cloud computing platforms (Fernandes et al., 2011), some function as standalone systems (Uwaoma & Mansingh, 2018). Given that smartphones are globally used for personal convenience, running healthcare applications on them does not only guarantee ease of use but also facilitate communication between patients and caregivers. Areas in which mHealth systems have been extensively deployed includes monitoring of chronic health conditions (Larson et al., 2017) and early detection of risk factors of such ailments (Uwaoma & Mansingh, 2019).

The drive to integrate mobile monitoring tools into traditional healthcare systems is anchored on simplifying the tasks of disease monitoring and control; and to encourage self-management of long-term health conditions. For instance, in (Uwaoma & Mansingh, 2018), smartphone was configured into a simple monitoring tool to assisting the detection of symptoms of respiratory distress during exercise. The tool is a standalone system that requires little or no effort from the user as it captures patient's data automatically, processes the data, and presents the feedback in real-time. The simplicity and affordability of mobile technology and digital healthcare systems have also been demonstrated in the management of disease outbreak.

Growth in world population, transport, communication, urbanization, and overcrowding conditions can be a catalyst to the spread of any form of viral infection such as Covid-19 pandemic (Li & Ray, 2010). With the increasing mobility of the global population, new emerging diseases are most likely to spread faster and therefore early awareness and proper preparation are considered effective tools for containing the spread of diseases especially among smaller communities that have difficulty preparing for emergencies. Implementation of eHealth and mHealth technologies are potential enablers for epidemic surveillance, mitigation, and response in the management of a pandemic (Mohanty et al., 2019).

Normally, physician reports are mostly the source of information for many surveillance systems. eHealth applications however, aid in reporting by providing evidence-based diagnosis and notification of a health risk to public health authorities. The study in (Li & Ray, 2010) describes an eHealth system – Health Alert Network (HAN) developed by Australian Government Department of Health and Ageing (DoHA), to enhance information gathering and dissemination in Australia. Despite its shortcomings, including slow response time, HAN functions as a supportive tool to Electronic Health Record (EHR) system by providing a secure platform for information sharing and interactions with other systems, as well as collaboration among stakeholders. These different interactions and reporting if done manually, could result in a waste of valuable time (Li & Ray, 2010).

There have been reports on the effectiveness of the use of SMS to increase preparedness and surveillance of a disease outbreak; as well as how mHealth can be used as an intervention tool to provide effective countermeasures. Basically, SMS messaging is one of the ways that mHealth contributes to pandemic management. Li & Ray (2010) in their work, highlight the use of FrontlineSMS - a text-message app that increases ease of communication between a hospital and the population in a certain region in Malawi. Rubin (2012), argues that mHealth has significant potential to bridge various capability gaps identified in the healthcare system in the United States such as funding, workforce, and community resiliency support. The article specifically identifies two major uses of mHealth in a wide-ranging pandemic namely, to improve communications with the public– i.e. dissemination of information; and to make "dispensing of medical countermeasures more effective" (Rubin, 2012).

There is no doubt that advanced capabilities of smartphones and large-scale usage globally, allows for effective communication which helps to disseminate preparedness information to the public during a pandemic. In this aspect, mHealth is mostly deployed in providing a unique way of sharing information and frequent reminders via text messaging and mobile apps. Earlier research reports have shown that reminder-base text messaging programs can promote behavior change among the citizens (Rubin, 2012). Mobile technology has also been used to provide medical countermeasures during epidemic crises. For instance, Denver public health services developed Handheld Automated Notification for Drugs and Immunization (HANDI) - a mobile app with the capabilities of capturing patient's data, and other standardized information automatically, with the use of scanning technology installed in the mobile device. This removes the need for manual data entry by a patient particularly, in critical situations (Rubin, 2012).

Studies in (Mohanty et al., 2019; Aslani et al., 2020) provide in-depth reviews of different categories of mobile technology solutions that have been previously adopted and already in-use for tackling global pandemic. Of significant interest among them are FluMob (Lwin et al., 2017) and Fever Coach (Kim et al., 2019). Both FluMob and Fever Coach apps are used for patient's data collection and management. Whereas FluMob was developed to assist healthcare workers to track and provide real-time report on Flu incidences in Singapore, Fever Coach app was designed to help parents and caregivers to provide real-time report on Flu activities among young children in South Korea. There are other mHealth applications that have been used for public health education and communication, as well as in the diagnosis and treatment of infections. For instance, the "Epidemic Tracker" and "ProMED-mails" apps are deployed in health education programs to provide users with update reports on diseases currently monitored, as well as information on outbreaks of new infections (Mohanty et al., 2019). And for disease diagnosis (Racine & Kobinger, 2019) and post-treatments; applications like Mobile Health Clinic (MHC) for Ebola survivors (Wadoum et al., 2017) and UniMovil" (Manusov et al., 2019), have been developed to provide primary care services to the medically underserved strata of the society.

Since the onset of COVID-19 pandemic, there has been the quest to gain more insight into the dynamics of the disease spread, and to predict subsequent outcomes so as to have better control of the disease infection and transmission. Containing the exponential spread of COVID-19 infection is the most difficult challenge particularly, in collecting exposure data, and determining the disease severity. This consequently undermines the efforts in providing accurate information on the impact, mostly in the areas of public health planning, and clinical management in real-time. Hence, the critical need for real-time data-capturing platform that will allow for a spectrum of subclinical and severe presentations of the disease to help identify the disparities in diagnosis, treatment, and clinical outcomes, as well as mitigation strategies that would help provide effective allocation of scarce medical resources for the management of the disease (Drew et al., 2020).

Physical distancing is considered as one the effective strategies for mitigating COVID-19 spread. And to avoid face-to-face contacts, mobile apps and web-based tools have become essential tools to enlighten the public of urgent health information (Brownstein et al., 2009). These tools have also been applied in research studies; while at the same time, providing platforms for single assessment of disease symptoms leading to personalized recommendations for treatment and further evaluations. (Drew et al., 2020).

Successful implementation of digital healthcare systems however, requires full participation of both clinicians and patients in the validation process, as well as long-tern integration of various components to ensure compliance to the acceptable standard of clinical practice (Uwaoma & Mansigh, 2018).

While the world waits for a formidable vaccine to prevent and manage COVID-19 infection, it is obvious there is heavy reliance on digital technologies to contain the ravaging impact of the disease.

The use of mobile apps and telemedicine has proven effective, but not near perfect in terms of reliability and scalability (Wicklund, 2020b). However, there are quite a number of on-going research efforts to address these factors. The next section provides broader insight into several mobile technology solutions developed by researchers and technologists through consolidated efforts, to curtail the rampaging effect of COVID-19 across the globe. The authors also highlight some challenges that may impede full implementation of these solutions on larger scales, and provide some recommendations.

DEPLOYMENT OF MOBILE DIGITAL TOOLS FOR MANAGING COVID-19

There are a number of mHealth solutions that have been developed to manage the COVID-19 outbreak. Table 1 outlines some of these mobile technology solutions and apps, their specific focus and purpose, as well as the segment of the society and target groups where they are deployed.

Table 1. Samples of mHealth solutions that have been developed to manage covid-19 outbreak

Application/Solution	Focus/Purpose	Segment/Target Group
Open Coronavirus	Monitoring, diagnosing and containing SARS-CoV-2 infection	Community-based Initiative/Transnational
COVID Symptom Study (Chan, 2020)	"To find out where the COVID hot spots are, new symptoms to look out for (can be used as a planning tool to target quarantines, send ventilators and provide real-time data to plan for future outbreaks)".	Public/UK
TraceCOVID-19	Provides effective way of interrupting possible transmission chains of COVID-19 in a community.	Community-based Initiative, Private/Portugal
Near Me (NHS NearMe, 2020)	"A video consulting service that enables people to have health and social care appointments from home or wherever is convenient".	Public/UK, Scotland
Pan-European Privacy-Preserving Proximity Tracing (PEPP-PT, n.d.)	"Makes it possible to interrupt new chains of SARS-CoV-2 transmission rapidly and effectively by informing potentially exposed people".	Private/Transnational
HOMECARE APP	Symptoms are queried in the app and the answers are transmitted in encrypted form to the Health Service division. Makes it possible to prioritize tests for people with the corresponding symptoms.	Public/Vienna, Austria

Source: (European mHealthHub, 2020)

Below are brief descriptions of some select COVID-19 mobile solutions and how they have benefited different segments of the society in coping with COVID-19 pandemic. Here, the authors described three categories of mobile solutions with some examples for each category.

COVID-19 Surveillance and Monitoring

This category of mobile health solutions covers strategies that allow public health institutions access to data for monitoring the spread of COVID-19. The apps provide real-time updates on the statistics of the populace identified to have been infected by the virus locally and globally. The surveillance and monitoring apps are "used by health authorities for public health planning and control", as well as for "public health education and communication", with the integration of existing social media apps like WhatsApp, and Twitter. (Ting et al., 2020). Examples include John Hopkin's online dashboard, South Korea CCTV footage, Singapore TraceTogether App (Ministry of Health, Singapore, 2020), Spain's Desescalapp, Switzerland's COVID Tracker, and Open Coronavirus (European mHealthHub, 2020). Figure 1 captures a demo on the use of the TraceTogether.

Figure 1. Singapore TraceTogether App
(Adapted from [Ministry of Health, Singapore, 2020])

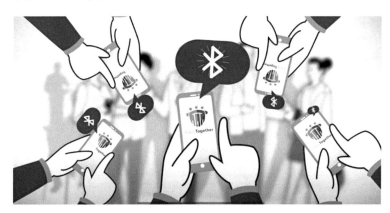

Preventing and Detecting COVID-19

Mobile applications in this category provide platform for raising awareness about the viral outbreak and preparing the public for protection measures. Some of the solutions have been developed to augment COVID-19 diagnosis by providing low-cost test particularly in developing countries that have limited resources to precisely differentiate COVID-19 symptoms from symptoms of related illnesses. They are used as initial screening tools for suspected cases in order to help physicians isolate, treat, and monitor patients (Ting et al., 2020). Key example apps for preventing and detecting COVID-19 infection include COVID-19 Alert!, Netherland's OLVG Corona Check, PEPP-PT, Austria's STOPP CORONA, etc. (European mHealthHub, 2020). An illustration of the STOPP CORONA app is shown in Figure 2.

Mitigating COVID-19 Impact on Healthcare Systems

While most of the digital solutions have focused on tackling the direct impact of COVID-19, there are indirect consequences of the disease on healthcare systems. Remote care is helpful in a time of pandemic such as with the coronavirus, in order to keep the hospitals decongested and to save patients from long

Figure 2. Austria's STOPP CORONA App
(Adapted from [Austrian Red Cross, 2020])

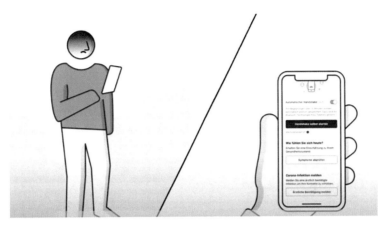

or short commuting. It also enables health workers to concentrate on more serious cases that require priority attention, and to give-one-on-one advice to a patient remotely monitored.

Some mobile applications have been developed to provide regular clinical services remotely to patients. This in so many ways, have helped reduce clinical loads of physicians and pressure on limited healthcare facilities. Examples of digital solutions in this category include AmWell (Amwell for Patients, 2020), Germany's Corona Datenspende, and UK's NearMe (European mHealthHub, 2020). Figure 3 highlights the focus and purposes of some of these apps.

Figure 3. NearMe and AmWell Apps
(Adapted from [NHS NearMe, 2020; Amwell for Patients, 2020])

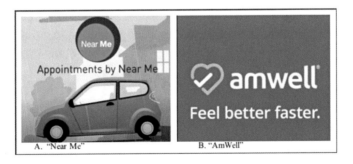

There is no doubt that these myriads of apps generate tons of data, which need to be put into proper use to improve public health by leveraging big data and intelligent analytics tools. In some cases, however, there is lack of transparency in how the data gathered on coronavirus by the mobile apps are verified and used for health management and control in this pandemic. While the use of the analytics tools on the digitally obtained data for prediction and surveillance of the disease is considered of great importance in curtailing COVID-19 outbreak; it is critical that these tools are used responsibly in compliance with regulations that govern data protection, and to acknowledge the need to respect people's privacy and confidential information (Ienca, & Vayena, 2020).

CHALLENGES AND FUTURE IMPLICATIONS

As the coronavirus pushes the health system into uncharted territory, existing medical infrastructures and healthcare systems need to be scaled up to accommodate increasing number of visits to hospitals. There are identifiable psychological, financial and social impacts of expanding mHealth and telehealth services to cover all cases (Gogia et al. 2016). Adoption of IT infrastructure for mHealth and telehealth might encounter serious resistance both on the part of patients and health institutions. This potential problem however, needs to be addressed from the onset (Wicklund, 2020b). In what follows, the authors highlight some of the challenges and future implications of using mhealth and telehealth services to manage disease outbreaks at global level.

Population Age Gap and Disease Severity

Using a mobile app for remote monitoring requires some level of self-efficacy on the part of the patient or caregiver. This might work well with the young adult population but can be challenging with the senior population unless data entries are made by a caregiver. For instance, if mild symptoms suddenly become life-threatening (as in the case of COVID-19 in which most patients are asymptomatic) and the patient becomes incapacitated and unable to make data entries into the app, the remote care would fail to offer the needed services (Gogia et al. 2016). Remote monitoring relies on caregivers for efficiency if the patient is aged. In such cases, hospitals should assign caregivers to patients who are remotely monitored (Heraeus Medical, n.d.).

Efficiency and Reliability

Since the phone is the principal system that collects data for the remote server used by the hospital for analysis, security issues or information overload such as phone notifications, calls, etc., might impede the efficiency of the monitoring app or distract the patient being monitored. While mobile phones generate a lot of data used in tracking movements of people especially through location monitoring, this option can be disabled on phones and therefore, becomes inefficient in obtaining data needed to fight against the virus (Ienca, & Vayena, 2020). The effectiveness of communication between the remote monitoring systems and the patient depends to a large extent, on the Internet signal strength or the bandwidth of the patient's home network. Poor Internet services could impede data sharing and upload from the client to the remote server (Gogia et al. 2016). So, it is necessary to ensure that the network services around the patient's home is stable.

Privacy and Security

Privacy and security issues need to be well addressed to win patients' confidence in the use of mobile apps or telehealth systems. Patients must be given the prerogative to decide whether to be placed on telehealth services or not. The physician might also use his discretionary power to decide when tele-health will yield the most benefits. In such scenario however, Wicklund (2020b) argues that the patient's consent must be duly obtained. There is also the need to use data in a way that is responsible in fighting the pandemic, by respecting privacy and confidentiality in order not to "undermine public trust that will make people less likely to follow public health advice or recommendations, which may lead to poorer health outcomes" (Ienca, & Vayena, 2020). However, it is worth noting here, that some of the digital solutions that have been developed to manage the pandemic incorporated security and privacy protection in the designs (Chan, 2020). Also, the new CDC digital contact tracing tools are designed to include case management tools that allow for automated notification and follow up, as well as sensing technologies that preserve personal privacy. However, these components are still under development (CDC Contact Tracing Resources, 2020).

To adopt mHealth and telehealth services as the new normal in addressing health challenges in a pandemic, stakeholders may consider the following approaches: (1) Adequate preparedness to implement digital transactions with a focus on plans to get the patients through the digital door; (2) It is important to make sure all online contents are from trusted sources. (3) Health institutions should consider outsourcing digital transactions and leverage cloud services to ensure the security of patients' medical data. Regulatory policies should be very strict on IT providers' partnership with health institutions.

As this pandemic has exposed the deficiencies in the current health care system, changes have to be made incrementally for a smooth transition to virtual care. Also, given that the healthcare system works with sensitive data, there is need to first put security measures in place before making any changes. Regulatory policies should include new ways of adapting to the changing times. The regulatory emergency authorizations occasioned by the COVID-19 also need to be made permanent after the crises (Ford, 2020; Wicklund, 2020a).

Lastly, there have been concerns about the misuse of public resources in the fight against this pandemic on how COVID-19 cases are manipulated for dubious reasons (Delić & Zwitter, 2020). To ensure transparency on how public funds are disbursed (Nicaise, 2020), there is need to have a centralized control on how data are collected and used for public health planning. Such strategy will help provide real-time notifications about who might be infected based on symptoms and locational movements, and do not involve data manipulation of any sort (Ienca, & Vayena, 2020).

CONCLUSION

The integration of digital technologies into healthcare systems plays essential roles in tackling major clinical challenges in a pandemic. In fact, COVID-19 outbreak has proven that mobile technology can augment traditional healthcare strategies such as clinical trials and data collection protocols existential in a clinical setting. For instance, the symptom tracking apps provide critical insight into population dynamics of the infection which is important for a pandemic epidemiology study. The data collected by various apps also underscore the potential benefits of real-time symptom tracking that can assist in the allocation of resources for testing, treatment, as well as procedures for easing lockdown in various locations. However, mobile technologies and apps inherently, are unable to provide sufficient representation and services across all population strata. This challenge, together with concerns for security, privacy, and scalability, need to be addressed in order to develop automated and more flexible personalized healthcare systems that are supplemental and reliable during a pandemic.

REFERENCES

Amwell for Patients. (2020). *Amwell*. Retrieved from https://amwell.com/cm/

Aslani, N., Lazem, M., Mahdavi, S., & Garavand, A. (in press). A Review of Mobile Health Applications in Epidemic and Pandemic Outbreaks: Lessons Learned for COVID-19. *Archives of Clinical Infectious Diseases*. Advance online publication. doi:10.5812/archcid.103649

Austrian Red Cross - Meet the STOPP CORONA App. (2020). *STOPP CORONA*. Retrieved from https://www.roteskreuz.at/site/meet-the-stopp-corona-app/

Brownstein, J. S., Freifeld, C. C., & Madoff, L. C. (2009). Digital disease detection—Harnessing the Web for public health surveillance. *The New England Journal of Medicine*, *360*(21), 2153–2157. doi:10.1056/NEJMp0900702 PMID:19423867

Buchan, P. G. (2020). *Australia Goes Hard and Goes Early on COVID-19*. Retrieved from https://www.csis.org/analysis/australia-goes-hard-and-goes-early-covid-19

Chan, A. (2020). *COVID Symptom Study*. Retrieved from https://covid.joinzoe.com/us

Contact Tracing Resources, C. D. C. (2020). *Guidelines for the Implementation and Use of Digital Tools to Augment Traditional Contact Tracing*. Retrieved from https://www.cdc.gov/coronavirus/2019-ncov/downloads/php/guidelines-digital-tools-contact-tracing.pdf

Delic, A., & Zwitter, M. (2020). *Opaque Coronavirus Procurement Deal Hands Millions to Slovenian Gambling Mogul*. Retrieved from https://www.occrp.org/en/coronavirus/opaque-coronavirus-procurement-deal-hands-millions-to-slovenian-gambling-mogul

Drew, D. A., Nguyen, L. H., Steves, C. J., Menni, C., Freydin, M., Varsavsky, T., Sudre, C. H., Cardoso, M. J., Ourselin, S., Wolf, J., Spector, T. D., & Chan, A. T. (2020). Rapid Implementation of Mobile Technology for Real-time Epidemiology of COVID-19. *Science*, *368*(6497), 1362–1367. Advance online publication. doi:10.1126cience.abc0473 PMID:32371477

European mHealthHub. (2020). *mHealth solutions for Managing the COVID-19 Outbreak*. Retrieved from https://mhealth-hub.org/mhealth-solutions-against-covid-19

Fernandes, B., Afonso, J. A., & Simões, R. (2011). Vital signs monitoring and management using mobile devices. In *6th Iberian Conference on Information Systems and Technologies (CISTI 2011)* (pp. 1-6). IEEE.

Ford, P. (2020). *COVID-19 Pandemic Opens Up New Frontiers for Health Data Privacy*. Retrieved from https://www.healthcareitnews.com/news/europe/covid-19-pandemic-opens-new-frontiers-health-data-privacy

Gogia, S. B., Maeder, A., Mars, M., Hartvigsen, G., Basu, A., & Abbott, P. (2016). Unintended consequences of tele health and their possible solutions. *Yearbook of Medical Informatics*, *25*(01), 41–46. doi:10.15265/IY-2016-012 PMID:27830229

Heraeus Medical. (n.d.). *How does the COVID-19 remote care solution work?* Retrieved from https://www.heraeus.com/us/hme/us_heraeuscare_covid19/us_covid_19_patient_monitoring

Ienca, M., & Vayena, E. (2020). On the responsible use of digital data to tackle the COVID-19 pandemic. *Nature Medicine*, *26*(4), 463–464. doi:10.103841591-020-0832-5 PMID:32284619

ITUNews Artificial Intelligence | Emerging Trends. (2020a). *COVID-19: How Korea is using innovative technology and AI to flatten the curve*. Retrieved from https://news.itu.int/covid-19-how-korea-is-using-innovative-technology-and-ai-to-flatten-the-curve/

ITUNews Artificial Intelligence | Emerging Trends. (2020b). *COVID-19: China's digital health strategies against the global pandemic*. Author. Retrieved from https://news.itu.int/covid-19-chinas-digital-health-strategies-against-the-global-pandemic/

Keesara, S., Jonas, A., & Schulman, K. (2020). COVID-19 and health care's digital revolution. *The New England Journal of Medicine*, *382*(23), e82. doi:10.1056/NEJMp2005835 PMID:32240581

Kim, M., Yune, S., Chang, S., Jung, Y., Sa, S. O., & Han, H. W. (2019). The Fever Coach Mobile App for Participatory Influenza Surveillance in Children: Usability Study. *JMIR mHealth and uHealth*, *7*(10), e14276. doi:10.2196/14276 PMID:31625946

Larson, E. C., Saba, E., Kaiser, S., Goel, M., & Patel, S. N. (2017). Pulmonary monitoring using smartphones. In J. Rehg, S. Murphy, & S. Kumar (Eds.), *Mobile Health* (pp. 239–264). Springer. doi:10.1007/978-3-319-51394-2_13

Li, J., & Ray, P. (2010). Applications of eHealth for pandemic management. In *Proceedings of 12th International Conference on e-Health Networking, Applications and Services* (pp. 391-398). IEEE.

Lwin, M. O., Yung, C. F., Yap, P., Jayasundar, K., Sheldenkar, A., Subasinghe, K., Foo, S., Gayantha, U., Xu, H., Chai, S. C., Kurlye, A., Chen, J., & Ang, B. S. P. (2017). FluMob: Enabling surveillance of acute respiratory infections in health-care workers via mobile phones. *Frontiers in Public Health*, *5*, 49. doi:10.3389/fpubh.2017.00049 PMID:28367433

Manusov, E. G., Diego, V. P., Smith, J., & Garza, J. R. (2019). UniMóvil: A Mobile Health Clinic Providing Primary Care to the Colonias of the Rio Grande Valley, South Texas. *Frontiers in Public Health*, *7*. PMID:31497586

Ministry of Health. Singapore. (2020). *TraceTogether*. Retrieved from https://www.healthhub.sg/apps/38/tracetogether-app

Mohanty, B., Chughtai, A., & Rabhi, F. (2019). Use of mobile apps for epidemic surveillance and response–availability and gaps. *Global Biosecurity*, *1*(2).

NHS Near Me - Video Consulting with Near Me. (n.d.). *NearMe*. Retrieved from https://www.nearme.scot.

Nicaise, G. (2020). *Covid-19 and Donor Financing*. Retrieved from https://www.u4.no/publications/covid-19-and-donor-financing.pdf

Pan-European Privacy-Preserving Proximity Tracing. (n.d.). *PEPP-PT*. Retrieved from https://www.pepp-pt.org

Racine, T., & Kobinger, G. P. (2019). Challenges and perspectives on the use of mobile laboratories during outbreaks and their use for vaccine evaluation. *Human Vaccines & Immunotherapeutics*, *15*(10), 2264–2268. doi:10.1080/21645515.2019.1597595 PMID:30893007

Rubin, S. (2012). The use of mhealth technology for pandemic preparedness. *Health Systems (Basingstoke, England)*, 21–24.

Ting, D. S. W., Carin, L., Dzau, V., & Wong, T. Y. (2020). Digital technology and COVID-19. *Nature Medicine*, *26*(4), 459–461. doi:10.103841591-020-0824-5 PMID:32284618

UN Department of Global Communications. (2020). *UN mobilizes global cooperation in science-based COVID-19 responses*. Retrieved from https://www.un.org/en/un-coronavirus-communications-team/un-mobilizes-global-cooperation-science-based-covid-19-responses

Uwaoma, C., & Mansingh, G. (2018). Certainty Modeling of a Decision Support System for Mobile Monitoring of Exercise-induced Respiratory Conditions. In *Proceedings of the 51st Hawaii International Conference on System Sciences* (pp. 2957-2966). HICSS. 10.24251/HICSS.2018.375

Uwaoma, C., Mansingh, G., Pepper, W., Lu, W., & Xiang, S. (2019). Estimation of Physical Activity Level and Ambient Condition Thresholds for Respiratory Health using Smartphone Sensors. In PECCS (pp. 113-120). SCITEPRESS. doi:10.5220/0008170001130120

Wadoum, R. G., Samin, A., Mafopa, N. G., Giovanetti, M., Russo, G., Turay, P., Tura, J., Kargbo, M., Kanu, M. T., Kargbo, B., Akpablie, J., Cain, C. J., Pasin, P., Batwala, V., Sobze, M. S., Potesta, M., Minutolo, A., Colizzi, V., & Montesano, C. (2017). Mobile health clinic for the medical management of clinical sequelae experienced by survivors of the 2013–2016 Ebola virus disease outbreak in Sierra Leone, West Africa. *European Journal of Clinical Microbiology & Infectious Diseases*, *36*(11), 2193–2200. doi:10.100710096-017-3045-1 PMID:28695354

Wicklund, E. (2020a). *Experts Weigh in on Post-COVID-19 Telehealth Rules and Policies*. Retrieved from https://mhealthintelligence.com/news/experts-weigh-in-on-post-covid-19-telehealth-rules-and-policies

Wicklund, E. (2020b). *Using Telehealth in a Pandemic: Focus on Flexibility and Scalability*. Retrieved from https://mhealthintelligence.com/news/using-telehealth-in-a-pandemic-focus-on-flexibility-scalability

Chapter 3
Early Detection of Cancer Using Smartphones

Kodieswari A.
Bannari Amman Institute of Technology, India

ABSTRACT

Cancer disease is the second largest disease in the world with high death mortality. Cancer is an abnormal growth of a normal cell. There are more than 100 types of cancer like blood cancer, brain cancer, small intestine cancer, lung cancer, liver cancer, etc. The type of cancer can be classified by the type of cell which is initially affected. When cancer grows it does not show any symptom. The symptom will appear when the cancer cell grows in mass and the symptom of cancer depends on the type of cancer. The cause of cancers is environmental pollutants, food habits, inherited genetics, tobacco, stress, etc., but in practice, it is not possible to prove the cause of cancer since various cancers do not have specific fingerprints. After the heart attack, cancer is a second killer disease in India. The death mortality is high in cancer because in most of the cases it is identified at the final stage which causes more death. According to ICMR, among 1.27 billion Indian populations, the incidence of cancer is 70-90 per 100,000 populations and 70% of cancer is identified in the last stage accounting for high morality. There are many types of treatment to treat cancer and they are surgery, radiation therapy, chemotherapy, targeted therapy, hormone therapy, stem cell transplant, etc. All cancer treatments will have side effects and the treatments will help only if the cancer cells are identified at the early stage. So time factor is important in diagnosing of cancer cells; hence, early detection of cancer will reduce the mortality rate. This chapter proposed the early detection of cancer cells using image processing techniques by the structure of circulating tumor cell. Early detection of cancer cells is very difficult because the concentration of cancer cells are extremely small and about one million malignant cell is encountered per billion of healthy cells. The circulating tumor cells, CTC, are shed into the bloodstream as a tumor grows, and it is believed these cells initiate the spread of cancer. CTC are rare, existing as only a few per one billion blood cells, and a highly efficient technology like chip-based biosensor platforms is required to capture the CTC, which in turn helps to detect cancer cell at an early stage before spreading. In proposed method, the circulating tumor cell has used a marker to detect cancer at early stage.

DOI: 10.4018/978-1-5225-6067-8.ch003

INTRODUCTION

Image processing technique plays a crucial role in the field of healthcare industries especially in the diagnosis of diseases.

The tumors can be classified into two types, they are, benign tumors and malignant tumors. The benign tumors remain in one place and do not appear to spread. The malignant tumors are more dangerous, spreads to other parts of the body through the blood stream or lymphatic system. When cancer spreads it is very hard to treat. Treatments for of cancer are surgery, chemotherapy, radiation and the advanced named Targeted treatment and Immunotherapy. The targeted treatment includes Erlotinib, Afatinib, Gefitinib, Bevacizumab, Crizotinib and Ceritinib. The immunotherapy treatment includes Monoclonal antibodies, Checkpoint inhibitors, Therapeutic vaccines and Adoptive T-cell transfers. But all these types of treatments may cause side effects. The cancer diagnosis highly requires histological examination of tissue abnormalities detected by radiological, clinical or endoscopic examination of patients. Even though the tests, technologies and treatments are available, if the cancer cells are not diagnosed at early stage, i.e., before Metastasis stage, then the possibility of life-saving is 30% only. Metastasis, spreading of cancer, is the cause of most cancer mortality. When primary tumors grow at the higher rate, the cells are released from the origin organ to others parts of the body through the blood stream or lymphatic system. These cells are named as circulating tumor cell. The circulating tumor cells, CTC, are shed into the bloodstream as the tumor grows and it is believed these cells initiate the spread of cancer. CTC, are rare, existing as only a few per one billion blood cells and highly efficient technology like chip based biosensor platforms is required to capture the CTC, which in turn helps to detect cancer cell at the early stage before spreading. Because by successful dissemination, the tumor cells surrounding around the primary tumor, intravasate into a blood and lymphatic vessels to form a metastasis. This CTC's when invading through the blood and lymphatic vessels it will get shed into the vasculature. Before forming to metastases when the CTC travels through the blood vessels the system is proposed to identify the cancer cell with its cell structure.

LITERATURE REVIEW

Cancer Detection Using CAD

Khosravi, F., et.al (2016) proposed a nanotube CTC chip to detect metastatic cancer. The researchers manufactured a 76-element single wall carbon nanotube array using photo lithography, metal deposition and etching techniques to identify the metastatic cancer cells in a small amount of blood drawn from cancer patient [6].The Nanochip –CTC chip is capable of detecting and capturing of cancer cells without any pre-labeling and processing steps. Blood is simply absorbed and by using electrical sensing and DTW (Dynamic Time Warping) the detection and stratification can be enabled. The electrical signal will be then confirmed using optical/confocal microscopy to hold spiked cancer cells. The nanotube–CTC chip has the potential for clinical translation by using higher information content both in detection and capture about the disease status.

Singh, S.P., Urooj, S., & Lay-Ekuakille, A. (2016) proposed Breast Cancer Detection Using CAD system. The X-ray image sensing is very challenging to visualize the abnormality. The human factor often causes the low degree of accuracy. Hence a Computer-aided detection is proposed to reduce the manual effect and to automize the diagnosis of breast cancer tissues by utilizing polar complex exponential transform moments. The CAD system is an automated system, to differentiate between benign and malignant tumor. With this system, the region of interest is only the manual input. Wavelet based Neural Networks is utilized to improve the accuracy of the CAD system. The main drawback of the system is, it does not handle with the color images.

Ulku, E. E., & Camurcu, A. Y. (2013) proposed Computer aided brain tumor detection with histogram equalization and morphological image processing techniques [12]. The Computer–aided Detection system in association with image processing helps to detect the brain tumor from brain MRI images. Bio-medical imaging processing is one of the most effective techniques to observe the human's health status. The CAD system used to detect unusual structures that may be the tumor and the system undergoes the preprocessing, segmentation, feature analysis, and classification. A histogram equalization technique is used to improve the quality of the digital medical image. The Region of Interest is determined by the masses in the image. The obtained ROIs are executed by classification algorithm and achieved 100% success result.

Rawat, J., et.al. (2015) proposed a Computer Aided Diagnostic System for Detection of Leukemia Using Microscopic Images [13]. The novel technique will differentiate the lymphoblast cells from healthy lymphocyte cells. The CAD system will identify leukemia based on gray level co-occurrence matrices and shape based feature extraction. The support vector machine binary classifier is used to identify the presence of leukemia cells. Leukemia and lymphocytes are the heterogeneous groups of cancers of the blood. All cancer cells are identified by the uncontrollable cell division. The abnormal growth of white cell division is called leukemia. The effective diagnosis of leukemia is possible by careful microscopic examination of a stained blood smear. Due to complex nature of white blood cells, the manual examination leads to inconsistent reports. Hence an automated CAD system to capable of handling the complex white blood cell by four different modules such as preprocessing, segmentation, feature extraction, and classification. The CAD system detects the acute lymphoblastic leukemia by analysis the shape and the texture.

Cancer Detection Using Lab-on-Chip

Zhang, J.et.al, (2016) proposed a Lab-on-chip technology which will separate the circulating tumor cells from other biological components by sorting a bio particles at Nano scale [4]. The technology can separate and detect particles as small as 20nm from smaller particles and exosome of size 100nm.Exosomes range in size from 20-140nm and contain the information about the health of the originating cell that they are shed from. A determined size, protein surface and a nucleic acid cargo carried by exosome can give essential information about the status of present and state of developing cancer and other diseases. The sorting can help to understand not only cancer but also viral disease like the flu. The technology called Nano-DLD, nanoscale deterministic lateral displacement developed a lab-on-chip technology which allows the liquid sample to pass in silicon chip containing asymmetric pillar array through continuous flow. The array sorts the particles by size down to tens of nanometers resolution. And also the array split the mixture of many different particles sizes into a spread of streams like a prism splits white light into different colors. The set of pillars in Nano-DLD will deflect larger particles while allowing smaller particles to flow through the gaps of pillar array without any damage. The IBM's nanoscale technology helps to detect the cancer disease before the symptoms appear.

Cai, H., et.al (2016), developed an optofluidic analysis system for detection of cancer DNA biomarkers in blood [7]. The system will process the biomolecular samples from whole blood, then analyzes and identifies multiple targets on the silicon based molecular based platform. Multiple targets are identified by using a spectral multiplexing technique based on wavelength-dependent multi-spot excitation on an antiresonant reflecting optical waveguide chip. Two types of melanoma biomarkers called BRAFV600E and NRAS from whole blood is extracted and the two targets are identified using spectral multiplexing technique. The optofluidic analysis system achieved 96% success rate in detection of cancer DNA.

C. Claussen, J. (2012) proposed Nanotechnology technology to Improve Lab on a Chip Devices [8] for medical diagnostics. Instead of sending the test samples to laboratories, the healthcare providers could send to LOC device, appoint-of-care facility to diminish analysis time from days to mins. The microsized LOC device is condensed with a modern chemistry laboratory, hence diagnostic testing is made possible in remote and resources poor location. The nanostructured surface is used to detect the target analytes from biological serum. The test fluid is passed through a capture region such as carbon nanotubes or graphene petals which are fabricated onto the microchip. The Biorecognition agents are attached physically/chemically to bind with the target analytes to initiate an electrical/optical transduction. The LOC device has given promising results and the main drawback with the device is an inability to detect low concentration levels, inability to multiplex and complex fabrication protocols that are costly and difficult to replicate.

Ziober, B. L., et.al (2007) proposed Lab-on-a-chip for screening and diagnosis of oral cancer[11]. Early detection is an important factor in determining the survival of patients with oral cancer because many patients continue to face a poor prognosis. Early detection will help the patient to facilitate the treatment earlier. The diagnostics techniques require an advanced laboratory, equipment's, skilled personnel and lengthy process. The lab-on-chip is a device which replaced this entire requirement with its miniaturized, integrated, automated and inexpensive technology. The device is a biomarker based identification of oral cancer. Nearly 40% of the oral cavity cancer accounted of head and neck including squamous cell carcinomas of the tongue, a floor of the mouth, buccal mucosa, lips, hard and soft palate, and gums.

Image Processing Techniques for Cancer Detection

Rejintal, A., & Aswini, N. (2016) generated an element to identify whether the cell is cancerous or non –cancerous cell and also to identify the type of leukemia [14]. Image processing normally use the element for processing the medical images like MRI,CT or any other acquired image using the image processing procedures representation, enhancement, segmentation and numerous more operations. K-means algorithm is used for image segmentation to detect the small and bright spot. Following the segmentation the feature extraction has been done to extract the nucleus using GLCM and GLDM.The proposed system has two parts training and testing which follows all the image processing steps from image acquisition to feature extraction. After feature extraction, the SVM classifier is used for classifying the cell type, cancerous or not.

Mehdy, M. M, Ng, P. Y., (2017) proposed a method for early detection of breast cancer by applying artificial neural network in image processing [15]. This method helps to enhance the detection technique. Image segmentation is a one of the techniques in image processing to detect the small and bright spot. After segmentation process, Artificial Neural Network (ANN) is used to differentiate the segmented objects, as either microcalcifications or nonmicrocalcifications. The accuracy of ANN is tested by determination of true positive (TP) and false positive (FP) detection rates from set of labelled test images.

Gabor wavelets and ANN are used to classify normal and abnormal tissues which have a good attribute in the field of image processing and computer vision. Mehdy, attempted to fulfill the vacuum in the field of image processing in the early detection of breast cancer.

Cancer Detection Using Smartphone

Im, H., Castro, C. M., et.al. (2015) developed a D3 system (digital diffraction diagnosis), smart phone based device to detect tumor and other diseases [1]. The system featured with a battery powered LED light clipped onto the smart phone that records high-resolution imaging data with its camera. It is capable of recording more than 1,00,000 cells than a traditional microscope. The data can be transmitted to a remote graphic processing server in a cloud service. The device will locate the diseases lacking with the latest medical technology. The technology used to make holograms to collect microscopic images for digital analysis of the molecular composition of cells and tissues. After a sample of blood collected, it is mixed with the micro beads attached with antibodies. The antibodies bind with the molecules of cancer cells and the mixture is placed on microscopic slide attached with the smart phone to take a picture. Initially, the researchers believed that they can differentiate cancerous and noncancerous cells simply if the beads bound to them. But the beads and cells diffracted the light which makes the image too distorted. This makes the researcher write an algorithm to reconstruct the images of bead bound cells from diffraction pattern. The device was tested for cervical cancer and found successful. It also helps to detect cancer from cell surface protein and to detect DNA.

Harald Fuchs, (2015), proposed a method to detect cancer cells before they form metastases [2]. Karlsruhe Institute of Technology developed a clinical method to detect single cancer cell in the blood sample. The microarray platform is used to detect the cancer cells from the blood sample before they form metastases. Polymer pen lithography, a surface is provided with a microscopically small structure using a plastic die were target cells adhere to these structures. The blood samples will be injected into the flat micro channel to cross the platform. When it crossed the platform the target cells will contact the array in a fish based structure at the top of the channel stirs up the passing liquid. While the tumor cells dock to the prepared locations according to the key-lock principle, the remaining cells are washed away.

Murat Baday1, Semih Calamak1 (2015), proposed an Integrating Cell Phone Imaging with Magnetic Levitation (i-LEV) for Label-Free Blood Analysis at the Point-of-Living [3]. The scientist designed a lantern sized device which can measure blood cell levels using magnetic levitation. The Smartphone was combined with the device to carry out a medical test. To proceed with the test, Smartphone is placed on the top of the lens so that the device's camera looks down the tube filled with the blood sample of 30 microliters. The users can also view the specimen with the help of mirrors and LED lights. The blood samples are laced with a gadobutrol (chemical), which is paramagnetic i.e., it is slightly attracted to magnetic fields. These samples are then placed between two long, thin magnets about the size of tooth-picks. The cells in the blood sample float up to different heights in the magnetic field depending on their density and type. These cell densities are accurately measured and separated based on their weight and magnetic forces. The Smartphone could see individual blood cells using i-LEV. Computer programs could then automatically count the number of blood cells seen in less than 30 seconds.

Ricard-Gauthier, D., et.al,(2015) proposed the Use of Smartphones as Adjuvant Tools for Cervical Cancer Screening in Low-Resource Settings[5].The International Agency for Research on Cancer (IARC) accounted 85% of death is caused by cervical cancer in the world and this high mortality rate is because of lack of efficient screening systems. Early detection and screening will help to reduce the mortality rate. A smartphone as an adjuvant tool was recommended for cervical cancer prevention and screening. Three hundred women's were screened using self-collected vaginal specimens. Digital images of the cervix were taken with the help of a smartphone and evaluated by health care providers in offsite. The progress of images in imaging devices, transfer, and quality of images has been allowed the use of cervical imaging for screening in low resource setting. It is assessed by the observers that 95.6% of all images are with good quality for interpretation purpose.

Sundberg, K., et.al (2017), proposed Early Detection and Management of Symptoms Using an Interactive Smartphone Application (Interaktor) During Radiotherapy for Prostate Cancer[10].an application called Interaktor for Smartphone and Tablets. Information and communication technology (ICT) is becoming an integral part of modern health care system. The ICT utilize digital technology access to eHealth (Internet-based programs) and use of mobile devices, for early detection reporting and management of symptoms, and concerns during treatment for prostate cancer. Based on the reports from two groups (Urban and Rural), the application has been developed.The reports via the application enable instant support from a nurse in early detection, management of symptoms and treatment for prostate cancer. The Interaktor, an app, is an efficient mHealth tool with its real-time communication enabling rapid management of symptoms when detected early.

SUMMARY

The medical community has been established to take care of human health with proficient experts like a clinician, chemist, hematopathologists, and many others specialized in health science. In manual diagnosis, the diagnosing time is high and accuracy rate is low. The advancement in technology provides faster and accurate automated medical tools for diagnosis and their future prognoses. This emerging need for portable, robust, inexpensive, and easy-to-use disease diagnosis and prognosis monitoring platforms to share health information at the point-of-living, including clinical and home settings. Recent advances in digital health technologies have improved early diagnosis, drug treatment, and personalized medicine. Nowadays, Smartphones are incredibly powerful portable computers that include handy devices such as multimega pixel cameras, and they can be found in both developing and developed countries. Making the smartphone, a hand held electronic machine as medical device will help to detect the cancer at early stage and save many lives

REFERENCES

Baday, Calamak, Durmus, Davis, Steinmetz, & Demirci. (2015). Proposed Integrating Cell Phone Imaging with Magnetic Levitation (i-LEV) for Label-Free Blood Analysis at the Point-of-Living. *Small Nano Micro*. Doi:10.1002mll.201501845

Cai, H., Stott, M. A., Ozcelik, D., Parks, J. W., Hawkins, A. R., & Schmidt, H. (2016, November). On-chip wavelength multiplexed detection of cancer DNA biomarkers in blood. In *Biomicrofluidics*. AIP Publishing. . doi:10.1063/1.4968033

Claussen, J. (2012). Using Nanotechnology to Improve Lab on a Chip Devices. *Journal of Biochips & Tissue Chips*. . doi:10.4172/2153-0777.1000e117

Fuchs. (2015, November 23). *Detecting cancer cells before they form metastases.* ScienceDaily. Retrieved July 10, 2017, Karlsruhe Institute of Technology from www.sciencedaily.com/releases/2015/11/151123103326.htm

Im, H., Castro, C. M., Shao, H., Liong, M., Song, J., & Pathania, D., … Lee, H. (2015, April 13). Digital diffraction analysis enables low-cost molecular diagnostics on a smartphone. Proceedings of the National Academy of Sciences. *Proceedings of the National Academy of Sciences.* 10.1073/pnas.1501815112

Khosravi, F., Trainor, P. J., Lambert, C., Kloecker, G., Wickstrom, E., Rai, S. N., & Panchapakesan, B. (2016, September 29). Static micro-array isolation, dynamic time series classification, capture and enumeration of spiked breast cancer cells in blood: the nanotube–CTC chip. In *Nanotechnology.* IOP Publishing. doi:10.1088/0957-4484/27/44/44lt03

Mehdy, M. M., Ng, P. Y., Shair, E. F., Saleh, N. I. M., & Gomes, C. (2017). Artificial Neural Networks in Image Processing for Early Detection of Breast Cancer. *Computational and Mathematical Methods in Medicine, 2017,* 1–15. doi:10.1155/2017/2610628 PMID:28473865

Rawat, J., Singh, A., Bhadauria, H. S., & Virmani, J. (2015). Computer Aided Diagnostic System for Detection of Leukemia Using Microscopic Images. *Procedia Computer Science, 70,* 748–756. doi:10.1016/j.procs.2015.10.113

Rejintal, A., & Aswini, N. (2016). Image processing based leukemia cancer cell detection. In *2016 IEEE International Conference on Recent Trends in Electronics, Information & Communication Technology (RTEICT).* IEEE. 10.1109/RTEICT.2016.7807865

Ricard-Gauthier, D., Wisniak, A., Catarino, R., van Rossum, A. F., Meyer-Hamme, U., Negulescu, R., … Petignat, P. (2015, October). Use of Smartphones as Adjuvant Tools for Cervical Cancer Screening in Low-Resource Settings. *Journal of Lower Genital Tract Disease.* . doi:10.1097/lgt.0000000000000136

Singh, S. P., Urooj, S., & Lay-Ekuakille, A. (2016). Breast Cancer Detection Using PCPCET and ADEWNN: A Geometric Invariant Approach to Medical X-Ray Image Sensors. *IEEE Sensors Journal, 16*(12), 4847–4855. doi:10.1109/JSEN.2016.2533440

Sundberg, K., Wengström, Y., Blomberg, K., Hälleberg-Nyman, M., Frank, C., & Langius-Eklöf, A. (2017, February 24). Early detection and management of symptoms using an interactive smartphone application (Interaktor) during radiotherapy for prostate cancer. In *Supportive Care in Cancer.* Springer Nature. . doi:10.100700520-017-3625-8

Ulku, E. E., & Camurcu, A. Y. (2013). Computer aided brain tumor detection with histogram equalization and morphological image processing techniques. In *2013 International Conference on Electronics, Computer and Computation (ICECCO).* IEEE. 10.1109/ICECCO.2013.6718225

Zhang, J., Chen, K., & Fan, Z. H. (2016). *Circulating Tumor Cell Isolation and Analysis. Advances in Clinical Chemistry.* Elsevier. doi:10.1016/bs.acc.2016.03.003

Ziober, B. L., Mauk, M. G., Falls, E. M., Chen, Z., Ziober, A. F., & Bau, H. H. (2007). *Lab-on-a-chip for oral cancer screening and diagnosis. Head & Neck.* Wiley-Blackwell. doi:10.1002/hed.20680

Chapter 4
Critical Issues in Mobile Solution–Based Clinical Decision Support Systems:
A Scoping Review

Nalika Ulapane
ⓘD https://orcid.org/0000-0003-3432-3943
Swinburne University of Technology, Australia

Nilmini Wickramasinghe
ⓘD https://orcid.org/0000-0002-1314-8843
Swinburne University of Technology, Australia & Epworth HealthCare, Australia

ABSTRACT

The use of mobile solutions for clinical decision support is still a rather nascent area within digital health. Shedding light on this important application of mobile technology, this chapter presents the initial findings of a scoping review. The review's primary objective is to identify the state of the art of mobile solution based clinical decision support systems and the persisting critical issues. The authors contribute by classifying identified critical issues into two matrices. Firstly, the issues are classified according to a matrix the authors developed, to be indicative of the stage (or timing) at which the issues occur along the timeline of mobile solution development. This classification includes the three classes: issues persisting at the (1) stage of developing mobile solutions, (2) stage of evaluating developed solutions, and (3) stage of adoption of developed solutions. Secondly, the authors present a classification of the same issues according to a standard socio-technical matrix containing the three classes: (1) technological, (2) process, and (3) people issues.

DOI: 10.4018/978-1-5225-6067-8.ch004

INTRODUCTION

The need for relevant data, pertinent information and germane knowledge as rapidly, complete and accurate as possible is essential to make sound an often lifesaving clinical decisions (Moghimi, De Steiger, Schaffer, & Wickramasinghe, 2013). Digital information can transform the quality and sustainability of health and care. National strategic plans have been put in place in recent years to enable the digital transformation of healthcare across the world, especially in Australia (Australia's National Digital Health Strategy, 2018). Investment in this interest is significant, and partnerships between governments, healthcare providers, and research institutions are evident (Digital Health CRC, 2020). The project CLOTS (Consultation on haematological Optimization and Thrombosis in Surgery) (Digital Health CRC, 2020), is a prime example for such investment and partnership relating to the digital transformation of healthcare.

A pivotal component playing a part in the digital transformation of healthcare is the use of mobile solutions for clinical decision support. On general observation, it is fair to comment that the state of the use of mobile solutions for clinical decision support, is still at a stage of nascency. A common consensus is that this is largely due to not a lack of technology solutions, but the fact that healthcare being quite a conservative domain. Clinical decision-making has been developed on a set of evidence-based practices (Clancy & Cronin, 2005), and is reinforced through regulation. This nature, along with a degree of reluctance shown by clinicians to adopt mobile technologies to assist their work (Jacob, Sanchez-Vazquez, & Ivory, 2019) may have been barriers preventing a strong entry for mobile solutions to support clinical decision-making to date. However, given the general adoption and diffusion of mobile solutions and the fact that clinicians are more and more time pressed at present, it is becoming essential for them to have quick, convenient and robust decision support solutions, and thus more attention is now being focused on mobile solutions to fill the void and address the needs of the sector (Blagec, Romagnoli, Boyce, & Samwald, 2016). As part of an ongoing research study (Digital Health CRC, 2020) relevant to the premise, focussing on designing and developing mobile decision support solutions for clinicians, the authors present in this chapter a preliminary scoping review, done via a survey of peer reviewed literature, in order to identify the state-of-the-art of using mobile solutions for clinical decision support, and the persisting issues that would require attention and improvement in this avenue. In doing so, authors begin to answer the research question: "How can we design and develop suitable mobile solutions to better support clinical decision making?"

The scope of this review as intended by the authors (prior to surveying literature), can be summarized as follows: Relates to solutions used inside hospitals (i.e., secondary and/or tertiary care); involves the use of mobile solutions (e.g., ubiquitous devices such as Tablets and mobile phones, as well as Apps that may or may not be supported by a cloud computation and/or database facility, in relation to electronic health records for instance); inputs to solutions may be fed by patients and/or clinicians only; and, serves as some form of a decision support tool for clinicians. In the subsequent sections of this chapter, the authors present how they performed a systematic review of literature covering the prior scoping the authors had formed, and discuss the findings. The objective of conducting this review can be presented to be two-fold: (1) Identifying the state-of-the-art of mobile solution based clinical decision support systems; (2) Identifying critical issues. What the authors identify as issues in this chapter, are the ones that have been raised in the Discussion and Limitations sections in recent literature. As such, the issues identified by the authors are quite likely ones that have not yet been solved at present. While the authors do not intend to propose solutions to such issues within this chapter, the authors intend to identify and list such persisting issues under some systematic matrices so that it would help researchers to survey such issues, and work towards addressing them.

As the main contribution of this chapter, the authors present the identified critical issues mapped onto two matrices. Firstly, the issues are classified (or mapped) according to a matrix the authors have developed. This matrix is indicative of the stage (or timing) at which the issues occur along the timeline of development of a mobile solution. Included in this matrix are the three classes: (1) Issues persisting at the stage of developing mobile solutions; (2) Issues persisting at the stage of evaluating developed solutions; and (3) Issues persisting at the stage of adoption of developed solutions. Secondly, the issues are classified according to a standard simple socio-technical matrix containing the three classes: (1) Technological Issues; (2) Process Issues; and (3) People Issues. As such mappings go on to list critical issues under categories, the mappings can help by revealing some form of a categorical roadmap that can guide the efforts to address the persisting issues, alongside the development of mobile solutions that better commensurate with the sector of healthcare.

The remainder of this chapter is arranged as follows: In the immediate subsequent section, the materials used and the methods followed to conduct the review are presented; in the subsequent section, the findings from this review are discussed; and in the final section, some conclusions that can be drawn from this review are summarized.

METHODOLOGY

Within the months of May and June of 2020, the authors conducted a systematic search of peer reviewed literature regarding the use of mobile solutions to support clinical decision-making. The authors search methodology was influenced by the PRISMA method for conducting systematic literature reviews (Moher, Liberati, Tetzlaff, Altman, & others, 2009). A university library database was used for the search. The summary details of the conducted database search are provided in Table 1.

The search resulted in 11,823 items. These items were narrowed down by selecting only those that have been published in Academic Journals. This narrowing resulted in 11,275 items. Then, 50 Subject areas were noted via automatic detection of Subject areas done by the search system. Those subject areas were classified by the authors to two categories named "Relevant" and "Exclude" (see Table 6 in the Appendix for the classification of the total 50 Subjects). The purpose behind this classification was to extract literature that are possibly most relevant for the work of this chapter; implying that the category titled "Relevant" would include the Subject areas that are more adjacent to this chapter. Out of 50 Subject areas, 30 ended up in the "Relevant" category. This classification was done manually based on the author's sense of judgement. The list of items was then made to narrow down to include only items that fall within the Subject areas listed in the "Relevant" category.

Narrowing likewise based on subject areas resulted in 4,402 items. From here onward, the authors' intention was to capture the items published in the highest impact forums. A logical approach to capture high impact forums was narrowing down the list further based on publishers. The Journal of Medical Internet Research (JMIR) is a prominent publisher known to hold 4 journals ranked among the top 8 according to Clarivate Medical Informatics / Digital Health journals category ranking as of 2019 (JMIR Publications, 2020). As per the 2019 standings, J Med Internet Res has been ranked #1 in the digital health category with a journal impact factor of almost 5 (4.945) and JMIR mHealth and uHealth has been ranked #2 with a journal impact factor of 4.301 (JMIR Publications, 2020). The JMIR journals have

Table 1. Summary details of the conducted database search for literature.

Date of Search	Saturday 2020/05/16
Source	The University of Melbourne library database. Note: This source is powered by the EBSCOhost platform. The library search facility is linked to major academic databases and search engines (such as, Scopus, Web of Science, MEDLINE, PubMed, Google Scholar, IEEE Xplore, etc.), and is able to retrieve items according to given keywords.
The search phrase	("clinical decision support tool*" OR "decision support tool*" OR "decision support*" OR "clinical decision support*" OR "clinical decision*") AND ("mobile device*" OR "ubiquitous device*" OR "mobile platform*" OR "mobile phone*" OR "smartphone*" OR "smart phone*" OR "smart device*" OR "iPhone*" OR "iPad*" OR "Tab" OR "Tabs" OR "Tablet" OR "Tablets" OR "app" OR "apps" OR "application" OR "applications") Note: The search phrase was articulated to have the emphasis on the use of mobile solutions for clinical decision support systems—the focus of this chapter.
Use of the search phrase	Note: The search phrase was used to scan the Titles and the Abstracts of research items, as those sections of a research item would be succinctly reflective of an item's content. An expression of the search criteria in Boolean logic can be presented in the following manner. List items that include, the following phrases within the Title: ("clinical decision support tool*" OR "decision support tool*" OR "decision support*" OR "clinical decision support*" OR "clinical decision*") AND ("mobile device*" OR "ubiquitous device*" OR "mobile platform*" OR "mobile phone*" OR "smartphone*" OR "smart phone*" OR "smart device*" OR "iPhone*" OR "iPad*" OR "Tab" OR "Tabs" OR "Tablet" OR "Tablets" OR "app" OR "apps" OR "application" OR "applications") OR the following phrases within the Abstract: ("clinical decision support tool*" OR "decision support tool*" OR "decision support*" OR "clinical decision support*" OR "clinical decision*") AND ("mobile device*" OR "ubiquitous device*" OR "mobile platform*" OR "mobile phone*" OR "smartphone*" OR "smart phone*" OR "smart device*" OR "iPhone*" OR "iPad*" OR "Tab" OR "Tabs" OR "Tablet" OR "Tablets" OR "app" OR "apps" OR "application" OR "applications").
Search constraints	Note: The five constraints (three restrictive, and two expansive) listed below were imposed on the search. 1) List only items that have accessible full texts—restrictive. 2) List only items that have been peer reviewed—restrictive. 3) List only items that have been published within the past five years (i.e., between 2015/01/01 and 2020/12/12). This constraint was imposed in the interest of capturing items that are reflective of the state-of-the-art—restrictive. 4) Search ALL databases accessible to the library in seek of items—expansive. 5) No restrictions on language (i.e., list items that have been published in any language)—expansive.

led the entire field and have remained ahead of other journals such as JAMIA (Journal of the American Medical Informatics Association) or IEEE Journal of Biomedical and Health Informatics. Based on such observations, authors decided to narrow down the search on the basis of publishers, to only include items from JMIR (JMIR Publications, 2020). This narrowing resulted in a listing containing 65 items. On duplicate items being removed, the list reduced to 32 items contained within journal such as: (1) Journal of Medical Internet Research (JMIR); (2) JMIR mHealth and uHealth (JMU); and (3) JMIR Medical Informatics (JMI)—all top-ranked journals in the Medical Informatics / Digital Health categories. The narrowed list of 32 items obtained likewise, is what the review carried out in this chapter focuses on.

RESULTS AND DISCUSSION

Further Narrowing Down of Literature Based on Relevance

On examining full texts of the 32 items, the availability of works related to different levels of care (i.e., primary, secondary, tertiary) was evident. Since the project (i.e., the CLOTS project (Digital Health CRC, 2020)) for which the authors attempt to form a scoping review deals with a tertiary care setting, authors excluded works relating to primary care and education from this review. The excluded works dealt with contributions such as: self-care and self-management by patients (8 research items); patient reported outcomes and post-care follow up (3 research items); education platforms (2 research items); ongoing studies—with further investigations pending (2 research items); development of information resources (1 research item), and tools designed for use by healthcare volunteers in the general community (1 research item). A total of 17 research items got excluded. These excluded items are available in Table 2. The 15 research items that remained following this exclusion led to the findings presented in the remainder of this chapter.

State-of-the-Art Contributions Made in the Literature

Due to the 5-year time window (i.e., 2015/01/01 to 2020/12/31) restriction imposed on this survey of literature, it is reasonable to mention that the contributions of the research items that made the cut for this chapter are representative of the state-of-the-art. Contributions made in the narrowed down 15 research items are presented in Table 3. According to the selection criteria the authors followed, these items ended being the filtered ones to be most aligned and relevant to the authors' work that relates to a project that aims to develop mobile solutions for a tertiary care setting.

The research items have focused on different aspects of care, and can be summarized as follows: Cancer (2 items); Emergency Department (4 items); some form of overall process in hospital care (3 items); risk assessment or prediction (2 items); psychiatric conditions (1 item); Chronic Kidney Disease (1 item); Diabetes (1 item), and Osteoporotic Fracture (1 item). These different aspects are highlighted in yellow as keywords in Column 2 of Table 3 for easy surveying along with the relevant references cited. Further, two well established mobile apps were identified in these works. The apps were: (1) Ottawa Rules App; (2) Concussion and Brain Bleed App. Both these apps are related to Emergency Department.

Notable Critical Issues

Critical issues were identified by reading the full texts of the 15 research items (i.e., those in Table 3). It should be recalled that what the authors have identified and listed as "issues" in this chapter, are those that have been mentioned in the "Discussion" and "Limitation" sections of the recent literature. As such, those issues are ones that are quite likely have not yet been solved, and stand as persisting issues to date. It is not the authors intention to propose solutions to such issues in this chapter. Instead, what the authors attempt is to identify and list such persisting issues in under some meaningful matrices so that would enable convenient surveying to researchers in order to address these issues. After identifying critical issues, the authors have attempted to present them classified (or mapped) according to two matrices (i.e., in Table 4 and Table 5). In the first column of Table 4, the identified issues are listed as topics and subtopics to be self-explanatory. Some keywords that summarize and reflect those issues are highlighted in yellow in Table 4. Table 5 then goes on to present these same keywords and issues under a mapping different to that of Table 4.

Table 2. Contributions made in research items that were excluded post full text review.

Contributions Made	Research Items
1. Tools for self-care and self-management by patients	(Con & De Cruz, 2016); (Wu, et al., 2017); (Lv, et al., 2017); (Woldaregay, et al., 2019); (Seto, et al., 2017); (Sandal, et al., 2019); (Ware, et al., 2020); (Pham, et al., 2018)
2. Tools for patient reported outcomes and post-care follow up	(Nhavoto, Grönlund, & Chaquilla, 2015); (Tran, et al., 2020); (van Kollenburg, de Bruin, & Wijkstra, 2019)
3. Education platforms	(Dafli, et al., 2015); (Barteit, et al., 2019)
4. Ongoing studies – with further investigations pending	(Camacho, Ch, Landis-Lewis, Douglas, & Boyce, 2018); (Jordan, McSwiggan, Parker, Halas, & Friesen, 2018)
5. Development of information resources	(Bogie, et al., 2018)
6. Tools designed for use by community healthcare volunteers	(van Heerden, Sen, Desmond, Louw, & Richter, 2017)

Firstly, the authors attempted to map the issues according to a matrix the authors developed for this chapter. This matrix (authors annotate it Matrix 1) may be useful for broader usage, for the purpose of identification and classification of critical issues in relevant contexts. The rationale underpinning this matrix is to be indicative of the stages (or timing) at which the issues arise and persist along the timeline of the development of a mobile solution. Aligning with this rationale, the authors present the matrix to be containing the following three classes, indicative of stages (or timing):

1. Issues persisting at the stage of developing mobile solutions.
2. Issues persisting at the stage of evaluating developed solutions.
3. Issues persisting at the stage of adoption of developed solutions.

The mapping of identified critical issues according to the proposed matrix is presented in Table 4.

Secondly, a mapping of the same issues onto a standard socio-technical matrix is presented. This socio-technical matrix (authors annotate it Matrix 2) classifies issues according to their type, and who (or what) is responsible for the issues should they occur. This matrix comprises the following classes, indicative of the type of an issue:

1. Technological Issues.
2. Process Issues.
3. People Issues.

The mapping of identified critical issues according to the socio-technical matrix is presented in Table 5.

Table 3. State-of-the-art contributions made in literature that did not get filtered out post full text review (Highlighted in bold are special keywords indicative of the application scenario and the specificity of the contribution).

Contribution	Condition	Research Items
1. Software framework for MRI based diagnosis	Paediatric **Cancer**	(Zarinabad N., Meeus, Manias, Foster, & Peet, 2018)
2. Qualitative case study to understand clinicians' roles in the adoption of a decision support app	Oncology, **Cancer**	(Jacob, Sanchez-Vazquez, & Ivory, 2019)
3. Evaluation of an App designed for assessing the requirement of diagnostic imaging ("**Ottawa Rules App**")	**Emergency Department** conditions	(Paradis, et al., 2018)
4. Evaluation of an improved App via survey; designed for assessing the requirement of diagnostic imaging ("**Ottawa Rules App**")	**Emergency Department** conditions	(Quan, et al., 2020)
5. Formative evaluation of an electronic Clinical Decision Support tool	**Emergency Department**, Head injury	(Melnick, et al., 2017)
6. Tablet-based patient-centred use of "**Concussion or Brain Bleed App**"	**Emergency Department**, Minor Head Injury	(Singh, et al., 2017)
7. Forecasting the adoption of Electronic Health Records in hospitals	N/A, **Overall Process**	(Kharrazi, Gonzalez, Lowe, Huerta, & Ford, 2018)
8. Discussing challenges in implementation of Machine Learning in Healthcare using the NASSS framework	N/A, **Overall Process**	(Shaw, Rudzicz, Jamieson, & Goldfarb, 2019)
9. Designing interactive visual displays to help clinicians interpret and compare the results of relevant Random Controlled Trials	N/A, **Overall Process**	(Bian, et al., 2018)
10. Prospective validation of a real-time Early Warning System (EWS) monitoring inpatients	Mortality **Risk** Assessment / Prediction	(Ye, et al., 2019)
11. Process development and outcomes of a Mobile Clinical Decision Support Tool	Paediatric Cardiovascular **Risk**	(Furberg, Williams, Bagwell, & LaBresh, 2017)
12. Evaluation of the use of a web and mobile phone-based application	**Psychiatric** conditions	(Berrouiguet, et al., 2017)
13. Reviewing the functionality of Mobile Apps	Chronic **Kidney Disease**	(Lee, Cui, Tu, Chen, & Chang, 2018)
14. Implementation and evaluation of a Digital Health Platform	**Diabetes**	(Abidi, Vallis, Piccinini-Vallis, Imran, & Abidi, 2018)
15. Illustration of a practical application of a clinical surveillance system	**Osteoporotic Fracture**	(Lin, et al., 2018)

CONCLUSION

A scoping review of the state-of-the-art was systematically conducted to identify critical issues that persist in the process of developing mobile solutions for healthcare (particularly the tertiary care setting). The identified issues were mapped onto two matrices. The first matrix was improvised by the authors. It is indicative of the stage (or timing) at which an issue occurs along the timeline of developing a mobile

Table 4. Listing identified critical issues under the Matrix 1 (based on the timing of the occurrence of issues)—Highlighted in yellow are keywords indicative of the specificity of the identified issues.

Issues	Research Items
1. Issues persisting at the stage of developing mobile solutions	
1.1 Complexity	
1.1.1 Complexity in translating written Clinical Practice Guidelines (CPGs) to Apps	(Furberg, Williams, Bagwell, & LaBresh, 2017)
1.2 Optimal Performance	
1.2.1 Requires improvement of algorithms	(Zarinabad N., Meeus, Manias, Foster, & Peet, 2018); (Lin, et al., 2018)
1.2.2 Requires more accessibility to Clinical Decision Rules (CDRs) and Electronic Medical Records (EMRs)	(Quan, et al., 2020)
1.2.3 Requires more ease of use and improved overall performance	(Jacob, Sanchez-Vazquez, & Ivory, 2019); (Abidi, Vallis, Piccinini-Vallis, Imran, & Abidi, 2018); (Melnick, et al., 2017)
1.3 Limited data	
1.3.1 Available data for training and testing algorithms is limited	(Zarinabad N., Meeus, Manias, Foster, & Peet, 2018); (Shaw, Rudzicz, Jamieson, & Goldfarb, 2019)
1.3.2 Lack of data to generalize models	(Ye, et al., 2019)
1.4 Validation	
1.4.1 Further validation of algorithms is required	(Zarinabad N., Meeus, Manias, Foster, & Peet, 2018)
1.4.2 Standardization of mobile solutions is required	(Lee, Cui, Tu, Chen, & Chang, 2018)
1.4.3 Founding mobile solutions on established scientific practices and peer reviewed literature is required	(Lee, Cui, Tu, Chen, & Chang, 2018)
2. Issues persisting at the stage of evaluating developed solutions	
2.1 Generalizability	
2.1.1 Lack of generalizability of user/participant opinions	(Quan, et al., 2020); (Jacob, Sanchez-Vazquez, & Ivory, 2019); (Paradis, et al., 2018); (Singh, et al., 2017)
2.2 Biases	
2.2.1 Familiarity biases of users/participants	(Quan, et al., 2020); (Paradis, et al., 2018); (Abidi, Vallis, Piccinini-Vallis, Imran, & Abidi, 2018)
2.2.2 Response biases of users/participants	(Quan, et al., 2020); (Abidi, Vallis, Piccinini-Vallis, Imran, & Abidi, 2018)
2.2.3 Self-selection biases of users/participants	(Singh, et al., 2017); (Abidi, Vallis, Piccinini-Vallis, Imran, & Abidi, 2018)
2.3 Validation	
2.3.1 More evidence on clinical impact of the use of mobile solutions in healthcare is required	(Quan, et al., 2020); (Singh, et al., 2017); (Bian, et al., 2018)
3. Issues persisting at the stage of adoption of developed solutions	
3.1 Workload	
3.1.1 Should not increase clinicians' workload	(Berrouiguet, et al., 2017); (Singh, et al., 2017); (Abidi, Vallis, Piccinini-Vallis, Imran, & Abidi, 2018)
3.2 Optimal performance	
3.2.1 Operation and stability	(Jacob, Sanchez-Vazquez, & Ivory, 2019)
3.2.2 Ease of use	(Abidi, Vallis, Piccinini-Vallis, Imran, & Abidi, 2018); (Melnick, et al., 2017)
3.2.3 Usefulness and meaningfulness of solution outcomes	(Shaw, Rudzicz, Jamieson, & Goldfarb, 2019)
3.3 Cost	
3.3.1 Potential requirement of advanced computation power	(Shaw, Rudzicz, Jamieson, & Goldfarb, 2019)
3.3.2 Requirement of additional staff	(Singh, et al., 2017)
3.4 Expandability	
3.4.1 Scepticism about black-box nature of certain Machine Learning algorithms	(Shaw, Rudzicz, Jamieson, & Goldfarb, 2019)
3.5 Privacy	
3.5.1 Privacy and consent concern the patients would have	(Shaw, Rudzicz, Jamieson, & Goldfarb, 2019)
3.5.2 Data security	(Shaw, Rudzicz, Jamieson, & Goldfarb, 2019)
3.6 Policy and legislative challenges	
3.6.1 Organizational support for technology uptake is required	(Abidi, Vallis, Piccinini-Vallis, Imran, & Abidi, 2018); (Shaw, Rudzicz, Jamieson, & Goldfarb, 2019)
3.6.2 Clear definition of professional roles and responsibilities of clinical staff is required	(Abidi, Vallis, Piccinini-Vallis, Imran, & Abidi, 2018); (Shaw, Rudzicz, Jamieson, & Goldfarb, 2019)
3.6.3 Adoption of mobile technologies in healthcare settings will remain slow without policy and legislative change	(Kharrazi, Gonzalez, Lowe, Huerta, & Ford, 2018)
3.7 Scalability	
3.7.1 Scepticism about linking algorithms to healthcare settings	(Quan, et al., 2020); (Shaw, Rudzicz, Jamieson, & Goldfarb, 2019)
3.8 Risks	
3.8.1 How bad can a mistake turn out to be?	(Shaw, Rudzicz, Jamieson, & Goldfarb, 2019); (Abidi, Vallis, Piccinini-Vallis, Imran, & Abidi, 2018)
3.8.2 Who is responsible and accountable in the event of mistakes?	(Shaw, Rudzicz, Jamieson, & Goldfarb, 2019); (Abidi, Vallis, Piccinini-Vallis, Imran, & Abidi, 2018)
3.9 Surveillance capitalism	(Shaw, Rudzicz, Jamieson, & Goldfarb, 2019)
3.10 Competence	
3.10.1 Competence of technology user	(Abidi, Vallis, Piccinini-Vallis, Imran, & Abidi, 2018)

Table 5. Listing identified critical issues under the Matrix 2 (based on the type of issue and who (or what) is responsible)—Highlighted in yellow are keywords indicative of the specificity of the identified issues

Technological Issues	Process Issues	People Issues
1.1 Complexity 1.1.1 Complexity in translating written Clinical Practice Guidelines (CPGs) to Apps 1.2 & 3.2 Optimal performance 1.2.1 Requires improvement of algorithms 1.2.2 Requires more accessibility to Clinical Decision Rules (CDRs) and Electronic Medical Records (EMRs) 1.2.3 & 3.2.2 Requires more ease of use and improved overall performance 3.2.1 Operation and stability 3.2.3 Usefulness and meaningfulness of solution outcomes 1.4 Validation 1.4.1 Further validation of algorithms is required 1.4.3 Founding mobile solutions on established scientific practices and peer reviewed literature is required 3.3 Cost 3.3.1 Potential requirement of advanced computation power	1.2 Complexity 1.1.1 Complexity in translating written Clinical Practice Guidelines (CPGs) to Apps 1.2 & 3.2 Optimal performance 1.2.1 Requires improvement of algorithms 1.2.2 Requires more accessibility to Clinical Decision Rules (CDRs) and Electronic Medical Records (EMRs) 1.2.3 & 3.2.2 Requires more ease of use and improved overall performance 3.2.1 Operation and stability 3.2.3 Usefulness and meaningfulness of solution outcomes 1.3 Limited data 1.3.1 Available data for training and testing algorithms is limited 1.3.2 Lack of data to generalize models 1.4 & 2.3 Validation 1.4.2 Standardization of mobile solutions is required 1.4.3 Founding mobile solutions on established scientific practices and peer reviewed literature is required 2.3.1 More evidence on clinical impact of the use of mobile solutions in healthcare is required 2.1 Generalizability 2.1.1 Lack of generalizability of user/participant opinions 3.1 Workload 3.1.1 Should not increase clinicians' workload 3.3 Cost 3.3.1 Potential requirement of advanced computation power 3.3.2 Requirement of additional staff 3.4 Expandability 3.4.1 Scepticism about black-box nature of certain Machine Learning algorithms 3.5 Privacy 3.5.1 Privacy and consent concern the patients would have 3.5.2 Data security 3.6 Policy and legislative challenges 3.6.1 Organizational support for technology uptake is required 3.6.2 Clear definition of professional roles and responsibilities of clinical staff is required 3.6.3 Adoption of mobile technologies in healthcare settings will remain slow without policy and legislative change 3.7 Scalability 3.7.1 Scepticism about linking algorithms to healthcare settings 3.8 Risks 3.8.1 How bad can a mistake turn out to be? 3.8.2 Who is responsible and accountable in the event of mistakes?	2.2 Biases 2.2.1 Familiarity biases of users/participants 2.2.2 Response biases of users/participants 2.2 3 Self-selection biases of users/participants 3.5 Privacy 3.5.1 Privacy and consent concern the patients would have 3.5.2 Data security 3.9 Surveillance capitalism 3.10 Competence 3.10.1 Competence of technology user

solution. The second matrix is of a standard socio-technical type. It is indicative of the type of an issue, and who (or what) is responsible should the issue occur.

According to the first matrix, it was evident that a majority of issues got mapped onto the stage of Adoption of mobile solutions in Healthcare. On the second matrix, the dominating class of issues happened to be the Process Issues class. It was evident that there is a significant overlap between "Adoption" issues (in the first matrix) and "Process Issues" (in the second matrix). This review also revealed that technological issues are not dominant.

These findings emphasize that, to reap out the optimal benefits from the introduction of mobile solutions to the sector of Healthcare, the two workflows: (a) Coordination to understand and address the issues with Process and Adoption, and (b) Development of mobile technological solutions, require to go hand-in-hand, and not in isolation.

REFERENCES

Abidi, S., Vallis, M., Piccinini-Vallis, H., Imran, S., & Abidi, S. (2018). Diabetes-related behavior change knowledge transfer to primary care practitioners and patients: Implementation and evaluation of a digital health platform. *JMIR Medical Informatics*, 6(2), e25. doi:10.2196/medinform.9629 PMID:29669705

Australia's National Digital Health Strategy. (2018). *Australia's national digital health strategy: safe, seamless and secure: evolving health and care to meet the needs of modern Australia.* Australian Government and Australian Digital Health Agency. Retrieved from https://conversation.digitalhealth.gov.au/australias-national-digital-health-strategy

Barteit, S., Neuhann, F., Bärnighausen, T., Bowa, A., Wolter, S., Siabwanta, H., & Jahn, A. (2019). Technology Acceptance and Information System Success of a Mobile Electronic Platform for Nonphysician Clinical Students in Zambia: Prospective, Nonrandomized Intervention Study. *Journal of Medical Internet Research*, 21(10), e14748. doi:10.2196/14748 PMID:31599731

Berrouiguet, S., Barrigón, M., Brandt, S., Nitzburg, G., Ovejero, S., Alvarez-Garcia, R., ... Lenca, P. (2017). Ecological assessment of clinicians' antipsychotic prescription habits in psychiatric inpatients: A novel web-and mobile phone–based prototype for a dynamic clinical decision support system. *Journal of Medical Internet Research*, 19(1), e25. doi:10.2196/jmir.5954 PMID:28126703

Bian, J., Weir, C., Unni, P., Borbolla, D., Reese, T., Wan, Y.-K., & Del Fiol, G. (2018). Interactive Visual Displays for Interpreting the Results of Clinical Trials: Formative Evaluation With Case Vignettes. *Journal of Medical Internet Research*, 20(6), e10507. doi:10.2196/10507 PMID:29941416

Blagec, K., Romagnoli, K. M., Boyce, R. D., & Samwald, M. (2016). Examining perceptions of the usefulness and usability of a mobile-based system for pharmacogenomics clinical decision support: A mixed methods study. *PeerJ*, *1671*. Advance online publication. doi:10.7717/peerj.1671 PMID:26925317

Bogie, K., Zhang, G.-Q., Roggenkamp, S., Zeng, N., Seton, J., Tao, S., Bloostein, A. L., & Sun, J. (2018). Individualized Clinical Practice Guidelines for Pressure Injury Management: Development of an Integrated Multi-Modal Biomedical Information Resource. *JMIR Research Protocols*, 7(9), e10871. doi:10.2196/10871 PMID:30190252

Camacho, J. Ch. A., Landis-Lewis, Z., Douglas, G., & Boyce, R. (2018). Comparing a Mobile Decision Support System Versus the Use of Printed Materials for the Implementation of an Evidence-Based Recommendation: Protocol for a Qualitative Evaluation. *JMIR Research Protocols*, 7(4), e105. doi:10.2196/resprot.9827 PMID:29653921

Clancy, C. M., & Cronin, K. (2005). Evidence-based decision making: Global evidence, local decisions. *Health Affairs*, 24(1), 151–162. doi:10.1377/hlthaff.24.1.151 PMID:15647226

Con, D., & De Cruz, P. (2016). Mobile phone apps for inflammatory bowel disease self-management: A systematic assessment of content and tools. *JMIR mHealth and uHealth, 4*(1), e13. doi:10.2196/mhealth.4874 PMID:26831935

Dafli, E., Antoniou, P., Ioannidis, L., Dombros, N., Topps, D., & Bamidis, P. (2015). Virtual patients on the semantic Web: A proof-of-application study. *Journal of Medical Internet Research, 17*(1), e16. doi:10.2196/jmir.3933 PMID:25616272

Digital Health, C. R. C. (2020). Retrieved from digital health CRC: https://www.digitalhealthcrc.com/

Furberg, R., Williams, P., Bagwell, J., & LaBresh, K. (2017). A mobile clinical decision support tool for pediatric cardiovascular risk-reduction clinical practice guidelines: Development and description. *JMIR mHealth and uHealth, 5*(3), e29. doi:10.2196/mhealth.6291 PMID:28270384

Jacob, C., Sanchez-Vazquez, A., & Ivory, C. (2019). Clinicians' Role in the Adoption of an Oncology Decision Support App in Europe and Its Implications for Organizational Practices: Qualitative Case Study. *JMIR mHealth and uHealth, 7*(5), e13555. doi:10.2196/13555 PMID:31066710

Jordan, S., McSwiggan, J., Parker, J., Halas, G., & Friesen, M. (2018). An mHealth App for decision-making support in wound dressing selection (wounDS): Protocol for a user-centered feasibility study. *JMIR Research Protocols, 7*(4), e108. doi:10.2196/resprot.9116 PMID:29691213

Kharrazi, H., Gonzalez, C., Lowe, K., Huerta, T., & Ford, E. (2018). Forecasting the maturation of electronic health record functions among US hospitals: Retrospective analysis and predictive model. *Journal of Medical Internet Research, 20*(8), e10458. doi:10.2196/10458 PMID:30087090

Lee, Y.-L., Cui, Y.-Y., Tu, M.-H., Chen, Y.-C., & Chang, P. (2018). Mobile health to maintain continuity of patient-centered care for chronic kidney disease: Content analysis of apps. *JMIR mHealth and uHealth, 6*(4), e10173. doi:10.2196/10173 PMID:29678805

Lin, F.-C., Wang, C.-Y., Shang, R., Hsiao, F.-Y., Lin, M.-S., Hung, K.-Y., ... Shen, L.-J. (2018). Identifying unmet treatment needs for patients with osteoporotic fracture: Feasibility study for an electronic clinical surveillance system. *Journal of Medical Internet Research, 20*(4), e142. doi:10.2196/jmir.9477 PMID:29691201

Lv, N., Xiao, L., Simmons, M., Rosas, L., Chan, A., & Entwistle, M. (2017). Personalized hypertension management using patient-generated health data integrated with electronic health records (EMPOWER-H): Six-month pre-post study. *Journal of Medical Internet Research, 19*(9), e311. doi:10.2196/jmir.7831 PMID:28928111

Melnick, E., Hess, E., Guo, G., Breslin, M., Lopez, K., Pavlo, A., Abujarad, F., Powsner, S. M., & Post, L. (2017). Patient-centered decision support: Formative usability evaluation of integrated clinical decision support with a patient decision aid for minor head injury in the emergency department. *Journal of Medical Internet Research, 19*(5), e174. doi:10.2196/jmir.7846 PMID:28526667

Moghimi, F. H., De Steiger, R., Schaffer, J., & Wickramasinghe, N. (2013). The benefits of adopting e-performance management techniques and strategies to facilitate superior healthcare delivery: The proffering of a conceptual framework for the context of Hip and Knee Arthroplasty. *Health and technology, 3*(3), 237–247. doi:10.100712553-013-0057-4

Moher, D., Liberati, A., Tetzlaff, J., & Altman, D. G. (2009). Preferred reporting items for systematic reviews and meta-analyses: The PRISMA statement. *PLoS Medicine, 6*(7), e1000097. doi:10.1371/journal.pmed.1000097 PMID:19621072

Nhavoto, J., Grönlund, Å., & Chaquilla, W. (2015). SMSaúde: Design, development, and implementation of a remote/mobile patient management system to improve retention in care for HIV/AIDS and tuberculosis patients. *JMIR mHealth and uHealth, 3*(1), e26. doi:10.2196/mhealth.3854 PMID:25757551

Paradis, M., Stiell, I., Atkinson, K., Guerinet, J., Sequeira, Y., Salter, L., Forster, A. J., Murphy, M. S. Q., & Wilson, K. (2018). Acceptability of a Mobile Clinical Decision Tool Among Emergency Department Clinicians: Development and Evaluation of The Ottawa Rules App. *JMIR mHealth and uHealth, 6*(6), e10263. doi:10.2196/10263 PMID:29891469

Pham, A., Bluett, E., Puthran, P., Sarkar, S., Kim, K., & Shankar, P. (2018). First 28: Design of a Mobile App for Neonatal Health Risk Assessment and Support for New Mothers. *Iproceedings, 4*(2), e11740. doi:10.2196/11740

Quan, A., Stiell, I., Perry, J., Paradis, M., Brown, E., Gignac, J., Wilson, L., & Wilson, K. (2020). Mobile Clinical Decision Tools Among Emergency Department Clinicians: Web-Based Survey and Analytic Data for Evaluation of The Ottawa Rules App. *JMIR mHealth and uHealth, 8*(1), e15503. doi:10.2196/15503 PMID:32012095

Sandal, L., Stochkendahl, M., Svendsen, M., Wood, K., Øverås, C., Nordstoga, A., ... Cooper, K. (2019). An App-Delivered Self-Management Program for People With Low Back Pain: Protocol for the self-BACK Randomized Controlled Trial. *JMIR Research Protocols, 8*(12), e14720. doi:10.2196/14720 PMID:31793897

Seto, E., Ware, P., Logan, A., Cafazzo, J., Chapman, K., Segal, P., & Ross, H. (2017). Self-management and clinical decision support for patients with complex chronic conditions through the use of smartphone-based telemonitoring: Randomized controlled trial protocol. *JMIR Research Protocols, 6*(11), e229. doi:10.2196/resprot.8367 PMID:29162557

Shaw, J., Rudzicz, F., Jamieson, T., & Goldfarb, A. (2019). Artificial Intelligence and the Implementation Challenge. *Journal of Medical Internet Research, 21*(7), e13659. doi:10.2196/13659 PMID:31293245

Singh, N., Hess, E., Guo, G., Sharp, A., Huang, B., Breslin, M., & Melnick, E. (2017). Tablet-based patient-centered decision support for minor head injury in the emergency department: Pilot study. *JMIR mHealth and uHealth, 5*(9), e144. doi:10.2196/mhealth.8732 PMID:28958987

Tran, C., Dicker, A., Leiby, B., Gressen, E., Williams, N., & Jim, H. (2020). Utilizing Digital Health to Collect Electronic Patient-Reported Outcomes in Prostate Cancer: Single-Arm Pilot Trial. *Journal of Medical Internet Research, 22*(3), e12689. doi:10.2196/12689 PMID:32209536

van Heerden, A., Sen, D., Desmond, C., Louw, J., & Richter, L. (2017). App-supported promotion of child growth and development by community health workers in Kenya: Feasibility and acceptability study. *JMIR mHealth and uHealth, 5*(12), e182. doi:10.2196/mhealth.6911 PMID:29208588 van Kollenburg, R., de Bruin, D., & Wijkstra, H. (2019). Validation of the Electronic Version of the International Index of Erectile Function (IIEF-5 and IIEF-15): A Crossover Study. *Journal of Medical Internet Research*, *21*(7), e13490. doi:10.2196/13490 PMID:31267983

Ware, P., Ross, H., Cafazzo, J., Boodoo, C., Munnery, M., & Seto, E. (2020). Outcomes of a Heart Failure Telemonitoring Program Implemented as the Standard of Care in an Outpatient Heart Function Clinic: Pretest-Posttest Pragmatic Study. *Journal of Medical Internet Research*, *22*(2), e16538. doi:10.2196/16538 PMID:32027309

Woldaregay, A., Årsand, E., Botsis, T., Albers, D., Mamykina, L., & Hartvigsen, G. (2019). Data-driven blood glucose pattern classification and anomalies detection: Machine-learning applications in type 1 diabetes. *Journal of Medical Internet Research*, *21*(5), e11030. doi:10.2196/11030 PMID:31042157

Wu, Y., Yao, X., Vespasiani, G., Nicolucci, A., Dong, Y., Kwong, J., Li, L., Sun, X., Tian, H., & Li, S. (2017). Mobile app-based interventions to support diabetes self-management: A systematic review of randomized controlled trials to identify functions associated with glycemic efficacy. *JMIR mHealth and uHealth*, *5*(3), e35. doi:10.2196/mhealth.6522 PMID:28292740

Ye, C., Wang, O., Liu, M., Zheng, L., Xia, M., Hao, S., ... Huang, C. (2019). A Real-Time Early Warning System for Monitoring Inpatient Mortality Risk: Prospective Study Using Electronic Medical Record Data. *Journal of Medical Internet Research*, *21*(7), e13719. doi:10.2196/13719 PMID:31278734

Zarinabad, N., Meeus, E. M., Manias, K., Foster, K., & Peet, A. (2018). Automated Modular Magnetic Resonance Imaging Clinical Decision Support System (MIROR): An Application in Pediatric Cancer Diagnosis. *JMIR Medical Informatics*, *6*(2), e30. doi:10.2196/medinform.9171 PMID:29720361

APPENDIX

Table 6. Classification of Subject topics into the two categories "Relevant" and "Exclude".

Relevant (Includes 30 Subject Areas)	Exclude (Includes 20 Subject Areas)
decision support systems	
decision making	
decision support system	
decision support	
decision support systems, clinical	
electronic health records	machine learning
artificial intelligence	data mining
telemedicine	company business management
decision making in clinical medicine	algorithms
mobile applications	big data
decision-making	algorithm
risk assessment	technology
mobile apps	sustainability
information storage & retrieval systems -- medical care	research funding
medical informatics	climate change
decision support techniques	research methodology
medical decision making	fuzzy logic
information technology	sustainable development
medical care	geographic information systems
diagnosis	descriptive statistics
decision-making -- analysis	artificial neural networks
clinical decision support	research article
mhealth	management
smartphone	computer simulation
evidence-based medicine	gis
optimization	
medicine	
therapeutics	
data analysis	
multiple criteria decision making	

Chapter 5
Comorbidities and Diabetes Type 2:
A Gender–Driven Probabilistic Estimate of Patient's Risk Factor

Chinedu I. Ossai

https://orcid.org/0000-0002-9749-3256

Swinburne University, Australia

Nilmini Wickramasinghe

https://orcid.org/0000-0002-1314-8843

Swinburne University, Australia

Steven Goldberg

INET International, Canada

ABSTRACT

The prevalence of diabetes type 2 among the population and the increasing rate of new diagnoses as well as other co-morbidities make it imperative that we develop a richer understanding of type 2 diabetes. An Australian survey of diabetes type 2 people for different co-morbidities was carried out to obtain information about the possible connections of the co-morbidities with type 2 diabetes. The analysis is done with the logit model and Pearson's chi-square and the results indicate that gender, age of the patients, and the duration of the diabetes type 2 diagnosis play a significant role in the exposure of individuals to different comorbidities. The influence of the duration of diagnosis and age of the patients is limited in comparison to the gender, which has females at a very high risk of developing the studied co-morbidities compared to males. The findings can improve diabetes type 2 management to boost high quality, proactive, and cost-effective caregiving for the patients.

DOI: 10.4018/978-1-5225-6067-8.ch005

1.0 INTRODUCTION

Diabetes is a chronic disease condition that results in the body's inability to effectively absorb the glucose it produces or when the pancreas is not able to produce sufficient insulin needed for the proper functioning of the body (WHO 2016). The menace can make it difficult for the body to effectively convert all monosaccharides and disaccharides sugar present in manufactured or cooked food including naturally occurring sugar in honey and fruits (WHO/FAO Expert Consultation 2003). Diabetes can be type 1 that is characterized by insufficient insulin production in the body (ADA 2005, Daneman 2006) or type 2, which results in the body's inability to effectively utilize the insulin produced by the pancreas (WHO 2016,ACCORD 2008). Type 1 diabetes is insulin-dependent and not preventable and exposes patients to excessive urination, taste, constant hunger, fatigue, weight loss, and vision impairments (WHO 2016). Diabetes type 2 has symptoms that are like type 1 but are not always pronounced hence, they may remain undiagnosed for an extensive period causing complications (WHO 2016).

In 2018, Over 500 million people are living globally with diabetes type 2 that has prevalence rate comparable among the poor and rich countries, but that is expected to increase over the next decade (Kaiser et al. 2018). Unfortunately, the ailment is a metabolic disease that is diagnosed on sustained hyperglycaemia and poses an elevated risk for heart problems, blindness, kidney failure, amputation, fractures, depression, arthritis, neuropathy, and cognitive decline (Kaiser et al. 2018, Laakso and Kuusisto 2007, Xie and Cheng 202, Coto-Segura et al. 2013, Solomon et al. 2011). The development of diabetes type 2 is associated with different environmental and genetic factors that increase insulin resistance. These factors could be linked to age, decreased exercise, and overweight especially the accumulation of intra-abdominal adiposity (WHO 2016, Gerich 2003, Kahn 2003, Xie and Cheng 2012).

The evidence of the increased risk factor of diabetes type 2 patients in the literature is numerous from many clinical trials. Goff Jr. *et al.* (2007) established the link between some of the comorbidities with the degree of hyperglycaemia by measuring the glycated haemoglobin level for 2 to 3 months. They concluded that a 1% increase in the glycated haemoglobin level resulted in 18% increase in the risk of cardiovascular diseases. Although the increase of glucose in diabetes type 2 patients can increase the chances of death, retinopathy, heart attack and stroke (WHO 2016, Laakso and Kuusisto 2007, Salvin et al. 2004), the use of intensive glycated haemoglobin reduction can result in the death of patients (ACCORD 2008). Juutilainen *et al.* (2005) investigated the risk of coronary heart disease mortality among diabetes type 2 patients without prior myocardial infarction and concluded that the risk of death among them is similar to non-diabetic type 2 patients with myocardial infarction. The authors also affirmed that the risk level is the same with men and women. However, women patients without coronary heart diseases such as myocardial infarction, angina pectoris, and ischemic ECG changes were at higher risk than non-diabetic patients with the same heart conditions (Juutilainen et al. 2005).

Other researchers have also associated diabetes type 2 with other diseases with Cheng *et al.* (2012) concluding that patients that suffer from psoriasis have a higher risk of developing diabetes type 2 more than those without the disease. Similarly, Coto-Segura *et al.* (2013) used metadata analysis to affirm that both psoriasis and psoriatic arthritis increase the risk of patients' susceptibility to diabetes type 2. Research has also shown that neuropathy is one of the common aftereffects of diabetes type 2 and impacts 1 in 6 patients (Daousi et al. 2004). Diabetic neuropathy affects the patients in the form of sensation loss and has been attributed to neuropathic ulcers and amputation (Poncelet 2003, Vileikyte et al. 2004). This finding concurs with the conclusions of Davies *et al.* (2006) that affirmed that chronic painful diabetic peripheral neuropathy negatively affected the quality of life of diabetes type 2 patients.

Again, Van Acker *et al.* (2009) showed that diabetic polyneuropathy with and without pains was predominant in diabetes type 2 patients and the severities increased with age and duration of diabetes. The authors further showed that neuropathy, obesity, low HDL cholesterol, and high triglyceride levels are associated with diabetic polyneuropathy that occurs with or without pains. Furthermore, Xie and Cheng (2012) showed that obesity and adipose tissue redistribution can enhance different health risks due to the potentials of diabetes type 2 patients' insulin resistance. To this end, the counseling of patients with obesity and adipose tissue redistribution will enhance their quality of life since prophylactic treatment is not recommended for all diabetes type 2 patients (Xie and cheng 2013).

Since diabetic peripheral neuropathy negatively affects the sensory functions with a consequent poor maximum grip strength, which negatively impacts hand dexterity, de Almeida Lima *et al.* (2017) developed a study to determine the response of diabetes type 2 patients to grip strength of the hand. They concluded that mild to moderate diabetic peripheral neuropathy impaired hand dexterity and control of individuals suffering from diabetes type 2. This condition can hamper the proficiency of daily live manipulation of tasks and can pose these individuals to safety risks from dropping handheld objects. On the other hand, a study has shown that the safety margin for handheld task performance of non-neuropathic diabetic individuals is lower than those of non-diabetic individuals (De Freitas et al. 2013). This suggests that these diabetic patients can be at risk of losing handheld objects because of their sensory impairment.

Although inflammatory conditions play a crucial role in chronic obstructive disease and have been associated with diabetes type 2 and asthma, there is limited evidence to link asthma to the increased risk of diabetes type 2 in women (Rana et al. 2004). This sentiment is also shared by Song *et al.* (2010) that concluded that asthma and chronic obstructive pulmonary disease did show individual and independent increased risk of diabetes type 2 after multivariate analysis of surveyed data of women of over 45 years of age. Other researchers have linked diabetes type 2 to vision loss via diabetic retinopathy, which is a microvascular complication of diabetes (ACCORD 2010). The risk of retinopathy and vision loss have been shown to increase due to the elevation of serum cholesterol and triglyceride (29- 29. Reichard et al. 1993,DCCTRG 1995,UPDSG 1998). However, clinical trials have shown that intensive control of glycaemic and blood pressure are playing a vital role in reducing the progression of retinopathy (Miljanovic et al. 2004).

Considering the various risk associated with diabetes type 2 patients, it is vital to understand the level of the impacts on the patients at different durations of the sickness and different ages. This will make it possible to have person-tailored management practices that will be efficient and cost-effective for improving the quality of life and reducing the effects of comorbidities.

2.0 AIM OF THE STUDY

This study aims to establish the risk of diabetes type 2 patients developing comorbidities such as arthritis, neuropathy, shaking and dexterity related problems, heart problems, vision loss problems, and asthma by extracting information from a selected group of individuals. We will use the information obtained from this sampled population to estimate the risk factors of both male and female patients diagnosed with diabetes type 2 by determining the chances of developing the listed comorbidities over the duration of suffering from diabetes. The risk level of the patients at different ages and duration of diabetes type 2 diagnosis will also be established while hypothesizing the influence of gender and the duration of the disease on the subjectiveness of patients to the listed comorbidities.

This knowledge will be vital for personalized management of diabetes type 2 at different durations of diagnosis seeing that one of the panaceas for enhanced quality of life of the sufferers is proper management. Since the elderly are most vulnerable to these risks (Van Acker et al. 2009), the understanding of the level of their vulnerability will provide useful information for developing early interventions that will help to reduce the financial burdens on the health system.

3.0 GENDER, DURATION OF DIAGNOSIS AND SUBJECTIVENESS TO COMORBIDITIES

The role of gender and the duration of diabetes type 2 diagnoses on the subjectiveness of patients to other diseases cannot be overemphasized as numerous researchers showed that genders (Rana et al. 2004, Song et al. 2010, Kautzky et al. 2016) and duration of suffering diabetes type 2 (Van Acker et al. 2009) can impact the vulnerability of patients to the comorbidities. For instance, diabetes type 2 diminishes the protection of females from developing cardiac sicknesses and nephropathy (Van Acker et al. 2009) and due to endocrine and behavioral factors, different genders have different effects and outcomes of disease interventions. Based on the above-stated information, it has been hypothesized that:

Proposition 1: "Gender of diabetes type 2 patients influences their subjectiveness to comorbidities"
Proposition 2: "The subjectiveness of patients to comorbidities is a function of the duration of diagnosis and gender."

4.0 RESEARCH METHODOLOGY

Data for this study was obtained from a survey that involved one hundred participants with twenty-one responses from diabetes type 2 patients drawn from Australia. They were asked to answer different questions relating to the time of diagnosis of diabetes type 2 and the various comorbidities they have been formally diagnosed by a physician. The participants were asked to answer yes, no, or don't know for the diagnosis of the diseases that included arthritis, asthma, heart problems, vision problems not helped by wearing corrective lenses, shaking and dexterity problems, and neuropathy. The questionnaire also requested them to provide information about their gender, duration of diabetes, and age. All the information was anonymously collected from the participants for the study.

To establish the probability of a diabetes type 2 patient suffering the diseases considered in this study, the logit model was used. This model is most appropriate for analysing variables that have the dependent parameter(s) varying dichotomously as a binary 'yes' or 'no' (1 and 0). As a predictive model, it describes the relationship between the dependent and independent variables and can also show how one dependent parameter varies with one or many nominal, ordinary, or ratio-level independent parameters. This model helps to estimate the probability of a female and male diabetic patient suffering the outlined diseases in consideration of their ages, duration of diabetes type 2, and gender. In the second stage of the analysis, we used Pearson's chi-square test because of the need to determine the likelihood that the acquired survey data for different categories of parameters are not chance events, hence, the goodness-of-fit test is used to establish how independent the distributions of the events are. The correlation between the genders and the demographic information of the respondents was established to measure the statistical significance of the associations at a 0.05 significant level.

5.0 RESULTS AND DISCUSSION

The summary of the demographic information of the respondents and the percentage that are diagnosed with different diseases are shown in Figure 1, which indicates that 24% of the respondents were diagnosed with arthritis and 71% were not. Asthmatic patients made up 14% of the sampled population, 19% suffered heart problems, 24% have vision loss that cannot be corrected with lenses, 14% have shaking and dexterity problems whereas 5% are not sure if they are suffering from arthritis, vision loss, and neuropathy.

Figure 1. Summary of the response of the sampled population and the proportion that suffer from different comorbidities

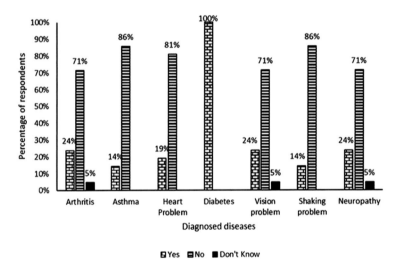

According to Figure 2, 48% of the respondents do not have any of the six comorbidities considered in this study while 5% of them have 3 and 5 other diseases they have been diagnosed. About 10% have 2 and 4 comorbidities and 24% have only one extra diagnosed disease. This result is not surprising because previous research by Iglay *et al.* (2016) indicated that 97.5% of adult diabetes type 2 patients have at least 1 comorbidity and the risk level increases with the patient's age.

The descriptive statistics of the respondents by gender and the percentage of respondents suffering the comorbidities are shown in Table 1.

The average duration of the time the male respondents have been diagnosed with diabetes type 2 is about 58% more than the average duration the female has been diagnosed and the female accounted for 43% of the participants (Table 1). However, the population of the female participants diagnosed with the studied comorbidities varied from 50% to more than 500% higher than the male. The duration of the patients' diabetes diagnoses and the comorbidity variabilities is shown in Figure 3. From Figure 3, all the patients suffering from diabetes type 2 for 10-15 years also suffer from asthma whereas only 13% of

Figure 2. Summary of the surveyed population with different comorbidities

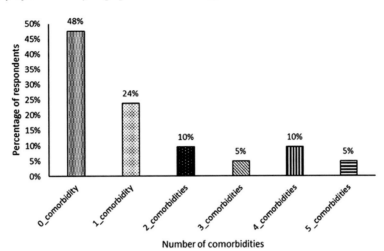

the participants diagnosed with asthma have suffered diabetes type 2 for 5-10 years. Similarly, 38% of patients that have diabetes type 2 for 5-10 years are suffering from neuropathy and 0%, 20%, and 17% of those that have suffered the disease for 10-15 years, >15 years, and < 5 years respectively were also diagnosed with neuropathy. There are 50% of the participants who suffer from diabetes type 2 between 5-10 years that are suffering from heart problems, arthritis, shaking and dexterity, and vision problems. Participants that have lived with diabetes type 2 for more than 15 years are more prone to heart problems

Table 1. Summary of Respondents by sex and other disease conditions

	Male	Female
Age (Years)		
Mean	50.83	51.67
STD	4.93	4.71
min	41	41
max	60	60
% respondent	57%	43%
Duration of Diabetes (years)		
Mean	5.92	3.75
STD	7.20	4.76
Comorbidity		
% Arthritis	8%	44%
% Asthma	0%	33%
% Heart problems	17%	22%
% Vision problems	8%	44%
% Shaking problems	8%	22%
%Neuropathy	17%	33%

Figure 3. Proportion of diabetes type2 patients diagnosed with other diseases for different durations of suffering diabetes type2

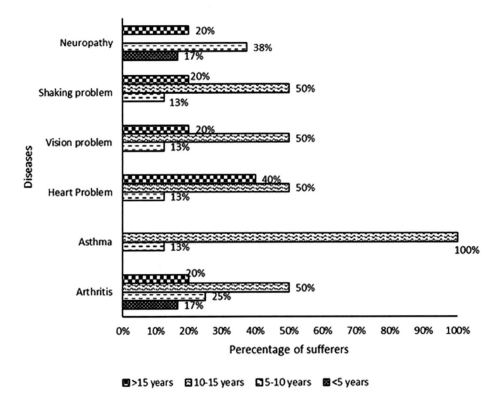

with 40% of respondents suffering different forms of heart diseases compared to 20% of these patients being impaired with vision problems, arthritis, neuropathy, and shaking and dexterity problems.

The summary statistics of the number of participants suffering from diabetes type 2 by different year groups and gender is shown in Table 2. Male sufferers with less than 5 years of diagnosis account for 0% to 17% of the comorbidities while the female is between 0% to 22%. For 5-10 years duration of diabetes type 2 diagnosis, the proportion of males suffering other diseases is from 0% to 8% whereas females are from 11% to 22%. The other age groups have male and female participants as 0 to 17% and 0 to 22% respectively.

The logit model estimated parameters for the development of comorbidities for different genders are determined with the percentage population of the sampled population that has been diagnosed with the comorbidity, the sex of the individual, the age, and the duration of the diabetes type 2 per Table 3.

The duration of diabetes type 2 diagnosis, age of the patients and their gender did not show statistical significance at 0.05 significant level. This may be attributed to the number of participants analysed or their age group. Nevertheless, the result in Table 3 shows that being a female diabetes type 2 patient increased the risk of developing comorbidities than a male patient. Females have the risk of subjectiveness to asthma extremely higher than the other comorbidities. The increase in age of the respondents didn't show a dramatic increase in the subjectiveness of the participants to the comorbidities as a unit change is age is expected only to result in between 1.09 to 1.36 increases in the chances of developing the comorbidities. This situation may be attributed to the narrow age bracket of the participants (41 to

Table 2. Summary of respondents by sex, comorbidity, and duration of diabetes

Duration of Diabetes	<5 Years	5-10 Years	10-15 Years	>15 Years
Male				
Age (years)				
Mean	49.00	50.00	0	55
STD	4.90	5.00	0	0
Min	41			
Max	60			
% respondent	42%	33%	0%	25%
% Arthritis	0%	0%	0%	8%
% Asthma	0%	0%	0%	0%
% Heart problems	0%	0%	0%	17%
% Vision problems	0%	0%	17%	8%
% Shaking problems	0%	0%	0%	8%
%Neuropathy	0%	8%	0%	0%
Female				
Age (years)				
Mean	55.00	52.50	55	45
STD	0.00	4.33	0	0
Min	41			
Max	60			
% respondent	11%	44%	22%	22%
% Arthritis	11%	22%	11%	0%
% Asthma	0%	11%	22%	0%
% Heart problems	0%	11%	11%	0%
% Vision problems	0%	11%	0%	11%
% Shaking problems	0%	11%	11%	0%
%Neuropathy	0%	22%	0%	0%

STD: standard deviation

60 years). Previous researchers (Van Acker et al. 2009, Iglay et al. 2016) have findings that support this result thereby making it emphatic that a comprehensive approach to managing diabetes type 2 patients with multimorbidity should be contextual in clinical decision making.

The risk probability for different genders as computed with the probability of developing the comorbidities at a mean age of participants and the average duration of the diabetes type 2 diagnosis has been shown in Figures 4 and 5.

Figure 4 buttresses the ascertain that women are more vulnerable to comorbidities than their male counterparts. As expected, the probability of developing the comorbidities increases with the length of the diabetes type 2 diagnosis except for arthritis and neuropathy that showed a slight decrease. Although this may not always be the case, proper management of diabetes type 2 could be a trigger for reducing

Table 3. Logit model estimated coefficients, Standard Error (SE), z_value, 95% Confidence Interval (CI) and the Odds-Rate (OR) of diabetes patients developing other diseases – arthritis, asthma, heart problems, shaking and dexterity, and neuropathy due to age, duration of diabetes and gender

	Estimate	SE	z_Value	Pr(>|z|)	95% CI		OR
Arthritis							
Duration of diabetes	-0.01	0.10	-0.06	0.95	-0.27	0.19	0.99
Age of Patient	0.06	0.11	0.56	0.57	-0.15	0.30	1.06
Sex (Female)	2.31	1.28	1.81	0.07	0.07	5.49	10.09
Asthma							
Duration of diabetes	0.10	0.25	0.42	0.68	-0.41	0.70	1.11
Age of Patient	0.18	0.23	0.78	0.43	-0.20	0.82	1.20
Sex (Female)	20.78	4551.53	0.01	1.00	-368.00	-	1.06E+09
Heart Problem							
Duration of diabetes	0.25	0.16	1.59	0.11	0.02	0.72	1.29
Age of Patient	0.31	0.20	1.51	0.13	-0.01	0.85	1.36
Sex (Female)	2.28	2.33	0.98	0.33	-1.21	9.35	9.79
Vision Problem							
Duration of diabetes	0.15	0.11	1.33	0.18	-0.05	0.46	1.16
Age of Patient	0.11	0.13	0.85	0.40	-0.12	0.42	1.11
Sex (Female)	3.06	1.92	1.59	0.11	0.20	8.75	21.22
Shaking and Dexterity Problems							
Duration of diabetes	0.11	0.12	0.89	0.37	-0.12	0.45	1.11
Age of Patient	0.21	0.17	1.25	0.21	-0.06	0.67	1.24
Sex (Female)	2.17	1.96	1.10	0.27	-0.92	8.27	8.72
Neuropathy							
Duration of diabetes	-0.05	0.10	-0.47	0.64	0.96	0.75	1.14
Age of Patient	0.19	0.13	1.44	0.15	1.21	0.97	1.69
Sex (Female)	1.25	1.15	1.09	0.28	3.49	0.38	43.03

susceptibility to comorbidities per previous research (Ose et al. 2009, Bogner et al.2012). The information further highlights the increasing need to enhance wellness among female diabetes type 2 patients since their vulnerability to the studied comorbidities can be high.

Figure 5 indicates that the increase in the age of patients results in an increased risk of developing comorbidities for a mean diabetes type 2 diagnosis duration of 8.67 years, with female patients being at higher risk than males. Similarly, a female patient is at a higher risk of developing arthritis at the age of 40 than any other comorbidity but the risk is almost the same for all the studied comorbidities when they get to 60 years. The male patients have the least risk of developing asthma followed by vision problems, arthritis, shaking and dexterity, heart problems, and neuropathy. This result is contrasted by previous work that showed that male patients are at higher risk of developing comorbidities (Iglay et al. 2016). The difference in the demography could be responsible for the difference in the findings since

Figure 4. The probability of a 52.08year-old diabetes type 2 patient developing other comorbidities over a 1 to 30 years duration of diagnoses – (a): arthritis, (b): asthma, (c): heart problems, (d): neuropathy, (e): shaking and dexterity problems, (f): vision problems.

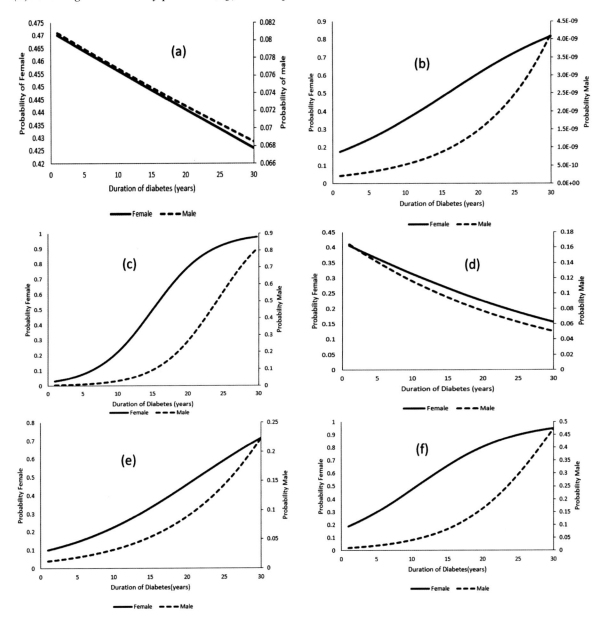

the researchers (Iglay et al. 2016) studied adults from 21 to over 75 years but this present study focused on 41 to 60 years of age.

Table 4 shows the result of Pearson's chi-square test for hypotheses that the gender of the patients influenced their subjectiveness to the comorbidities.

Table 4 shows that the gender of the diabetes type 2 patients influenced their subjectiveness to the studied comorbidities seeing that no statistically significant difference existed between the average propor-

Figure 5. The probability of a diabetes type 2 patient diagnosed for 8.67 years developing other co-morbidities between the ages of 40 to 60 years – (a): arthritis, (b): asthma, (c): heart problems, (d): neuropathy, (e): shaking and dexterity problems, (f): vision problems

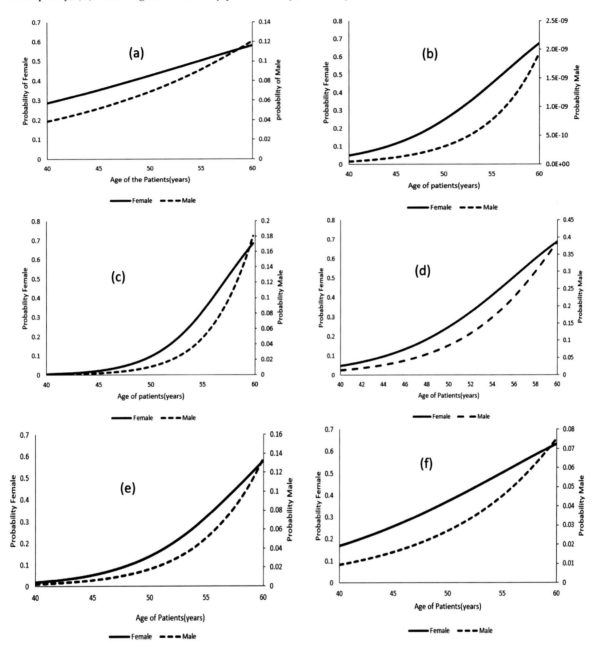

tion of the male and female populations diagnosed with the various comorbidities hence, proposition 1 is accepted. This result is further supported by previous findings (Van Acker et al. 2009, Heraclides and Chandola 2012) that indicate that various genders of diabetes type 2 patients are distinctively influenced by the comorbidities they suffer. There is also no significant difference existing between the genders of the patients and their subjectiveness to the comorbidities for the following durations of diabetes type 2

Table 4. Summary of Pearson's chi-squared test result for testing the influence of gender and the duration of diabetes type 2 diagnosis on the subjectiveness of patients to comorbidities.

H0: Null Hypothesis	P-Value	Chi-Squared (χ^2)	Statistical Significance	Remarks
The gender of diabetes type 2 patients influenced their subjectiveness to comorbidities.	0.2873	5.00	No statistical difference	H0 is accepted
The subjectiveness of patients with less than 5 years of diabetes type 2 diagnosis is a function of their gender.	0.1258	2.34	No statistical difference	H0 is accepted
The subjectiveness of patients with 5 to 10 years of diabetes type 2 diagnosis is a function of their gender.	0.04979	6.00	statistical difference	H0 is not accepted
The subjectiveness of patients with 10 to 15 years of diabetes type 2 diagnosis is a function of their gender.	0.01735	12.00	Statistical difference	H0 is not accepted
The subjectiveness of patients with more than 15 years of diabetes type 2 diagnosis is a function of their gender.	0.06999	8.67	No statistical difference	H0 is accepted

diagnosis: < 5years and > 15 years. Therefore, proposition 2 is accepted for the two durations, which implies that patients' gender plays a good role in their risk of developing comorbidities. This assertion is shared by some researchers that have shown that male and female diabetes type 2 patients have different levels of exposure to different diseases (Rana et al. 2004, Song et al. 2010). On the other hand, for the duration: 5 – 10 years and 10-15 years, there is a significant difference between the comorbidities for the genders, hence proposition 2 is rejected. This means that for the patients with the duration of their diabetes type 2 diagnosis within the stated times, the effect of gender on the comorbidities cannot be established. This finding could mean that some of the comorbidities have not been diagnosed because their symptoms are still latent seeing that endocrine and behavioural factors cause the difference in the health outcomes for both male and female genders (Kautzky-Willer et al. 2016).

6.0 CONCLUSION AND FUTURE RESEARCH

The importance of this study cannot be overstated because it holds great values for understanding the vulnerability of diabetes type 2 patients to the studied comorbidities because the level of exposure at different ages and duration of diagnosis is shown. We analysed the risk of developing comorbidities such as arthritis, asthma, heart problems, vision loss that is not corrected by using lenses, shaking, and dexterity and neuropathy by surveying a population of Australian residents suffering from diabetes type 2. By collecting information about the duration of the diagnosis of diabetes type 2, the age of the patients, the comorbidities diagnosed, and the gender of the respondents, vital information for establishing the risk of patients' susceptibility to the diseases was determined probabilistically with the logit model. Pearson's chi-square was also used to test the hypotheses that focused on the influence of gender and the duration of diabetes type 2 diagnoses on the risk of patients developing the studied co-morbidities.

The study found that gender plays a significant role in the probability of patients developing co-morbidities with females being more susceptible than males. The risk probabilities also varied with the comorbidities, age of the patients, and the duration of diabetes type 2 diagnosis but the risk posed by gender is far greater. The risk of heart problems and vision loss was found to be more pronounced with the increase in the duration of diabetes type 2 diagnosis than the other comorbidities while the risk of developing arthritis and vision problems at the age of 40 is higher than the other diseases. The chances of developing the comorbidities at 60 years are almost the same for the female patients but varied dramatically for the male.

This work is expected to continue to collect data from more people to further validate the trend established in the current analysis. This is vital for gaining more understanding about the changing gender-driven risk of developing the comorbidities while enhancing the potentials of developing a management plan that will be tailored to different genders. There is also a higher tendency of using the management framework to target the age of the patients and the duration of diabetes type 2 diagnosis. More data from diabetes type 2 diagnosis of fewer than 5 years and between 10 to 15 years will be needed to establish how gender did not influence the risk of the patients developing the studied comorbidities.

REFERENCES

ACCORD Study Group and ACCORD Eye Study Group. (2010). Effects of medical therapies on retinopathy progression in type 2 diabetes. *The New England Journal of Medicine, 363*(3), 233–244. doi:10.1056/NEJMoa1001288 PMID:20587587

Action to Control Cardiovascular Risk in Diabetes (ACCORD) Study Group. (2008). Effects of intensive glucose lowering in type 2 diabetes. *The New England Journal of Medicine, 358*(24), 2545–2559. doi:10.1056/NEJMoa0802743 PMID:18539917

American Diabetes Association (ADA). (2005). Clinical practice recommendations 2005. *Diabetes Care, 28*, S1. PMID:15618109

Bogner, H. R., Morales, K. H., de Vries, H. F., & Cappola, A. R. (2012). Integrated management of type 2 diabetes mellitus and depression treatment to improve medication adherence: A randomized controlled trial. *Annals of Family Medicine, 10*(1), 15–22. doi:10.1370/afm.1344 PMID:22230826

Cheng, J., Kuai, D., Zhang, L., Yang, X., & Qiu, B. (2012). Psoriasis increased the risk of diabetes: A meta-analysis. *Archives of Dermatological Research, 304*(2), 119–125. doi:10.100700403-011-1200-6 PMID:22210176

Coto-Segura, P., Eiris-Salvado, N., González-Lara, L., Queiro-Silva, R., Martinez-Camblor, P., Maldonado-Seral, C., García-García, B., Palacios-García, L., Gomez-Bernal, S., Santos-Juanes, J., & Coto, E. (2013). Psoriasis, psoriatic arthritis and type 2 diabetes mellitus: A systematic review and meta-analysis. *British Journal of Dermatology, 169*(4), 783–793. doi:10.1111/bjd.12473 PMID:23772556

Daneman, D. (2006). Type 1 diabetes. *Lancet, 367*(9513), 847–858. doi:10.1016/S0140-6736(06)68341-4 PMID:16530579

Daousi, C., MacFarlane, I. A., Woodward, A., Nurmikko, T. J., Bundred, P. E., & Benbow, S. J. (2004). Chronic painful peripheral neuropathy in an urban community: A controlled comparison of people with and without diabetes. *Diabetic Medicine, 21*(9), 976–982. doi:10.1111/j.1464-5491.2004.01271.x PMID:15317601

Davies, M., Brophy, S., Williams, R., & Taylor, A. (2006). The prevalence, severity, and impact of painful diabetic peripheral neuropathy in type 2 diabetes. *Diabetes Care*, 29(7), 1518–1522. doi:10.2337/dc05-2228 PMID:16801572

de Almeida Lima, K. C., da Silva Borges, L., Hatanaka, E., Rolim, L. C., & de Freitas, P. B. (2017). Grip force control and hand dexterity are impaired in individuals with diabetic peripheral neuropathy. *Neuroscience Letters*, 659, 54–59. doi:10.1016/j.neulet.2017.08.071 PMID:28867590

De Freitas, P. B., & Lima, K. C. A. (2013). Grip force control during simple manipulation tasks in non-neuropathic diabetic individuals. *Clinical Neurophysiology*, 124(9), 1904–1910. doi:10.1016/j.clinph.2013.04.002 PMID:23643574

Diabetes Control and Complications Trial Research Group. (1995). The effect of intensive diabetes treatment on the progression of diabetic retinopathy in insulin dependent diabetes mellitus. *Archives of Ophthalmology*, 113(1), 36–51. doi:10.1001/archopht.1995.01100010038019 PMID:7826293

Gerich, J. E. (2003, April). Contributions of insulin-resistance and insulin-secretory defects to the pathogenesis of type 2 diabetes mellitus. *Mayo Clinic Proceedings*, 78(4), 447–456. doi:10.4065/78.4.447 PMID:12683697

Goff, D. C. Jr, Gerstein, H. C., Ginsberg, H. N., Cushman, W. C., Margolis, K. L., Byington, R. P., Buse, J. B., Genuth, S., Probstfield, J. L., & Simons-Morton, D. G.ACCORD Study Group. (2007). Prevention of cardiovascular disease in persons with type 2 diabetes mellitus: Current knowledge and rationale for the Action to Control Cardiovascular Risk in Diabetes (ACCORD) trial. *The American Journal of Cardiology*, 99(12), S4–S20. doi:10.1016/j.amjcard.2007.03.002 PMID:17599424

Heraclides, A. M., Chandola, T., Witte, D. R., & Brunner, E. J. (2012). Work stress, obesity and the risk of Type 2 Diabetes: Gender-specific bidirectional effect in the Whitehall II study. *Obesity (Silver Spring, Md.)*, 20(2), 428–433. doi:10.1038/oby.2011.95 PMID:21593804

Iglay, K., Hannachi, H., Joseph Howie, P., Xu, J., Li, X., Engel, S. S., Moore, L. M., & Rajpathak, S. (2016). Prevalence and co-prevalence of comorbidities among patients with type 2 diabetes mellitus. *Current Medical Research and Opinion*, 32(7), 1243–1252. doi:10.1185/03007995.2016.1168291 PMID:26986190

Juutilainen, A., Lehto, S., Rönnemaa, T., Pyörälä, K., & Laakso, M. (2005). Type 2 diabetes as a "coronary heart disease equivalent": An 18-year prospective population-based study in Finnish subjects. *Diabetes Care*, 28(12), 2901–2907. doi:10.2337/diacare.28.12.2901 PMID:16306552

Kahn, S. E. (2003). The relative contributions of insulin resistance and beta-cell dysfunction to the pathophysiology of type 2 diabetes. *Diabetologia*, 46(1), 3–19. doi:10.100700125-002-1009-0 PMID:12637977

Kaiser, A. B., Zhang, N., & Van der Pluijm, W. (2018). *Global prevalence of type 2 diabetes over the next ten years (2018-2028)*. American Diabetes Association. Available from https://diabetes.diabetesjournals.org/content/67/Supplement_1/202-LB

Kautzky-Willer, A., Harreiter, J., & Pacini, G. (2016). Sex and gender differences in risk, pathophysiology and complications of type 2 diabetes mellitus. *Endocrine Reviews*, 37(3), 278–316. doi:10.1210/er.2015-1137 PMID:27159875

Laakso, M., & Kuusisto, J. (2007, August). Cerebrovascular disease in type 2 diabetes. In *International Congress Series* (Vol. 1303, pp. 65–69). Elsevier.

Miljanovic, B., Glynn, R. J., Nathan, D. M., Manson, J. E., & Schaumberg, D. A. (2004). A prospective study of serum lipids and risk of diabetic macular edema in type 1 diabetes. *Diabetes*, *53*(11), 2883–2892. doi:10.2337/diabetes.53.11.2883 PMID:15504969

Ose, D., Wensing, M., Szecsenyi, J., Joos, S., Hermann, K., & Miksch, A. (2009). Impact of primary care–based disease management on the health-related quality of life in patients with type 2 diabetes and comorbidity. *Diabetes Care*, *32*(9), 1594–1596. doi:10.2337/dc08-2223 PMID:19509007

Poncelet, A. N. (2003). Diabetic polyneuropathy. Risk factors, patterns of presentation, diagnosis, and treatment. *Geriatrics (Basel, Switzerland)*, *58*(6), 16–18. PMID:12813869

Rana, J. S., Mittleman, M. A., Sheikh, J., Hu, F. B., Manson, J. E., Colditz, G. A., Speizer, F. E., Barr, R. G., & Camargo, C. A. (2004). Chronic obstructive pulmonary disease, asthma, and risk of type 2 diabetes in women. *Diabetes Care*, *27*(10), 2478–2484. doi:10.2337/diacare.27.10.2478 PMID:15451919

Reichard, P., Nilsson, B. Y., & Rosenqvist, U. (1993). The effect of long-term intensified insulin treatment on the development of microvascular complications of diabetes mellitus. *The New England Journal of Medicine*, *329*(5), 304–309. doi:10.1056/NEJM199307293290502 PMID:8147960

Selvin, E., Marinopoulos, S., Berkenblit, G., Rami, T., Brancati, F. L., Powe, N. R., & Golden, S. H. (2004). Meta-analysis: Glycosylated hemoglobin and cardiovascular disease in diabetes mellitus. *Annals of Internal Medicine*, *141*(6), 421–431. doi:10.7326/0003-4819-141-6-200409210-00007 PMID:15381515

Solomon, D. H., Massarotti, E., Garg, R., Liu, J., Canning, C., & Schneeweiss, S. (2011). Association between disease-modifying antirheumatic drugs and diabetes risk in patients with rheumatoid arthritis and psoriasis. *Journal of the American Medical Association*, *305*(24), 2525–2531. doi:10.1001/jama.2011.878 PMID:21693740

Song, Y., Klevak, A., Manson, J. E., Buring, J. E., & Liu, S. (2010). Asthma, chronic obstructive pulmonary disease, and type 2 diabetes in the Women's Health Study. *Diabetes Research and Clinical Practice*, *90*(3), 365–371. doi:10.1016/j.diabres.2010.09.010 PMID:20926152

UK Prospective Diabetes Study Group (UPDSG). (1998). Tight blood pressure control and risk of macrovascular and microvascular complications in type 2 diabetes: UKPDS 38. *British Medical Journal*, *317*(7160), p.703.

Van Acker, K., Bouhassira, D., De Bacquer, D., Weiss, S., Matthys, K., Raemen, H., Mathieu, C., & Colin, I. M. (2009). Prevalence and impact on quality of life of peripheral neuropathy with or without neuropathic pain in type 1 and type 2 diabetic patients attending hospital outpatients clinics. *Diabetes & Metabolism*, *35*(3), 206–213. doi:10.1016/j.diabet.2008.11.004 PMID:19297223

Vileikyte, L., Rubin, R. R., & Leventhal, H. (2004). Psychological aspects of diabetic neuropathic foot complications: An overview. *Diabetes/Metabolism Research and Reviews*, *20*(S1), S13–S18. doi:10.1002/dmrr.437 PMID:15150807

WHO/FAO Expert Consultation. (2003). *WHO Technical Report Series 916 Diet, Nutrition, and the Prevention of Chronic Diseases*. Geneva: WHO. Available from http://health.euroafrica.org/books/ dietnutritionwho.pdf

World Health Organization (WHO). (2016). *Global report on diabetes: executive summary* (No. WHO/ NMH/NVI/16.3). World Health Organization. Available from https://apps.who.int/iris/bitstream/ handle/10665/204871/9789241565257_eng.pdf?sequence=1

Xie, L. J., & Cheng, M. H. (2012). Body adipose distribution among patients with type 2 diabetes mellitus. *Obesity Research & Clinical Practice, 6*(4), e270–e279. doi:10.1016/j.orcp.2012.09.003 PMID:24331587

Chapter 6
Depression Reduction for Patients With Type 2 Diabetes via E–Health Interventions

Cynthia Wong
Monash University, Australia

ABSTRACT

Diabetes is one of the most significant global health emergencies affecting populations in the 21st century, where one out of 15 adults has type II diabetes. Impaired glucose tolerance contributes to more than half of all causes of diabetes. Further, depression has adverse economic and health outcomes. The condition also contributes to poor outcomes in screening efforts among type II diabetes patients. E-health intervention is one of the means for reducing depression. There is, therefore, a need to investigate whether the strategy effectively reduces depression among patients with type II diabetes. The research examined the e-health interventions, which include personal health records (PHRs), diabetes mobile apps, patient portals, information repositories, telehealth, and electronic health records (EHRs). The research findings indicated that e-health would significantly help in reducing depression among people with type II diabetes.

INTRODUCTION

Certainly, diabetes in the twenty-first-century world has become a significant health concern leading the health disease burned among noncommunicable diseases (Atlas, 2015). The prevalence of diabetes, particularly type II, is that one out of fifteen adults has the condition. Impaired glucose tolerance adversely affects the mental health of the patients (Badescu et al., 2016). Type II diabetes contributes to more than half of all the causes of depression compared to any other stressor or factor (Darwish et al., 2018; Badescu et al., 2016). Some of the factors that contribute to a positive relationship between type II diabetes and depression include frailty from the advanced duration of having the condition, distress associated with the diseases, poor self-management, and low levels of physical activities (Bai et al., 2017; Darwish et al., 2018). Depression is also another factor that contributes to poor outcomes in the screening of risks

DOI: 10.4018/978-1-5225-6067-8.ch006

linked with type II diabetes (Darwish et al., 2018). Given the adverse impacts resulting from the correlation between diabetes and depression, clinical interventions that can be used to manage such highly comorbid conditions is necessitated. According to Deady et al. (2015), depression burdens individuals and healthcare systems globally; unfortunately, recognising and addressing the psychological problems associated with diabetes mellitus remains a significant clinical challenge. E-health applications such as diabetes mobile apps, teleconference with patients, and m-health intervention provide means that can be used to reduce depression among patients with type II diabetes.

ELECTRONIC HEALTH RECORDS (EHRS)

According to Holt (2014), there is a noticeable level of efficiency in terms of health outcomes in treating depression among patients with type II diabetes. First, it is necessary to employ EHR in screening diabetics for depression because timely detection, as well as management, minimise the risks of disease exacerbation and severity. Employing or applying EHRs in the primary setting proffers physicians with not only precise but also timely information for functional disease management strategies. Unfortunately, most data in EHRs is incomplete as information such as those of depression is not entered into EHRs when compared to laboratory data and vital signs (Madden et al., 2016). Routinely recording depression information on patients with type II diabetes will proffer healthcare providers with adequate information pivotal in not only decision-making but also the development of effective evidence-based interventions, and thus, promote quality care and safety among patients with type II diabetes (Patel et al., 2015).

An additional benefit of EHRs is ensuring a structured follow-up process and improved monitoring (Falck et al., 2019). Further, type II diabetics' wellbeing is fundamental because it not only bolsters the patients' quality life but also reduces their chances of developing complications associated with the disease. Monitoring and structured follow-up will thus, empower the physician with knowledge and understanding whether the implemented interventions are effective in reducing the level of depression or if new strategies need to be laid down and applied.

DIABETES MOBILE APPS

One of the widely used e-health technologies in diabetes management is mobile applications. There primarily exist several applications that have been created to assist patients in controlling their conditions. Some of these apps include mySugr, Zero Fasting Tracker, MyFitnessPal, and 7 Minute Workout. According to Ebert et al. (2018), mobile health applications are used in treating depression with a focus on CBT (Cognitive Behavioural Therapy)-oriented self-management and behavioural health coaching on depression. The use of mobile apps is effective because of the extensive evidence indicating the effectiveness of the psychological intervention in treating depression among patients with diabetes (Rathbone & Prescott, 2017). Corroborating this assertion is Markowitz et al. (2011), whose systematic review ascertains that research on psychosocial interventions such as CBT and collaborative care has proven their efficiency in treating depression in type II diabetics. Reiterating are Xie and Deng (2017), whose randomised controlled meta-analysis research revealed that psychosocial interventions such as CBT are efficacious in treating comorbid depression in Type II diabetes patients. Thus, novel technological interventions such as diabetes mobile apps bolster healthy behaviours through a collaborative approach while simultaneously curbing glycaemic levels.

Unfortunately, there are gaps between the evidence-based recommendation and functionality of the wide selection of mobile apps available in the market for people with diabetes (Chomutare et al., 2011). There is minimal information about the best practices when selecting and using a mobile application for self-management care. Therefore, there is a need for critical evaluation of the features of the mobile application to ensure that they have the most appropriate features and contents that will facilitate the treatment of depression. The diabetes apps have attracted a significant number of healthcare stakeholders, such as providers of care, consumers, and payers. The market value is projected to hit 742 million U.S. dollars by the year 2022 (Kebede & Pischke, 2019). The findings are a reflection of the opportunities presented by using diabetes-targeted apps in managing or controlling the condition. Studies by Ye et al. (2018) showed that out of fifty-six apps presented in the iTunes store and eighty-one in Google Play Store, only two were designated for types I and II diabetes. The study contradicts previous findings. Particularly, the mobile apps selected should be capable of promoting self-managed depression and reducing the symptoms through strategies such as problem-solving therapy, which consequently helps in reducing depression among patients with type II diabetes.

PATIENT PORTALS

Patient portals are an internet-based interactive portal providing patients and healthcare providers with a platform where they can actively collaborate in the healthcare process (Fraccaro et al., 2017). Patient portals facilitate communication between healthcare providers and patients, and it has several functions such as a portion of medical records, all of which are necessary to developing and enhancing a patient-centred care system, which is necessary when managing depression among patients with diabetes. Some sub-clinical depression type II diabetes patients are associated with worst self-care behaviour, which includes blood glucose monitoring, medication, exercise, and diet (Hermanns et al., 2013; Kok et al., 2015). People with type II diabetes can perform numerous self-care activities that enhance the management of the condition. Patient portals will provide type II diabetes patients with regular yet vast information about the events that they need to perform to improve the management of their conditions. The use of patient portals differs considerably among individuals. The use of the portal is dependent on factors such as gender and age, with more females using the service, and patients aged seventy-one years and above are less likely to adopt such use from the demographic analysis of MyChart, and Epic Inc (Oest et al., 2018). Children aged eleven and above years have shown increased activity in activating the patient portal, similar to the adult population (Oest et al., 2018). Data from the 2017 National Cancer Institute survey shows that fifty-two per cent of patients accessed their medical records, up from forty-two per cent in the year 2014 (Heath, 2018). The patient portals can further be enhanced with dashboards that allow patients to share testimonies on the activities that help them to manage the disease. The sharing of testimonies will enable the patients to encourage one another to perform self-care activities that reduce depression.

INFORMATION REPOSITORIES

Information repositories constitute tools that are used for the storage of information typical for sharing and collaboration between users. Clinical data repositories consolidate data and information from different sources such as lab systems and electronic medical records to proffer a comprehensive understanding of the care accorded to a patient (Keator et al., 2016). They are simply databases containing information such as diagnoses, admissions, transfers, demographics, and lab results, among others. All the information collected in clinical data repositories is typical to patients with diabetes and comorbid depression. Unfortunately, data repositories are inefficient because they lack analytical tools for examination of the data, they have sizeable, costly margin errors, reports and tools used are not standardised, and that data is not always secure (Campbell, 2014; Haarbrandt et al., 2016). Therefore, the clinical repositories application may not provide adequate assistance in depression treatment among people with diabetes. However, Keator et al. (2016) and Bauer et al. (2016) find that research programs can benefit significantly with approved data sharing repositories. Information repositories have particularly transcended off the backdrop of an increasing number of available diabetes databases. The American Diabetes Association supported efforts by researchers to increase access to their data from January 1st, 2019. Clinical data repositories can, therefore, be developed to collect vast information about diabetes and comorbid depression to facilitate research necessary for identifying the causes of depression as well as intervention programs that will effectively treat the condition.

TELEHEALTH

While diabetes affects people from both urban and rural areas, rural dwellers are seventeen per cent more prone to type II diabetes (Massey et al., 2010). Consequently, the prevalence of depression among the population is relatively higher. Despite their prevalence, the people in rural areas face distinct challenges that are exacerbated by longer travel times to hospitals, worse public transport, and less car ownership (Oliver, 2017). Further, rural areas are characterised by single occupier households and social isolation, all of which can worsen the state of depression among the patients.

Olson and Thomas (2017) posit that telehealth technology is fundamental as it helps in breaking the barrier between specialty and primary care, especially in medically underserved areas. Therefore, broadening the use of telehealth constitute communication and information technologies, which enhances the abilities to provide long-distance medical assistance as well as health administration, personal and public health education. The features of telehealth are fundamental as they can increase the management of depression for people in rural areas as well as urban areas. Applying telehealth as a diabetes management intervention has gained prominence according to findings by Malasanos and Ramnitz (2013). The researchers report that the telemedicine program saves $27,860 per year, and its use since implementation has been well-received by patients, where 90% expressed satisfaction in the use of the technology.

Some notable telehealth strategies include store-and-forward, video conferencing, e-consult, m-health, and remote patient monitoring. The delivery mechanism facilitates the exchange of crucial medical information not only between healthcare providers and patients but also between the providers. These communications enable healthcare providers to encourage and provide a suitable intervention program for managing depression among diabetics with comorbid depression (Mochari-Greenberger et al., 2016).

M-Health

M-health technology is the application of mobile-based technologies such as iPads, smartphones, tablets, wireless devices, personal digital assistance, and patient monitoring devices to enhance medical and public health practice. The use of M-Health continues to increase in different health sectors because of the associated benefits. The application of M-health in treating depression among diabetics is promising in ensuring effective reduction. Yasmin et al. (2016) researched the application of M-health on people living with HIV and found that simple text messages increase adherence to antiretroviral drugs. Similarly, the use of M-Health can increase patient adherence to the intervention programs necessary for managing the level of depression as well as encourage the patients to refrain from activities that are likely to worsen their conditions.

M-health technology has real-time health analytics and biometric hardware, which provides physicians with increased chances of detecting signs of depression and monitoring progress. Consequently, a healthcare provider will implement strategies to ensure that patients experience positive progress in their levels of depressions. For instance, information obtained from m-health can be used by the medical team to titrate medications and educate the patients without necessarily having a face to face interaction.

Video Conferencing

Video conferencing technology provides two-way live interactions between providers and patients that use audio-visual communication (Uscher-Pines et al., 2019). Video conferencing is useful in bridging the geographical gap between healthcare providers and the patients and thus increases the dissemination of medical education (Olson & Thomas, 2017). In the past, continuous medical interventions were provided to patients from medical centres; however, video conferences have facilitated the routinely broadcast of the information to distant locations (Olson & Thomas, 2017). Management of depression would require patients to continuously have access to the education necessary for effective management of depression. Fundamentally, health education is central in psychological counselling – a psychosocial intervention proven by Xie and Deng (2017) to be effective in managing comorbid depression in type II diabetes patients.

Remote Patient Monitoring

Remote patient monitoring technology facilitates the sending of medical and personal data of a patient and sent to the providers at different locations (Uscher-Pines et al., 2019) who can then use the information to enhance care delivery for management of depression.

E-Consult

The E-Health technology enables the primary care providers to take advantage of the video conferencing to consult with a specialist (Uscher-Pines et al. 2019). The strategy is particularly important in the treatment of depression as providers can discuss and come with the most effective approach for treating diabetes and its comorbidities.

Store-and-Forward

The technology stores medical information such as pre-recorded videos, documents, and digital images, which are then sent to the provider using electronic communication systems. The health provider can then use the information to evaluate cases and plan outside live interactions (Uscher-Pines et al., 2019). The technology, as applied in the management of depression among diabetics, provides physicians with medical information which they can use to treat and advise patients on proper strategies to manage depression at later hours which thus counters the challenge of the fact that healthcare providers may not always be available to offer real-time assistance to the patients.

PERSONAL HEALTH RECORDS (PHRS)

PHR is descriptively an application that allows patients to control their health data in a confidential, secure, and private environment. The PHR is different from the EHR as the individual patient manages the former, and the patient manages the latter. The PHR contains information entered by an individual patient as well as data from other sources such as care providers, labs, and pharmacies (Lin et al., 2006). Personal health records are fundamental E-Health tools that can enhance the management of depression among type II diabetics.

Clinically depressed diabetics often have poor self-care of diabetes, lower medication adherence, and increased complications (Lin et al., 2006). Enhanced self-care and treatment of depression will improve the management of the disease. PHR provides a means for patients with diabetes mellitus to communicate their comorbid conditions to the healthcare provider consistently. The communications include the multi-disciplinary clinical pathways and follow-ups of diabetes as well as components such as monitoring of diabetes and depression, coping and stress resources, medical history, and complications in treatment (Satoh-Asahara et al., 2016). Researchers have projected that the use of patient health records is expected to increase with seventy-five percent of adults utilising the application by 2020 (Landi, 2016). With the components, the patients with diabetes mellitus can manage communication and healthcare tasks, which consequently help in the reduction of depression and continuous improvement of quality care.

CONCLUSION

The depression prevalence among patients with impaired glucose tolerance in Australia and across the world is burdensome to healthcare systems, individual patients, and families, among others. Intervention measures to reduce the level of depression among the patient are an essential factor as it eases the management of type II diabetes. There is no doubt that E-Health is ultimately transforming the delivery of healthcare to patients, behavioural change interventions, and education on self-management. The different E-Health strategies such as telehealth, clinical data repositories, electronic health records, mobile apps, and personal health records are fundamental as they can be used to reduce depression levels among patients with diabetes. However, there is insufficient information about the efficacy and safety of using the different E-Health tools in the management of diabetes. There are few standardised E-Health tools at a national level. Therefore, users should critically evaluate the tools before implementing, and research needs to be conducted to examine the appropriateness of using the different devices.

REFERENCES

Atlas, D. (2015). *International diabetes federation.* IDF Diabetes Atlas.

Badescu, S. V., Tataru, C., Kobylinska, L., Georgescu, E. L., Zahiu, D. M., Zăgrean, A. M., & Zăgrean, L. (2016). The association between diabetes mellitus and depression. *Journal of Medicine and Life, 9*(2), 120–125. PMID:27453739

Bai, J. W., Lovblom, L. E., Cardinez, M., Weisman, A., Farooqi, M. A., Halpern, E. M., ... Keenan, H. A. (2017). Neuropathy and presence of emotional distress and depression in longstanding diabetes: Results from the Canadian study of longevity in type 1 diabetes. *Journal of Diabetes and Its Complications, 31*(8), 1318–1324. doi:10.1016/j.jdiacomp.2017.05.002 PMID:28599823

Bauer, C. R. K. D., Ganslandt, T., Baum, B., Christoph, J., Engel, I., Löbe, M., ... Winter, A. (2016). Integrated data repository toolkit (IDRT). *Methods of Information in Medicine, 55*(2), 125–135. doi:10.3414/ME15-01-0082 PMID:26534843

Campbell, T. (2014). *Clinical data repository versus a data warehouse — which do you need?* https://www.healthcatalyst.com/insights/clinical-data-repository-data-warehouse

Chomutare, T., Fernandez-Luque, L., Årsand, E., & Hartvigsen, G. (2011). Features of mobile diabetes applications: Review of the literature and analysis of current applications compared against evidence-based guidelines. *Journal of Medical Internet Research, 13*(3), e65. doi:10.2196/jmir.1874 PMID:21979293

Darwish, L., Beroncal, E., Sison, M. V., & Swardfager, W. (2018). Depression in people with type 2 diabetes: Current perspectives. *Diabetes, Metabolic Syndrome and Obesity, 11,* 333–343. doi:10.2147/DMSO.S106797 PMID:30022843

Deady, M., Choi, I., Calvo, R. A., Glozier, N., Christensen, H., & Harvey, S. B. (2017). eHealth interventions for the prevention of depression and anxiety in the general population: A systematic review and meta-analysis. *BMC Psychiatry, 17*(1), 310. doi:10.118612888-017-1473-1 PMID:28851342

Ebert, D. D., Van Daele, T., Nordgreen, T., Karekla, M., Compare, A., Zarbo, C., ... Kaehlke, F. (2018). Internet-and mobile-based psychological interventions: Applications, efficacy, and potential for improving mental health. *European Psychologist, 23*(3), 167–187. doi:10.1027/1016-9040/a000318

Falck, L., Zoller, M., Rosemann, T., Martínez-González, N. A., & Chmiel, C. (2019). Toward standardized monitoring of patients with chronic diseases in primary care using electronic medical records: Systematic review. *JMIR Medical Informatics, 7*(2), e10879. doi:10.2196/10879 PMID:31127717

Fraccaro, V., Balatsoukas, B., & Peek, V. D. V. (2017). Patient portal adoption rates: A systematic literature review and meta-analysis. *Studies in Health Technology and Informatics, 245,* 79–83. PMID:29295056

Haarbrandt, B., Tute, E., & Marschollek, M. (2016). Automated population of an i2b2 clinical data warehouse from an open EHR-based data repository. *Journal of Biomedical Informatics, 63,* 277–294. doi:10.1016/j.jbi.2016.08.007 PMID:27507090

Heath, S. (2018). *Patient portal access use reaches 52% of healthcare consumers.* https://patientengagementhit.com/news/patient-portal-access-use-reach-52-of-healthcare-consumers

Hermanns, N., Caputo, S., Dzida, G., Khunti, K., Meneghini, L. F., & Snoek, F. (2013). Screening, evaluation, and management of depression in people with diabetes in primary care. *Primary Care Diabetes*, *7*(1), 1–10. doi:10.1016/j.pcd.2012.11.002 PMID:23280258

Holt, R. I., de Groot, M., & Golden, S. H. (2014). Diabetes and depression. *Current Diabetes Reports*, *14*(6), 491. doi:10.100711892-014-0491-3 PMID:24743941

Keator, D. B., van Erp, T. G., Turner, J. A., Glover, G. H., Mueller, B. A., Liu, T. T., ... Toga, A. W. (2016). The function biomedical informatics research network data repository. *NeuroImage*, *124*, 1074–1079. doi:10.1016/j.neuroimage.2015.09.003 PMID:26364863

Kebede, M. M., & Pischke, C. R. (2019). Popular diabetes apps and the impact of diabetes app use on self-care behaviour: A survey among the digital community of persons with diabetes on social media. *Frontiers in Endocrinology*, *10*, 135. doi:10.3389/fendo.2019.00135 PMID:30881349

Kok, J. L. A., Williams, A., & Zhao, L. (2015). Psychosocial interventions for people with diabetes and comorbid depression. A systematic review. *International Journal of Nursing Studies*, *52*(10), 1625–1639. doi:10.1016/j.ijnurstu.2015.05.012 PMID:26118440

Landi, H. (2016). *Study: 75% of adults will use personal health records by 2020, exceeding M.U. targets.* https://www.hcinnovationgroup.com/policy-value-based-care/news/13026586/study-75-of-adults-will-use-personal-health-records-by-2020-exceeding-mu-targets

Lin, E. H., Katon, W., Rutter, C., Simon, G. E., Ludman, E. J., Von Korff, M., Young, B., Oliver, M., Ciechanowski, P. C., Kinder, L., & Walker, E. (2006). Effects of enhanced depression treatment on diabetes self-care. *Annals of Family Medicine*, *4*(1), 46–53. doi:10.1370/afm.423 PMID:16449396

Madden, J. M., Lakoma, M. D., Rusinak, D., Lu, C. Y., & Soumerai, S. B. (2016). Missing clinical and behavioural health data in a large electronic health record (EHR) system. *Journal of the American Medical Informatics Association*, *23*(6), 1143–1149. doi:10.1093/jamia/ocw021 PMID:27079506

Malasanos, T., & Ramnitz, M. S. (2013). Diabetes clinic at a distance: Telemedicine bridges the gap. *Diabetes Spectrum*, *26*(4), 226–231. doi:10.2337/diaspect.26.4.226

Markowitz, S. M., Gonzalez, J. S., Wilkinson, J. L., & Safren, S. A. (2011). A review of treating depression in diabetes: Emerging findings. *Psychosomatics*, *52*(1), 1–18. doi:10.1016/j.psym.2010.11.007 PMID:21300190

Massey, C. N., Appel, S. J., Buchanan, K. L., & Cherrington, A. L. (2010). Improving diabetes care in rural communities: An overview of current initiatives and a call for renewed efforts. *Clinical Diabetes*, *28*(1), 20–27. doi:10.2337/diaclin.28.1.20

Mochari-Greenberger, H., Vue, L., Luka, A., Peters, A., & Pande, R. L. (2016). A tele-behavioural health intervention to reduce depression, anxiety, and stress and improve diabetes self-management. *Telemedicine Journal and e-Health*, *22*(8), 624–630. doi:10.1089/tmj.2015.0231 PMID:26954880

Oest, S. E., Hightower, M., & Krasowski, M. D. (2018). Activation and utilization of an electronic health record patient portal at an academic medical centre—Impact of patient demographics and geographic location. *Academic Pathology*, *5*, e2374289518797573. doi:10.1177/2374289518797573 PMID:30302394

Oliver, D. (2017). David Oliver: Challenges for rural hospitals—the same but different. *BMJ (Clinical Research Ed.)*, *357*, 17–31. doi:10.1136/bmj.j17 PMID:28400387

Olson, C. A., & Thomas, J. F. (2017). Telehealth: No longer an idea for the future. *Advances in Pediatrics*, *64*(1), 347–370. doi:10.1016/j.yapd.2017.03.009 PMID:28688597

Patel, V., Reed, M. E., & Grant, R. W. (2015). Electronic health records and the evolution of diabetes care: A narrative review. *Journal of Diabetes Science and Technology*, *9*(3), 676–680. doi:10.1177/1932296815572256 PMID:25711684

Rathbone, A. L., & Prescott, J. (2017). The use of mobile apps and SMS messaging as physical and mental health interventions: Systematic review. *Journal of Medical Internet Research*, *19*(8), e295. doi:10.2196/jmir.7740 PMID:28838887

Satoh-Asahara, N., Ito, H., Akashi, T., Yamakage, H., Kotani, K., Nagata, D., Nakagome, K., & Noda, M. (2016). A patient-held medical record integrating depression care into diabetes care. *Japanese Clinical Medicine*, *7*, 19–22. doi:10.4137/JCM.S39766 PMID:27478395

Uscher-Pines, L., Bouskill, K., Sousa, J., Shen, M., & Fischer, S. H. (2019). *Experiences of Medicaid programs and health centres in implementing telehealth*. RAND. doi:10.7249/RR2564

Xie, J., & Deng, W. (2017). Psychosocial intervention for patients with type 2 diabetes mellitus and comorbid depression: A meta-analysis of randomized controlled trials. *Neuropsychiatric Disease and Treatment*, *13*, 2681–2690. doi:10.2147/NDT.S116465 PMID:29123401

Yasmin, F., Banu, B., Zakir, S. M., Sauerborn, R., Ali, L., & Souares, A. (2016). Positive influence of short message service and voice call interventions on adherence and health outcomes in case of chronic disease care: A systematic review. *BMC Medical Informatics and Decision Making*, *16*(1), 46. doi:10.118612911-016-0286-3 PMID:27106263

Ye, Q., Khan, U., Boren, S. A., Simoes, E. J., & Kim, M. S. (2018). An analysis of diabetes mobile application features compared to AADE7™: Addressing self-management behaviors in people with diabetes. *Journal of Diabetes Science and Technology*, *12*(4), 808–816. doi:10.1177/1932296818754907 PMID:29390917

Chapter 7
Developing a Personalised Diabetic Platform Using a Design Science Research Methodology

Shane Joachim

Swinburne University of Technology, Australia

Prem Prakash Jayaraman

Swinburne University of Technology, Australia

Abdur Rahim Mohammad Forkan

https://orcid.org/0000-0003-0237-1705

Swinburne University of Technology, Australia

Ahsan Morshed

CQUniversity, Australia

Nilmini Wickramasinghe

https://orcid.org/0000-0002-1314-8843

Swinburne University of Technology, Australia & Epworth HealthCare, Australia

ABSTRACT

Type II diabetes is a rapidly growing non-communicable chronic disease that is causing significant concern to healthcare systems around the world. As there is no foreseeable cure, the most effective solution is to focus on strategies to control blood glucose levels by regular monitoring of diet, exercise, and when necessary, medication management. In today's environment, to do so effectively necessitates the need for a personalised self-management technology solution which can help patients take control of their diabetes. This chapter presents initial data from a research in progress study focused on designing a personalised diabetic application. The authors proffer a design science research methodology (DSRM)

DOI: 10.4018/978-1-5225-6067-8.ch007

approach to design, develop, and ultimately, evaluate a patient-centric diabetes platform. This application is not only a smart patient empowering solution which serves to guide patients and assist their care team with regard to diet, exercise, medication and their respective impacts on blood sugar levels but is also designed to be culturally sensitive.

INTRODUCTION

Diabetes Mellitus (aka Diabetes), a prominent chronic disease, affects individuals of all genders and ages across the globe (International Diabetes Federation, 2019). About 425 Million people were directly affected by both Type I and II diabetes in 2017 (International Diabetes Federation, 2019). This has rapidly grown to 463 Million in 2019 as reported by IDF Diabetes (International Diabetes Federation, 2019). The number is expected to grow further, to at least 578 Million individuals by 2030 (International Diabetes Federation, 2019) given the continuing increase of Type II diabetes in most countries due to a combination of issues including drastic change of lifestyle, diet and lack of regular exercise (Kharroubi & Darwish, 2015). Currently in Australia, over 1.3 million individuals have type 2 diabetes and this figure continues to grow exponentially (Shaw & Tanamas, 2012). If this growth continues, up to 3 million Australians over the age of 25 will have diabetes by the year 2025 (Shaw & Tanamas, 2012).

The most common complications of diabetes include damage to: (i) the large blood vessels leading to heart attack, stroke or circulation problems in the lower limbs; (ii) the small blood vessels causing problems in the eyes, kidneys, feet and nerves and (iii) issues with the skin, teeth and gums (National Diabetes services scheme, Diabetes-related complications June 2016); thus making it an unpleasant chronic condition that requires further invasive, ongoing and expensive healthcare attention if left unchecked.

As there is no effective cure for diabetes at this time, typical patient care focusses on maintaining appropriate blood glucose levels by focusing on appropriate diet, exercise and when necessary medication management (Khan et al., 2019). Critical to this approach is to empower patients with diabetes to actively engage in self-management regimens (Wickramasinghe et al., 2019). In this way, it is possible to avoid the nasty complications that can develop with uncontrolled diabetes and, in some cases, type II diabetes can be permanently reversed (Khan et al., 2019). Self-management generally involves daily monitoring of blood glucose levels and blood pressure and keeping these within the target ranges; eating a healthy diet focusing on foods with a low glycaemic index (GI); engaging in regular exercise, at least 30 minutes on most days; reducing weight if it is above the recommended range and quitting smoking (National Diabetes services scheme, Diabetes-related complications June 2016). Based on research conducted by inet International Inc., it was demonstrated that the majority of people with diabetes find self-management regimens difficult to follow on an on-going basis (Wickramasinghe et al., 2019).

Not only are the consequences of poor self-management potentially devastating for an individual with diabetes but also the pressures on the healthcare system with the alarming rising figures of individuals with diabetes is unsustainable (Shaw & Tanamas, 2012). For example, in Australia, 40% ($55 billion) of healthcare costs are for chronic conditions while $2 billion of that is paid by private health insurers. Moreover, hospitals see more patients for preventable operations and these individuals have higher risks of adverse events while GPs payments are shifting towards patient outcomes. Hence, there is an urgent need to develop technological solutions to support and coach people with diabetes in self-management and monitor their medication adherence.

Given this exponential increase in the numbers of individuals developing diabetes, coupled with the fact that there remains no cure for this non-communicable chronic condition, it becomes essential to focus on designing and developing solution for better management and personalised care (Forkan et al., 2015). In particular, it is important to focus on 24/7 support and patient empowerment. With this in mind, the researchers set out to investigate the research question,

How can we develop a smart patient empowerment solution for patients with Diabetes?

This chapter provides a review of the extant literature in addressing the challenge of diabetes. The researchers present a design science research methodology inspired approach for co-designing and co-developing a diabatic platform for patients with diabetics that provides self-management and personalization to fit the context of the patient with diabetes. The rest of the chapter is organized as follows, with a detailed presentation of the methodology and initial results, followed by the discussion and finally the conclusion and future works.

BACKGROUND

Type II Diabetes

Type II Diabetes, the most common form of diabetes, accounts for around 90% of all diabetes worldwide (International Diabetes Federation, 2019). In Type II diabetes, reaching hyperglycaemia, is when the body cells fail to respond to insulin, making the individual insulin resistant (International Diabetes Federation, 2019). It is known that Type II diabetes present similar symptoms to Type I diabetes (excessive thirst, blurred vision, frequent urination, sudden weight loss etc.), but often in a much less intense fashion. Sometimes individuals go symptomless (International Diabetes Federation, 2019). This causes uncertainty around the start of the Type II diabetes, which results in one-third to one-half of people with type II diabetes undiagnosed for a long time (International Diabetes Federation, 2019).

With over 416 million people effected by Type II diabetes, researches are still trying to understand many aspects related to cause and impact around this disease (International Diabetes Federation, 2019). However, one area that is very clear is the strong correlation between being overweight, clinically obese, increasing age, ethnicity and even family history when it comes to having a high propensity for being affected by type II diabetes (International Diabetes Federation, 2019). Further, lifestyle factors such as physical inactivity, smoking and alcohol consumption also are all key contributing factors to developing type II diabetes (Wu, Y., Ding, Y. et al, 2014).

Thus, the most frequently recommended treatment and prevention for patients with type II diabetes is an intervention on their current lifestyle (International Diabetes Federation, 2019). This includes a push for more physical activity, which alone is known to contribute to 30-50% to the reduction in the development of type II diabetes, healthy eating, and obesity management (Wu, Y., Ding, Y. et al, 2014). This needs to be a sustained lifestyle change, meaning that the patients would need to implement a self-management routine by eating right and increasing their physical activity load in an ongoing fashion to keep their diabetes under control. Hence, pushing for a change in lifestyle without any assistance makes it quite difficult to stay on and motivated to the assigned self-management routines.

In recent times, the popularity and availability of smartphones has allowed them to leverage the quality of lifestyle and health of individuals through mobile health (mHealth) applications (Cortez, N. G. et al 2014, Dorsey, R. et al 2017). These applications have been hailed as the perfect answer for improving overall health outcomes while reducing medical errors, avoiding expensive interventions, and supporting chronic disease self-management (Cortez, N. G. et al 2014). Further, smartphones enable improved monitoring of chronic conditions such as diabetes; the integrations of sophisticated algorithms in a smartphone allows for the improved management of acute episodes and symptoms caused by these chronic disease, and this in return also reduces physical clinician visits (Cortez, N. G. et al 2014).

Hence, the need for diabetes management support solutions, which offer a variety of self-management features such as tracking blood sugar levels, fitness information, nutritional information and more.

Related Works

In this section, the researchers describe the current work in the literature that has been designed and developed to address the issues faced by patients with diabetes in relation to self-management of their chronic illness.

With more than 300,000 mHealth applications currently active in the iOS and Android market, there appears to be a slow adoption rate of these applications as compared to other industries (Huang, Z. et al. 2018, Jimenez, Lum, & Car, 2019). For experienced and adaptive smartphone users, adoption of mHealth platforms and applications is seen to help adjust their lifestyle changes, to better suit their chronic disease management (Huang, Z. et al. 2018). However, there is still a poor perception of mHealth applications due to *third party* developed software and algorithms for handling an individual's current health condition data (Huang, Z. et al. 2018); this not only raises questions around patient privacy but also legal liabilities of any damages caused by the app (Cortez, N. G. et al 2014).

In addition, the lack of regulations and support from authoritative bodies makes it problematic for clinicians to select mHealth technologies for patients to incorporate as a part of their *clinically approved* diabetes self-management routine (Huang, Z. et al. 2018). Further, the lack of regulations and authoritativeness has enabled commercially available mHealth platforms and applications to provide diabetes management capabilities without any medical or research-based evidence which can make them potentially dangerous to an individual's health (Villalba-Mora, Elena. et al 2017). Moreover, many of these apps have been identified to have a limited number of functionalities (providing an atomistic experience, rather than an holistic experience), poor usability, and accessibility experience, lack personalisation features, and fail to incorporate with a current clinician support system, which further questions the credibility of *third party* diabetes self-management applications (Cortez, N. G. et al 2014, Huang, Z. et al. 2018, Villalba-Mora, Elena. et al 2017).

Hence, the researchers conducted this study on iOS and Android diabetic management applications, where they focused on 10 applications for analysis with the following traits: *I)* Total user downloads, *II)* Standard set of features, *III)* Standout unique features. Apple's App Store and Google Play were utilised to search for diabetes management mobile applications. Keywords such as "diabetes", "management", "self-management", "adherence" were applied in the search and the primary goal was to choose applications with the most downloads. Applications were further categorised and chosen manually in order to filter this down further to 10 key applications.

It must be highlighted that the number of ratings were considered. Since Apple's App Store does not publicly present the number of downloads of any application, the number of ratings was taken into consideration when selecting applications from the App Store. Hence, applications with more than 4 stars were selected for the current study. Additionally, selecting freely available applications in the market can be regarded as a limitation of the current study. Table 1 shows features of the applications. The table marks the existence and completeness of the features through three symbols; *Tick* (✓): The described feature exists or is complete; *Cross* (✗): The described feature does not exist or is incomplete; Strike (–): The feature is partially present or uses an external application to cater for this.

In the review of these 10 applications, based on qualitative data, it can be understood that there are gaps that can be addressed. By referring to Table 1, the following information is extracted and grouped by a set of taxonomy.

Taxonomy

The following have been identified as some of the key factors that influence diabetes. Hence, a diabetes self-management application should ideally contain the following defined set of taxonomy.

Medication

- **Log medication:** A method to keep track and log any intake of medication including dosage.
- **Medication search:** Ability to search and log medication from a library.
- **Custom medication:** Ability to create a medication based on various input.

Outcome: *80%* of the reviewed applications had some form of medication logger. However, they were all custom medication trackers, while only *10% of* them offered the ability to search and select a medication from an existing library/selection.

Blood Glucose

- **Log blood glucose levels:** A method to keep track and log a blood glucose reading with a timestamp.
- **Blood glucose visualisation:** A visualisation that presents the logged blood glucose data.
- **Set blood glucose thresholds:** Ability to set a minimum and maximum goal to help visualise the progress.
- **Blood glucose statistics:** A section which provides insightful information on based on the logged blood glucose data

Outcome: All the applications reviewed contained a comprehensive blood glucose logger, some form of visualisation and rolling statistics. *20%* of these applications failed to allow the user to set any diabetics related goals or thresholds. For example, setting the minimum and maximum ranges for mmol\L for the blood glucose entries and visualisations.

Fitness

- **Log Fitness Activity:** A method to keep track and log fitness activity.
- **Add Custom Activity:** Ability to enter a customised activity with relevant fields such as duration, intensity etc.
- **Calorie estimator:** Feature which estimates total calories burned for the logged activity.

Outcome: Only *30%* of the applications allowed for the users to enter fitness related information.

Nutrition

- **Log Nutrition:** A method to keep track and intake of nutritional content.
- **Search Online for Nutritional Content:** Ability to search for meals, drinks, snacks etc, through an online entity.
- **Custom Nutritional Content:** Ability to manually create and log items that was consumed.
- **Nutritional Information on Meals:** Feature which displays a comprehensive list of nutritional information (ingredients, kcal, protein etc.) based on a selected meal
- **Nutrition planner:** A feature that allows for a list of pre-planned meals ready for logging
- **Nutrition recommender:** A personalised nutrition recommender feature, which suggests meals based on a range of context parameters

Outcome: *80%* of all applications contained meal logging. In that, only *30%* offered the ability to search and select meals from an online source and provide nutritional information. While *none* of the applications offered a fully comprehensive nutrition planner and meal recommender system.

Clinical

- **Support Network:** A method for the patients to reach out for further support through the app e.g. diabetes coach.
- **Remote Clinician Monitoring:** Ability for Clinicians to monitor and view the progress of the assigned patient remotely.
- **Assigned Clinician Information:** Feature which enables the patient to view the details of their assigned Clinician.

Outcome: Only *10%* application offered options for clinical support. While *20%* offered a paid support network through a diabetic coach as an option. The other *80%* failed to cover this area.

Type II diabetes is typically directly correlated with poor lifestyle and nutrition management (International Diabetes Federation, 2019), yet none of these applications cater for these areas completely. There are clear gaps in the areas of *Clinical* support, *Nutrition (planner + meal recommender)* and *Fitness* logger to be addressed. As there are applications such as *'Glucose buddy diabetes tracker'* which cater for *Fitness* features and *'Diabetes:M'* that comprehensively cover the *clinical* features, there is no single personalised Diabetes self-management application that covers all the vital features outlined as a part of this review. In addition, findings suggest that none of these solutions catered for cultural or ethnic nuances. This highlights the requirement of including the users perspective; thus the researchers take a

Table 1. Taxonomy comparison of existing diabetes applications

Name	Medication			Blood Glucose (BG)				Fitness			Nutrition (Meals, Snack Drinks etc.)						Clinical		
	Log Medication	Add Medication by Search	Custom Medication	Log BG Levels	BG Visualisation	Set BG Goals/ Thresholds	BG Statistics	Log Fitness Activities	Add Custom Activities	Calories Burned Estimator	Log Nutrition Content	Search Online for Meals	Custom Meals	Nutritional Info of Meals	Nutrition Planner	Meal Recommender	Support Network (Coach etc.)	Assigned Clinician Info	Remote Clinician Monitoring
MySugr	✓	✗	✓	✓	✓	✓	✓	✗	✗	✗	✓	✗	✓	✗	✗	✗	✗	✗	✗
Blood Sugar Log	✓	✗	✓	✓	✓	✗	✓	✗	✗	✗	✗	✗	✗	✗	✗	✗	✗	✗	✗
Glucose Tracker & Diabetic Diary	✓	✗	✓	✓	✓	✓	✓	–	✗	✗	–	✗	✗	✗	✗	✗	✗	✗	✗
Diabetes:M	✓	–	✓	✓	✓	✓	✓	✗	✗	✗	✓	✓	✓	✗	✗	✗	✓	✓	✓
Glucose buddy diabetes tracker	✓	✗	✓	✓	✓	✗	✓	✓	✓	–	✓	–	✓	✓	✗	✗	✗	✗	✗
One drop diabetes management	✓	–	✓	✓	✓	✓	✓	–	–	–	✓	✓	✓	✓	–	✗	✓	✗	✗
Blood sugar monitor by Dario	✗	✗	✗	✓	✓	✓	✓	–	✗	✗	✓	✓	✓	✓	✗	✗	✗	✗	✗
Blood Glucose Tracker	✓	✗	✓	✓	✓	✓	✓	✗	✗	✗	✓	✗	✓	✗	✗	✗	✗	✗	✗
forDiabetes: diabetes self-management app	✓	✗	✓	✓	✓	✓	✓	–	–	–	–	✗	✗	✗	✗	✗	✗	✗	✗
Glucose - blood sugar tracker (iOS only)	–	✗	–	✓	✓	✓	✓	✗	✗	✗	–	✗	✗	✗	✗	✗	✗	✗	✗

Design Science Research Methodology approach to design and develop a personalised diabetes application validated through rigorous evaluation strategies, to address a key void in diabetes self-management care support.

DESIGN SCIENCE RESEARCH METHODOLOGY (DSRM): A SYNOPSIS

Developed by Hevener, DSRM is an important research inquiry approach in information systems (Gregor & Hevner, 2013). Specifically, DSRM involves building various socio-technical artefacts, such as new software, processes, algorithms, or systems in order to improve or solve an identified problem (Myers & Venable, 2014; Jayaram et al 2020; Morshed et al 2017). Importantly, Hevner and Wickramasinghe (2017) adapted DSRM for healthcare contexts noting that in healthcare contexts use of DSRM is especially prudent when fine tuning innovative solutions to ensure high user satisfaction and adoption. Given this, DSRM approach was incorporated into the methodology. In particular, the researchers follow the seven guidelines noted by Hevener et al (2004) for understanding, executing, and evaluating design science research. Various studies (Nguyen and Wickramasinghe 2017; John et al 2016; Arnott & Pervan 2012; Xu, Wang, Li, & Chau 2007) have used these guidelines for building algorithms and systems. The improved four-cycle model of IS design science research for capturing the dynamic nature of IS artefact design is illustrated in Figure 1.

Figure 1. Four-cycle model of IS design science research
(Drechsler & Hevner, 2016)

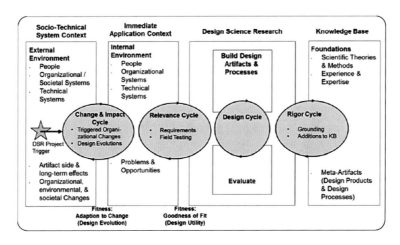

The four-cycle model was employed to structure the actions taken for the design phase of this longitudinal project. The application of the DSRM model is as follows:

- **The Change and Impact Cycle** ensures that the solution would be fit for purpose in the Australian Healthcare context. Taking things into consideration such as the solution in its entirety, the mobile devices(s) used and the patients and/or clinicians which may use the solution.

- **The Relevance Cycle** assists us with the identification of key requirements of the patients and clinicians by understanding the problems faced in their environment through a wide array of discussions such as interviews, focus groups and other techniques.
- **The Design Cycle I, II & III** is where the design and development of the artefacts such as the paper prototype and mobile solution itself took place, coupled with a range of evaluation strategies which ensure the nature of the application caters the targeted problem domain.
- **The Rigor Cycle** allows us to verify and populate the *knowledge base,* with our contributions to this space. The contributions are extracted from the *artefacts* developed during the *Design cycles,* which could be scientific theories, artefact evaluations – capturing what works and what does not, but also experience and expertise (Drechsler & Hevner, 2016).

USING DSRM TO DESIGN A DIABETIC PLATFORM FOR SELF-MANAGEMENT OF DIABETES

In this section, the researchers first present the adaptation of the DSRM guidelines, followed by the integration of the DSRM cycles with the self-management of diabetes context.

DSRM Guidelines

The DSRM guidelines used in the design of the diabetes platform is discussed below:

Guideline 1: *Design as an Artefact***:** A diabetic platform for both patients and clinicians (e.g. nurses), that allow for self-management of their diabetes journey. This further could support a 'value-based' care agenda, as it can potentially increase the quality of care received and the timeliness of feedback yet not impact cost of care delivery.

Guideline 2: *Problem Relevance***:** To cater the requirement of continuous and superior monitoring and management of patient's diabetes. The ability to provide in a timely fashion, anywhere, at any given time, the information required to make better decisions in relation to their diabetes; also providing a sufficient technological solution that can drive and support self-management of diabetes for both patients and clinicians.

Guideline 3: *Design Evaluation***:** There was the integration of both clinicians and potential patient users at different stages of the design and testing of the solution. Furthermore, representatives from hospitals were consulted to ensure the solution complied with government regulations and requirements for technology solutions interacting with patients in medical research. This was an iterative process which reached a conclusion when legal, clinical, and patient users were satisfied with the artefact that was produced and that it served its purpose.

Guideline 4: *Research Contributions***:** In this study, users' perspectives of the mediating role of the solution are explored.

Guideline 5: *Research Rigor***:** Theoretical foundations and conceptual models drawn from information systems, chronic disease management protocols, healthcare quality and safety were used to inform the development cycles to evaluate the solution in clinical contexts.

Guideline 6: *Design as a Search Process***:** In this project, the design had to be correct to meet with ethics requirements for running of a clinical trial and securing patient data.

Guideline 7: *Communication of Research*: **(I)** *Internal communication*: Present the technology and clinically oriented users through focus groups, simulations exercises, brainstorming meetings, as well as technical and managerial meetings. **(II)** *External communication*: Progress and findings are to be reported in relevant peer review outlets including international conferences and professional peer-reviewed journals in relevant disciplines.

DSRM Cycles

Here the researchers present the adoption and actualisation of the DSRM cycles presented in Figure 1 and the aforementioned guidelines in the development of a personalised self-management diabetes platform.

Change and Impact Cycle

The change and impact (CI) cycle allows us to identify the External Environmental factors (with the context of *Australian Healthcare* and *Patient Environment*) which has the potential to influence both patients and clinicians in a wider context. To do this, the researchers partnered with *healthcare professionals* with extensive industry knowledge about health care in Australia yet had a strong foundation in diabetes. The CI Cycle also inherits a *design evolution fitness model*. Which enable us to validate the artefacts designed, and make sure that the research grounding still has the intended effects to the External Environmental factors. In contrast, this also enables us to validate our artefact, when there are any changes made to the state or process of the identified External Environmental factors.

Relevance

The aim of the relevance cycle was to help recognise *requirements* that were crucial for the diabetic management solution. This was initiated by identifying factors of the *Internal Environment* which directly influence the diabetes platform. The identified factors are as follows: **I)** Patients with diabetes; **II)** Healthcare professionals; **III)** Diabetes platform (proposed artefact); **IV)** Mobile devices used to interact with the platform.

The researchers conducted a range of semi structured interviews and workshops involving *patients with diabetes* and *healthcare professionals respectively*. This allowed for the identification of desirable features which are intended to help manage their diabetes. Further, our relevance cycle, incorporates a *Design Utility* model. This allows us to make sure that the platform stays fit for purpose by conducting a joint evaluation of the identified requirements and the data from the user studies once conducted.

In one of the workshops, there was an engagement of a group discussion, caused by a problem-solving strategy 'Working backwards'. As the name suggests, the concept of this method is to start off with a large/desired end goal, and demystify the steps required to achieve that goal by working backwards (Portnov- Neeman, Yelena & Amit, Miriam, 2016). This activity was run iteratively over a predefined set of key objectives and topics that were noted as most important by healthcare domain experts. The results are presented in Table 2.

Participating *healthcare professionals - Physicians, Nurses, Dietitians and Endocrinologists,* were selected to provide a wide variety of domain expertise on diabetes and had prior experience in managing patients with diabetes. Identifying requirements involving both the patients and clinicians provided a more holistic overview on the features that were desired but also made clear some *problems and opportunities* that needed to be addressed.

Problem and Opportunities

With the identified Internal Environment factors in mind, below are the problems and opportunities for each:

Patients with Diabetes:

- How can the patient ensure consistency in using the diabetes self-management platform?

Table 2. Relevance cycle results for diabetes management solutions

Topic Area	Requirement	Solution
Lifestyle	Searching for meals	Ability to find meals based of name search.
	Meal plans	Picking a meal from a defined meal plan.
	View meal information	View ingredients and nutrition information of a selected meal.
	Log meals	Add meals consumed to a log.
	Meal preferences	Ability to set culture specific cuisines and other preferences as priority during search.
	Log fitness activities	Add any physical activity with duration undertaken.
Medication management	Log medication	Add any medication taken for a given day.
Resources	Type II diabetes information	Provide FAQ information from Diabetes Australia.
	Support group	N/A
	Hospital contact	Provide contact details of their hospital/GP from in app.
Miscellaneous	General Statistics	To view how the patient is tracking with their diabetes journey. - Avg, highest, lowest mmol\L - Overall progress
	Log blood sugar levels	Ability to log mmol\L levels at a given time.
	View blood sugar in an interactive chart	A line chart which contains all the blood sugar entries for a given timeframe.

Figure 2. Example application design concepts and mock-up designs

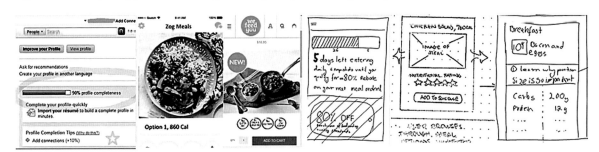

- How can the clinician keep the patient motivated in their journey through the diabetes self-management platform?

Healthcare Professionals:

- How can the patient receive effective feedback on their progress from the clinician?

Diabetes Platform:

- How can we ensure accurate data is entered by the patient?
- How can the platform cater for patient-clinician communication pipeline?

Mobile Devices:

- How can we ensure accurate data is entered by the patient?
- How can the clinician verify that the data collected through the devices are accurate?

Co-Design Cycle I

The co-design cycle is an iterative process. In our scenario, the designing and the development of the artefacts was split into three parts, followed by thorough evaluation methods affirming the artefacts developed. I) In the first iteration of the design cycle, a set of mock-up pages was created. These mock-ups were inspired by existing applications but were adapted for the requirements of the diabetic platform. Examples of current diabetic management application found in the literature and/or the Internet. Their mock-up designs are presented in Figure 2. Following the creation of the application mock-up, the patients and clinicians were asked questions to evaluate them.

Co-Design Cycle II

Following the evaluation of the first iteration, the results were reflected in the revised the mock-up. The results reflected many *Tick* (ü) & *Cross* (Ò) dominant sections of Table 1. In particular, tailoring more around patient and clinician requirements were added. For patients, this refers to features that allow for them to set preferences around their diet and exercise. While the clinician requirements highlighted the need of a simple visual graphing system, with patient blood glucose being the context. This led way for the second iteration of the same cycle. II) Creation of the Paper Prototype. Given the initial set of mock-ups and the corresponding evaluation results, the paper prototype acted as the successor. The paper prototype contained all the requested changes and mapped out the User Interface for the whole application in a more detailed fashion. Allowing the patients and clinicians to evaluate the design choices and functional elements.

Co-Design Cycle III

After the evaluation of the *paper prototype* took place with the patients and clinicians, the design and the flow of the application was finalised. With this knowledge, the process of developing the application was started. Throughout the artefact development process, there was a scheduled bi-weekly meeting with clinicians and stakeholders to evaluate and validate the state of the application at that given time. This ensured the development process was continuously being validated and is verified to be on track to address the original problem domain as intended. The output of the developed application can be found in Figure 3.

Figure 3. DSRM Artefact

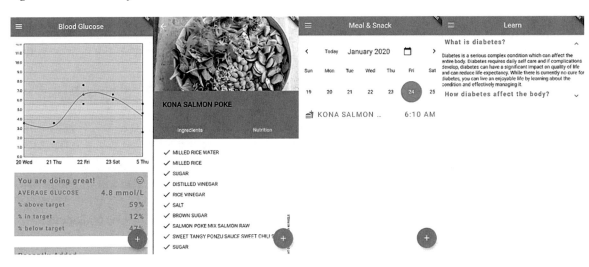

Rigor Cycle

The rigor cycle helped us to verify and populate the knowledge base with our contributions. Here, our contributions include the usage of *DSRM and Co-design for diabetes self-management platforms* to identify the requirements of the platform as well as validate UI design elements, further use of co-design for improved *health platform evaluation strategies*, general contributions to *Experience & Expertise* and finally the designed and developed artefact itself.

The use of DSRM and Co-design approach proved vital in identifying the requirements for the diabetes platform. By merging the context of not only the patient, but the clinician as well, the approach to designing the requirements was greatly impacted. The clinical care team were able to offer advice on how diabetes can be treated while the patients provided the valuable input regarding what they look for in a platform to make sure their experience is adequate.

The co-design approach has also changed the way the platform was evaluated. With the addition of the healthcare professionals, the platform can be evaluated in a more clinical fashion, which provides the grounding for a medically safe and clinically sound technology, while meeting the needs of the patients as well.

An example of this is the suggestions of a culturally sensitive diet preference for an individual. Higher consumption of white rice is associated with a significant increased risk of Type 2 diabetes (Hu, E. A. et al, 2012), however, at the same time, white rice is a staple in a lot of Asian cuisines. Hence asking for a patient with an Asian background to completely disregard this item is quite unreasonable. But with the help of a dietitian (*healthcare professional*), the researchers were able to understand that eating rice at certain time of day significantly reduces the impact on diabetes; in return, allowing us to design the platform to make improved personalised meal recommendations based on information as such.

DISCUSSION

Using the four-cycle model of the DSRM and a co-design approach, the researchers were able to identify core requirements and develop a holistic diabetes self-management platform. Based on the information collected through numerous interviews and workshops with both patients and clinicians during *relevance cycle* of DSRM, allowed for the identification and outlining of the key requirements that was considered important by both context groups. Features outlined in table 2.

These results further affirm on the existing evidence recognised and outlined in the *related works* section as well as the *taxonomy comparison of existing diabetes application – table 1*. The results attained through the DSRM and co-design approach highlights the necessity of having a capable set of *Nutrition* management features and *Clinical* support features, as it was identified as a priority by both patients with diabetes and clinicians. With this knowledge, when compared how well these features are covered in existing diabetes management technologies, it can be see that there are only partial implementations, or in most cases, specifically for *clinical* support, they were not covered at all. This further place the emphasis on the integral addition of the co-design principles with DSRM, which ensures the developed platform incorporates clinician and patient needs; and thus, is more likely to have significant and sustained uptake, usefulness, and usability.

Hence, the inclusion of the co-design approach allowed for us to gain a view on a unique blend of patient-clinician context when identifying requirements and further developing artefact evaluation strategies. Through the patient-clinician context, the researchers were able to obtain insights from both a technical standpoint on what was required for the patients, and what the patients with diabetes wanted. With the merging of the technical and non-technical contexts, further allowed for us to identify requirements for the platform more accurately and with assurance. Assuming that the patient input data is accurate, the patient-clinician communication pipeline has also been improved; as now healthcare professionals can relay real clinical input and feedback on the patient's current progress, straight back to the patient. This improves the chances on minimizing medical and clinical oversight on validated information, providing personalised care through the platform, enabling for a true patient centric experience and promotes patient empowerment.

The development of the diabetes self-management platform using DSRM and co-design cycles allowed for regular evaluation of the *artefacts* to take place, however a formal clinical pilot trial involving semi structured interviews and workshops will still need to be conducted, once the researchers obtain ethics approval from the hospital.

Further, the four-cycle model and co-design approach were strictly followed to ensure that a systematic and rigorous approach was adhered to address the identified problem and from this build a solution that is fit-for-purpose.

LIMITATIONS

During the development of the conceptual prototype, the researchers had only a limited number of patients provide feedback due to the time factors for patients. Thus, the patient feedback is clearly only indicative and not fully representative of the whole diabetic population at the hospital. Given this, the researchers are confident that the vast clinical knowledge of the patient population did supplement the paucity of patient input at this stage. Further, there are plans to have a much larger cohort included for the next phase, clinical trial so this will not be an issue.

CONCLUSION AND FUTURE WORKS

This research in progress adopted DSRM to enable the design and development of a diabetes platform that supports patient self-empowerment around diet, exercise, and medication regarding the impact on blood glucose as well as offering cultural sensitivity regarding preferences presented. By placing an emphasis on the Four-cycle IS DSRM approach, the researchers were able to better understand the problem domain from the relevant stakeholders, in a rigorous and systematic fashion. The diabetic platform reported (Design Cycle III) has been developed and tested internally for functionality. The next key steps include testing the developed solution in a clinical trial to establish usability, usefulness, desirability, and feasibility.

Most of the future development revolves around improving and enhancing the application to make personalised recommendations of meals and exercise based on several parameters including their reported/captured blood glucose level, eating habits, medication, and fitness habits etc. The researchers also aim to extend the current nutrition planner features (that recommends meals) to take into consideration patients personalisation's inputs. This can be achieved by understanding how certain meals, medication, fitness habits effect the blood sugar levels of that given individual. By doing so, this technology would attempt to predict and recommend the ideal meals completely personalised to the given individual, in turn this would help to make sure that the patients' blood sugar levels do not fluctuate erratically.

ACKNOWLEDGMENT

The researchers are very grateful to the input and support provided during the study from Dr Michael Kirk, Dr John Zelcer, Professor Penelope Schofield and Professor Peter Brooks. The researchers would also like to thank AWS, Northern Health and all the patients and clinicians who participated in the study. All necessary ethical permissions were secured.

REFERENCES

Arnott, D., & Pervan, G. (2014). A Critical Analysis of Decision Support Systems Research Revisited: The Rise of Design Science. *Journal of Information Technology, 29*(4), 269–293. doi:10.1057/jit.2014.16

Cortez, N. G., Cohen, I. G., & Kesselheim, A. S. (2014). FDA regulation of mobile health technologies. *The New England Journal of Medicine, 371*(4), 372–379. doi:10.1056/NEJMhle1403384 PMID:25054722

Dorsey, Chan, Feng. McConnell, Shaw, Trister, & Friend. (2017). The Use of Smartphones for Health Research. *Academic Medicine, 92*(2), 157-160. doi:10.1097/ACM.0000000000001205

Drechsler, A., & Hevner, A. (2016). A four-cycle model of IS design science research: capturing the dynamic nature of IS artifact design. Academic Press.

Forkan, A. R. M., Khalil, I., Ibaida, A., & Tari, Z. (2015). BDCaM: Big data for context-aware monitoring—A personalized knowledge discovery framework for assisted healthcare. *IEEE Transactions on Cloud Computing, 5*(4), 628-641.

Gregor, S., & Hevner, A. R. (2013). Positioning and Presenting Design Science Research for Maximum Impact. *MIS Quarterly, 37*(2), 337-355.

Hevner, A., March, S., Park, J., & Ram, S. (2004). Design science in information systems research. *Management Information Systems Quarterly, 28*(1), 75–105. doi:10.2307/25148625

Hevner, A., & Wickramasinghe, N. (2017). *Design Science Research Opportunities in Healthcare.* Theories for Health Informatics Research.

Hu, E. A., Pan, A., Malik, V., & Sun, Q. (2012). White rice consumption and risk of type 2 diabetes: Meta-analysis and systematic review. *BMJ (Clinical Research Ed.), 344*(3), e1454. doi:10.1136/bmj.e1454 PMID:22422870

Huang, Z., Soljak, M., Boehm, B. O., & Car, J. (2018). Clinical relevance of smartphone apps for diabetes management: A global overview. *Diabetes/Metabolism Research and Reviews, 34*(4), e2990. doi:10.1002/dmrr.2990 PMID:29431916

International Diabetes Federation. (2019). *IDF Diabetes Atlas* (9th ed.). Available at: https://www.diabetesatlas.org

Jayaraman, P. P., Forkan, A. R. M., Morshed, A., Haghighi, P. D., & Kang, Y. B. (2020). Healthcare 4.0: A review of frontiers in digital health. *Wiley Interdisciplinary Reviews. Data Mining and Knowledge Discovery, 10*(2), e1350. doi:10.1002/widm.1350

Jimenez, G., Lum, E., & Car, J. (2019). Examining Diabetes Management Apps Recommended From a Google Search: Content Analysis. *JMIR mHealth and uHealth, 7*(1), e11848. doi:10.2196/11848 PMID:30303485

John, B. M., Goh, D. H. L., Chua, A. Y. K., & Wickramasinghe, N. (2016). Graph-based Cluster Analysis to Identify Similar Questions: A Design Science Approach. *Journal of the Association for Information Systems, 17*(9), 590.

Khan, M., Chua, Z., Yang, Y., Liao, Z., & Zhao, Y. (2019). *From Pre-Diabetes to Diabetes: Diagnosis, Treatments and Translational Research*. Medicina. Available at https://www.mdpi.com/1010-660X/55/9/546

Kharroubi, A. T., & Darwish, H. M. (2015). Diabetes mellitus: The epidemic of the century. *World Journal of Diabetes*, *6*(6), 850–867. doi:10.4239/wjd.v6.i6.850 PMID:26131326

Morshed, A., Jayaraman, P. P., Sellis, T., Georgakopoulos, D., Villari, M., & Ranjan, R. (2017). Deep osmosis: Holistic distributed deep learning in osmotic computing. *IEEE Cloud Computing*, *4*(6), 22–32. doi:10.1109/MCC.2018.1081070

Myers, M. D., & Venable, J. R. (2014). A set of ethical principles for design science research in information systems. *Information & Management*, *51*(6), 801–809. doi:10.1016/j.im.2014.01.002

National Diabetes Services Scheme. (2016). *Diabetes-related complication*. Available at: https://www.ndss.com.au/

Nguyen, L., & Wickramasinghe, N. (2017). An examination of the mediating role for a nursing information system. *AJIS. Australasian Journal of Information Systems*, *21*, 1–21. doi:10.3127/ajis.v21i0.1387

Portnov-Neeman, Y., & Amit, M. (2016). *The Effect of the Explicit Teaching Method on Learning the Working Backwards Strategy*. Academic Press.

Shaw, J., & Tanamas, S. (2012) *Diabetes the silent pandemic and its impacts on Australia*. Available at: https://static.diabetesaustralia.com.au/s/fileassets/diabetes-australia/e7282521-472b-4313-b18e-be84c3d5d907.pdf

Villalba-Mora, E., Peinado, I., & Guerrero, D. P. F. (2017). eHealth and diabetes: Designing a novel system for remotely monitoring older adults with type 2 diabetes. Diabetes in Old Age, Fourth Edition. doi:10.1002/9781118954621.ch14

Wickramasinghe, N., John, B., George, J., & Vogel, D. (2019). Achieving Value-Based Care in Chronic Disease Management: The DiaMonD (diabetes monitoring device) Solution. *JMIR Diabetes*, *4*(2), e10368. doi:10.2196/10368 PMID:31066699

Wu, Y., Ding, Y., Tanaka, Y., & Zhang, W. (2014). Risk factors contributing to type 2 diabetes and recent advances in the treatment and prevention. *International Journal of Medical Sciences*, *11*(11), 1185–1200. doi:10.7150/ijms.10001 PMID:25249787

Xu, J., Wang, G. A., Li, J., & Chau, M. (2007). Complex problem solving: Identity matching based on social contextual information. *Journal of the Association for Information Systems*, *8*(10), 525-545.

Chapter 8

Lifetime Enhancement and Reliability in Wireless Body Area Network

Saranya Vasanthamani

Sri Krishna College of Engineering and Technology, India

S. Shankar

Hindusthan College of Engineering and Technology, India

ABSTRACT

The wireless body area network (WBAN) consists of wearable or implantable sensor nodes, which is a technology that enables pervasive observing and delivery of health-related information and services. The network capability of body devices and integration with wireless infrastructure can result in pervasive environment deliver the information about the patients to health care service providers. WBAN has a major part in e-health observing system. Due to sensitivity and critical of the data carried and handled by WBAN, reliability becomes a critical issues. WBAN loads a high degree of reliability as it openly affects the quality of patient observing. A main requirement is that the health care professionals receive the monitored data correctly. Thus reliability can be measured to achieve reliable network are fault tolerance, QoS, and security. As WBAN is a special type of WSN. The objective is to achieve a reliable network with minimum delay and maximum throughput while considering power consumption by reducing unnecessary communication.

1. INTRODUCTION

Wireless technology has advanced to be become a vital part of our lives starting from mobile communication to health care departments. Recently, there has been growing interest from system inventors application and researchers on a newly designed type of network architecture usually known as body sensor networks (BSNs) or body area networks (BANs), one made feasible by novel advances on ultra-low-power, lightweight, small-size and intelligent observing wearable sensors. In BANs, sensors are

DOI: 10.4018/978-1-5225-6067-8.ch008

used to constantly monitor human's functional activities and movements, such as health position and movement pattern. A wireless healthcare application offers and brings many benefits and challenges to the healthcare sector. These benefits provide a convenient-environment that can monitor the daily lives and medical situations of patients at any time, anywhere and without limitations. The Figure 1 shows how WBAN provides a wireless connection between these devices and a Personal digital assistant (PDA) or a smartphone, which is responsible for the connection with other networks. For example, the obtained data can be forwarded to a hospital server.

Figure 1. Data transmission in WBSN

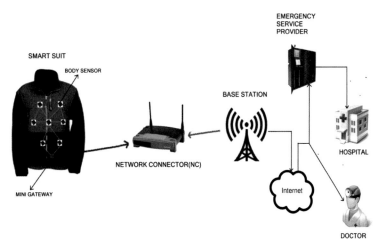

1.1 Wireless BSN Scenario

Wireless BSN applications are in great demand in medical care [1-3], sports and entertainment [4], the military-industrial sector [7], and the social public field [8-10], and BSNs have gradually become a research hotspot. BSNs is a type of WSN which is formed by physiological factors of sensors placed in the human body or on the body surface or around the body. The key performances it covers are sensors, data fusion, and network communication. It focuses on the advancements in universal health care, disease monitoring, and prevention solution, but also an essential component of the so-called Internet of Things. Its foremost purpose is to make available an integrated ubiquitous computing hardware, software, and wireless communication technology platform, and a vital situation for the imminent improvement of ubiquitous healthcare observing systems [11].BSNs initiated from WSNs, so there are many resemblances between them. However, the features are consistently different as of their different application resolutions. Initially, allowing for network deployment, WSNs can be deployed to the unreachable environments, such as forests, swamps or mountains. Several redundant nodes are positioned in the positions indicated above to resolve the problem of node failures, so node density is greater, however, BSN nodes are positioned in, on or around the human body, so the total number of nodes is usually up to a few dozens. Each node confirms the correctness of observing consequences by its robustness [12]. Moreover, considering attributes, nodes in WSNs accomplish the similar functions and have the identical properties. The size of nodes is not very critical. Formerly the node is deployed, it will probably no longer need to be relocated.

Agreeing to the dissimilar physical signals collected, BSN applications ensure different sensor types [13]. Furthermore, the necessities of BSN node design are comparatively high. The node dimensions must be small enough, and the nodes must have high wearability and high biocompatibility [14]. Due to the locations, the nodes are deployed, they will move as the human body moves. Furthermore, considering energy supply, WSNs and BSNs can be battery-powered. The earlier, positioned outdoors, can also be powered by wind energy or solar energy, while the latter can also be powered by kinetic energy and heat [15]. Lastly, allowing for data transmission, the transfer rates of WSNs are almost the same, but those of BSNs are different, as the data type and channel task are different among nodes on the body surface and in the BSNs [13]. Additionally, BSN deployed in the human body are for observing human physiological data, which are subject to user's personal safety and privacy protection issues. Therefore, QoS and the real-time prosperity of data transmission must be considered [17,18,19].

1.1.1 Implanted Node

Implanted nodes are used to analyze the health factors with the biosensors which in need to be in the close touching base with the skin, and every now and then even inside the human body. Implantable biosensors are an important class of biosensors constructed on their capability to continuously measure metabolite levels, without the prerequisite for patient intervention and irrespective of the patient's physiological state (sleep, rest, *etc.*) For example, implantable biosensors symbolize an extremely necessary proposition for diabetes management which presently relies on data obtained by using test strips blood from finger pricking, a practice which is not only painful, but as well is incapable of reflecting the global direction, trends, and patterns related with daily habits.

Figure 2. Representations of Implanted Sensors

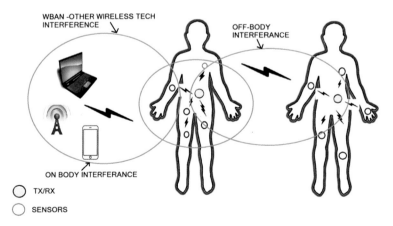

A startup of a broad research effort predictable at developing implantable biosensors for continuous observing of multiple biologically relevant metabolites, but not wearable sensors. Additional classes of implantable devices which ensure be situated intensively investigated comprise of sensors for nerve stimulation can ease acute pain sensors to the detecting electric signals in brain and sensors to monitor biological analysis in the brain with implanted drug delivery systems for controlled delivery at the site of pain and stress [33].

In the course of the end of the last era, there has been a major increase in the number of various wearable health observing devices, extending from simple pulse monitors, activity monitors, and portable Holter monitors, to sophisticated and exclusive implantable sensors. IWBANs(Implantable Wireless Body Area Networks) are more desirable than WWBAN(Wearable Wireless Body Area Network) for numerous advantages. WWBANs have some disadvantages: they limit the mobility of the patients; in accumulation, they can cause skin infections, thus donating poor health conditions. Regardless of the wireless connection is not an essential requirement for observing physiological parameters from implanted sensors. This problem is measured as one of the main incentives for the trend in modern biomedical implanted systems to use wireless technology [33]. In[34] explored a vision of the near future when one single device will be able to create a WSN with a large number of nodes, which are put on inside and outside the body may be one or the other predetermined or aimlessly, in accord with the application. This visualization can only be achieved over a broad communication standard for wireless telemetry link. Typical hardware and software architecture can support compatible devices, which are predictable to meaningfully affect the succeeding generation of healthcare systems. Certain of these devices can then be incorporated into the wireless body area network, providing novel opportunities for technology to monitor the health status.

1.1.2 Non Implanted Node

WSN technology has the would be to offering a wide range of welfares to patients, medical staff, and society through uninterrupted observing in an ambulatory setting, premature detection of abnormal circumstances, vision rehabilitation, and potential discovery of knowledge through data mining of all assembled information. This part shows exactly how to use the planning and mechanism of WWBANs as well as main arrangement enabling unobtrusive, continuous, daily observing of health. In accumulation, this section defines some important implementation issues.

Figure 3. Non-Implanted Sensors Nodes

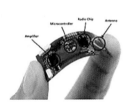 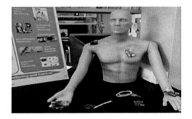

Wearable health observing systems agree the individual follow closely the changes in her or his vital functions and provide feedback for maintaining optimal health status. If integrated into the telemedicine system, such systems can alert medical personnel when serious changes occur. In accumulation with medical centers, patients could be benefited for uninterrupted long-term observing as a portion of a diagnostic practice. We can accomplish optimal maintenance of a chronic condition or can be monitored during the recovery period after the critical event or surgical procedure. Durable health observing can capture the diurnal and circadian variations in physiological signals. These changes, for example, are a very good indicator of cardiac recovery of patients after myocardial infarction [35]. Long-term observing can also confirm adherence to treatment guidelines or help monitor the effects of drug therapy. Other patients may also benefit from these systems; for example, monitors can be used during physical restoration after hip or knee surgeries, stroke restoration, or brain trauma restoration.

The practice of wearable sensors for observing several health-related biometric parameters in daily activities is attracting more interest in recent times. Several individuals are familiar with the use of devices such as wearable heart rate monitors and pedometers for medical reasons or as part of a fitness administration. Importance of the use of such wearable systems for personal health and restoration has increased as part of a wider initiative for increasing the input of the individual or patient in their private care. It is understood that this could help in reducing the strain put on healthcare systems of elderly populations, rising costs and increasing incidence of chronic diseases requiring extensive term care.

The architecture includes the major stage to cover the number of wireless nodes of medical sensor that are integrated into WWBANs. Respectively, each sensor node sense, sample, and process one or more physiological signals. For example, an electrocardiogram sensor can be used to monitor heart action, an electromyogram sensor for observing muscle activity, an electroencephalogram sensor for observing brain electrical activity, a blood pressure sensor for observing blood pressure, a tilt sensor for observing trunk situation, and a breathing sensor for observing breathing; and motion sensors can be used to categorize the user's status and to estimate her or his level of activity.

1.2 Topology of the Node Deployment

The deployment of nodes for the data transmission in a network is based on the Energy level of the nodes and the node with the maximum energy is considered as a SINK node.

Figure 4. Data Communication using SINK

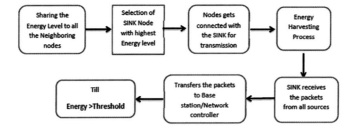

Initially, the energy level of all the neighboring nodes is analyzed for the selection of a SINK node which holds the highest energy level. After the selection of the SINK, all the other nodes get connected with the SINK till the energy level reaches the minimum threshold level. The packet transmission takes place with the assistance of the SINK acting as an intermediate with the network controller. The same process is repeated till the SINK energy level decreases. Even after reaching the minimum energy level the transmission has to be continued then reelection of another SINK node will to processed for a long-term communication with the same procedure to be continued.

2. LIFETIME ENHANCEMENT METHODS

2.1 Concept of Network Lifetime

In WBANs, energy is consumed mainly on transmission, sensing and unusual energy unused including idle listening, collision, and overhearing. Wireless Body Area Network (WBAN) is a collection of low-power, miniaturized, invasive/non-invasive lightweight wireless sensor nodes that monitor the human body functions and the surrounding environment

2.2 Network Model

Figure 5. Network Model

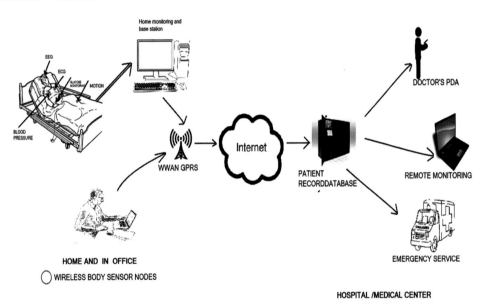

WBAN devices are implanted inside the body or might be surface-mounted on the body in a fixed position or else may be accompanied devices which humans can carry in dissimilar positions, in dress pockets, by hand or in bags. Whereas there is a development of tiny devices, in specific, networks consisting of several tiny body sensor units (BSUs) organized with a particular body central unit (BCU).The observing is done in both the places at home and office with these nodes. The development in WBAN technology implements communications on, near, and around the human body and they can transfer information through gateways to reach longer ranges. Through gateway devices, it is possible to connect the wearable devices on the human body to the internet. This way, medical professionals can access patient data online using the internet independent of the patient location.

2.3 Energy Consumption Model

Medical information collected by sensors on the patient's body (WPAN-Wireless Personal Area Networks) is displayed on a bedside monitor. This information is also transmitted to another hospital location for remote monitoring, e.g., a nurses' station) In case of emergency, when the patient is moved from his/her room to the intensive care unit, these communications need to be maintained.

Figure 6. Energy Consumption and Node Deployment using WPAN

di,j: the distance between each pair of sensor nodes and the distance between sensor nodes and the controller.

p_t: *the transmission path state (LOS/NLOS-Line of Sight/Non Line of Sight) between each pair of nodes including the controller.*

ETXelec, ERXelec, Eamp: the energy consumption parameters.

P_L: *the packet length in the network.*

E_s: *the energy storage condition of each sensor node in the network.*

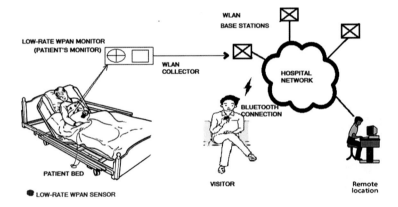

The energy cost to guarantee reliable transmission during transmitting and receiving are described in Equations (1) and (2) as follows:

Figure 7. Three Tier communications in WBAN

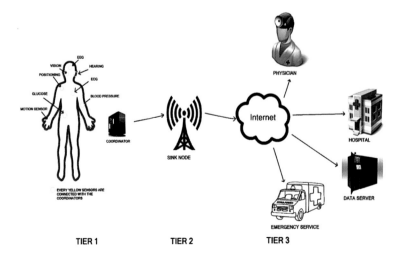

$$Etx(P_L, d, p_t) = ETXelec \cdot P_L + Eamp \cdot P_L \cdot d\,p_t, \tag{1}$$

$$Erx(k) = ERXelec \cdot P_L. \tag{2}$$

The model takes d n as energy costs due to a channel variation and the path loss in respect with distance d between sender and receiver. Etx represents the transmission energy, Erx the receiver energy, ETXelec and ERXelec the energy the radio dissipates to run the circuitry for the transmitter and receiver, respectively, and Eamp is the energy for the transmitter amplifier. The specific values of these parameters are hardware dependent. In addition, k represents the number of bits sent for the transmission. n is path loss coefficient related to shadow effect.

The tier 1 of communication in the wireless body area sensor network is based on a number of smart nodes, each accomplished of detecting, sampling, processing, and creating interactive functional signals. Every sensor node obtains initialization guidelines and responds to queries from the personal server. A Coordinator which collects the information from each sensing node and transfers to the SINK node. The tier 2 is the private server that interfaces WBAN sensor nodes, be responsible for the graphical user interface, and communicates with services at the top tier. The private server is classically implemented on a PDA or a cell phone, but instead, it can run on a home private computer. This is predominantly suitable for in-home monitoring of elderly patients. The private server interfaces the WBAN nodes through a network coordinator (NC) that implements ZigBee or Bluetooth connectivity. To interconnect with the medical server, the private server employs mobile telephone networks (2G, GPRS, 3G) or WLANs to reach an Internet access point.

The tier 3, concentrated on a medical server, is enhanced to check hundreds or thousands of discrete users and incorporates a composite network of unified services, medical personnel, and healthcare professionals. Each user wears a number of sensor nodes that are intentionally placed on her/his body. The medical server preserves electronic medical records of enumerated users and delivers several facilities to the users, medical personnel, and informal caretakers. It is the responsibility of the medical server to verify users, receive health monitoring session uploads, design and introduce the particular session data into equivalent medical records, analyze the data patterns, identify serious health variances in order to communicate with emergency caretakers, and forward original directions to the users, such as physician recommended daily workouts. The patient's physician can access the data from his/her work through the Internet and observe it safeguard the patient is within probable health metrics (heart rate, blood pressure, activity), guarantee that the patient is responding to a treatment given by the physician or that a patient has been carrying out the given exercises. A server agent may examine the uploaded data and generate an alert in the case of a latent medical condition. A larger amount of data collected through these services can also be used for knowledge discovery through data mining. Integration of the collected data into exploration databases and measurable analysis of conditions and patterns could demonstrate the precious information to the researchers trying to link symptoms and diagnosed with chronological changes in health status, physiological data, or supplementary factors (e.g., gender, age, weight). It could significantly contribute to monitoring and studying of drug therapy effects for the patients during unavoidable emergency situations.

2.4 Effective Methods

As the total number of sensor nodes in a WBAN is not large, $d_{i,j}$ can be measured manually after the sensor nodes have been deployed as well as p_t, e.g., the transmission path state of each pair of nodes according to the location of each node. Furthermore, the energy consumption parameters are obtained depending on the transceiver types of sensor nodes in the networks. K is identified by the communication protocol and is simply known by WBAN manipulators. E_s can be known by two means depending on two conditions: (A) if the transmit selection is appealed at the network initialization where each sensor node is filled with energy, we can directly achieve the energy storage information from the sensor node form and battery-operated information; (B) if the transmit selection is appealed at a resume from a network recovery, the controller can set a appeal flag in the inspiration frame in order to inform each sensor node to report its residual energy situation in the transmitting time slots. Once all of the parameter values are gained, the controller records this information in its memory and has the ability to execute the relay selection scheme. Then, we illustrate how to implement our relay selection scheme in dual cases. In the principal case where a WBAN is at the initialization stage, the controller will directly execute the relay selection scheme at the beginning of the first frame since it has all values needed to execute the relay selection scheme and load the relay allocation results and the corresponding timeslot allocation in the ideal frame. Then, in the ideal transmission slot, the controller broadcasts the ideal frame to all of the sensor nodes in the network. As each node must listen and receive this ideal frame, all of the sensor nodes in the network will know their transmission strategy and their relay nodes, if needed. In the succeeding case, e.g., a WBAN restarts, where the energy storage condition of sensor nodes is unknown, the controller sets a request flag in the ideal frame at the beginning of the first frame and allocates timeslots for each sensor node in the network to report their energy storage conditions. As a result, in the first frame, sensor nodes send their energy storage information to the controller in their allocated report slots. After the controllers have received all of the report frames, it invokes the proposed relay selection scheme and loads the results and the corresponding timeslot allocation in the next ideal frame, which will be broadcasted in the second frame. Then, in the second frame, each node will know its transmission strategy and their relay nodes. It should be emphasized that the low complexity of the rapid solution in our proposed scheme guarantees that the controller can finish the algorithm in the interval between the point when the controller has received all the energy storage reports to the slot for broadcasting the next ideal frame. Furthermore, it should be noticed that the implementation discussed here does not involve the detailed interaction procedures between the controller and sensor nodes that will be further studied in the future.

3. RELIABILITY

WBANs, which promise significant improvement in the reliability of observing and treating people's health, comprise a number of sensors and actuators that may either be implanted or mounted on the surface of the human body, and which are capable of wireless communication to one or more external nodes that are in close proximity to the human body. Achieving minimal energy consumption, with the required level of reliability is critical for the proper functioning of many wireless sensor and body area networks. Additionally, anyway of the traffic appearances, the methods we introduce to understand reliable wireless sensor networks using (occasionally) unreliable components (wireless sensor nodes).

- **Cooperative communications** enable efficient consumption of **communication** resources, by permitting nodes or terminals in a **communication network** to cooperate with each other in information transmission. It is a promising technique for yet to come **communication** systems. The energy efficiency of cooperative systems in wireless body area network (WBAN) to outage the performance of three transmission patterns, specifically direct transmission, single-relay cooperation, and multi-relay cooperation.

At any node ni, the reliability estimator module is responsible to measure the average link reliability LRi,j of link $Li-j$ for neighbor node nj. If N successful is the number of successful transmissions and N total is the number of total transmissions, then the average probability P average of successful transmission over a time window δt can be calculated as

P average= N successful / N total.

4. MEDICAL APPLICATIONS OF WIRELESS BODY SENSOR NETWORKS

In recent times, interest in wireless systems for medical applications has been promptly growing. By a number of benefits in wired alternatives, comprises of ease of use, reduced possibility of infection, reduced the possibility of failure, reduce patient uneasiness, improve mobility and low cost of precaution conveyance, wireless applications convey exciting potentials for new applications in the medical market. Portable devices such as heart rate monitors, pulse oximeters, spirometers and blood pressure monitors are essential instruments in intensive care. Usually, the sensors for these utensils are implanted to the patient by wires and the patient will consecutively turn into bed-bound. On every occasion patient needs to be moved, all intensive care devices have to be disconnected and then reconnected later. Currently, all of these time-consuming works could be terminated and patients could be liberated from instrumentation and bed by wireless technology. Integrated wireless technology, these wireless devices could communicate with a gateway that connects to the medical center's network and transmits data to health data stores for monitoring, control, or evaluating in real time or offline after storage.

The data acquisition begins with the physical property to be measured. Data interpretation and decision making are done based on the data acquisition measured and also treatment is based on the acquisition.

New and improved healing devices in figure 8 are continuously introduced to identify vital signals and present them in an appropriate format for health care supporters. The interpretation can be regarded as a data compression and data conformity process. The general practitioner make a treatment recommendation based on the patient's medical history and current experimental reports by referring the evidence-based database, pharmacological handbook, and other resources

5. CONCLUSION

The essentiality of Lifetime Enhancement and Reliability in Wireless Body Area Network is discussed in this chapter. Which describes types of WBAN and the usage of it based on our requirement and patients problem. Then the transmission path state of each pair of nodes is located according to the location of

Figure 8. Applications of WBAN

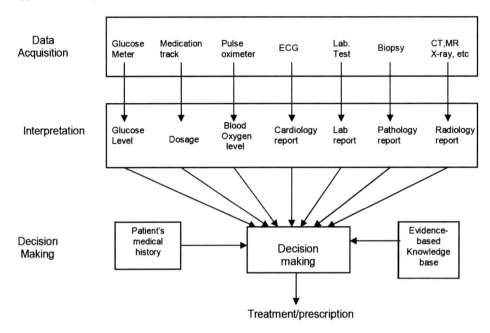

each node. Moreover, the energy consumption parameters are acquired depending on the transceiver types of sensor nodes in the networks. Reliability is maintained by the cooperative communication between the nodes. Thus a prolonged network lifetime achieves a reliable network with minimum delay and maximum throughput while considering power consumption by reducing unnecessary communication.

REFERENCES

Akyildiz, I. F., Su, W., Sankarasubramaniam, Y., & Cayirci, E. (2002). "A Survey on Sensor Networks," proc. *IEEE Communications Magazine, 40*(Aug), 102–114. doi:10.1109/MCOM.2002.1024422

Almashaqbeh, G., Hayajneh, T., & Vasilakos, A. V. (2014). A cloud-based interference-aware remote health observingsystem for non-hospitalized patients. *Proceedings of the IEEE 12th global communication conference (IEEE Globecom'14).*

Almashaqbeh, G., Hayajneh, T., Vasilakos, A. V., &Mohd, B. J. (2014). QoS-aware health observingsystem using cloud-based WBANs. *Journal of Medical Systems, 38*(121), 1–20. doi:10.1007/s10916-014-0121-2

Ben Elhadj, H., Chaari, L., & Kamoun, L. (2012). A survey of routing protocols in wireless body area networks for healthcare applications. *Int. J. of E-Health and Medical Commun., 3*(2), 1–18.

Binkley, P., Frontera, W., Standaert, D. G., & Stein, J. (2003). Predicting the potential of wearable technology. *IEEE Engineering in Medicine and Biology Magazine, 22*(3), 23–24. doi:10.1109/MEMB.2003.1213623 PMID:12845813

Carrano, R., Passos, D., Magalhaes, L., & Albuquerque, C. (2013). Survey and taxonomy of duty cycling mechanisms in wireless sensor networks. IEEE Commun. Surveys Tutorials, 1–14.

Chiti, F., Fantacci, R., & Lappoli, S. (2010). Contention delay minimization in wireless body sensor networks: A game theoretic perspective. *IEEE Global Telecommunications Conference*, 1-6. 10.1109/GLOCOM.2010.5683753

Conroy, L., Ó'Conaire, C., Coyle, S., Healy, G., Kelly, P., O'Connor, N., Caulfield, B., Connaghan, D., Smeaton, A., & Nixon, P. (2009). TennisSense: A Multi-Sensory Approach to Performance Analysis in Tennis. *Proceedings of the 27th International Society of Biomechanics in Sports Conference 2009.*

Emmanuel, D., Kola, S., & Mohana, J. (2014). A Survey on wireless Body Area Networks. International Journal of Scientific and Research Publications, 4(3), 1-7.

Fallahzadeh, R., Ma, Y., & Ghasemzadeh, H. (2016). Context-Aware System Design for Remote Health Monitoring: An Application to Continuous Edema Assessment. *IEEE Trans. Mob. Comput.*

Fareeha. (2012). Review of Body Area Network technology and wireless medical monitoring. *International Journal of Information and Communication Technology Research, 2*(2).

FCC-Medical Body Area Networks - small entity compliance guide. (2013). http://www.fcc.gov/document/medical-body-area-networks

Filipe, L., Fdez-Riverola, F., Costa, N., & Pereira, A. (2015). Wireless body area networks for healthcare applications: Protocol stack review. *International Journal of Distributed Sensor Networks, 11*(10), 1–23. doi:10.1155/2015/213705

Garth, Tirthankar, Renita, & Craig. (2012). Wireless Body Area Networks for Healthcare: A Survey. *International Journal of Ad hoc, Sensor & Ubiquitous Computing, 3*(3).

Gonza'lez-Valenzuela, S., Liang, X., Cao, H., Chen, M., & Leung, V. C. (2013). *"Body area networks," in Autonomous Sensor Networks.* Springer.

Gravina, R., Alinia, P., Ghasemzadeh, H., & Fortino, G. (2016). Multi-sensor fusion in body sensor networks: State-of-the-art and research challenges. *Information Fusion, 35,* 68–80. doi:10.1016/j.inffus.2016.09.005

Hadda, E. B., Lamia, C., & Lotfi, K. (2012). A Survey of routing protocols in Wireless Body Area Networks for healthcare applications. International Journal of Ehealth and Medical Communications, 3(2), 1-18.

Jamil & Mehmet. (2010). Wireless Body Area Network (WBAN) for Medical Applications. *New Developments in Biomedical Engineering, 1,* 591-628.

Kavitha, Balapriya, & Sundrarajan. (2016). A Survey of routing protocols in Wireless Body Area Networks. *South Asian Journal of Engineering and Technology, 2*(21), 44-51.

Khan, J. Y., & Yuce, M. R. (2010). Wireless body area network (WBAN) for medical applications. In C. Domenico (Ed.), *New Developments in Biomedical Engineering* (pp. 591–627). Intech Publishing.

Khan, Z. A., Sivakumar, S., Phillips, W., Robertson, B., & Javaid, N. (2015). QPRD: QoS-aware peering routing protocol for delay-sensitive data in hospital body area network. *Mobile Information Systems, 2015*, 16. doi:10.1155/2015/153232

Liu, Y., Liu, A., Hu, Y., Li, Z., Choi, Y.-J., Sekiya, H., & Li, J. (2016). FFSC: An Energy Efðciency Communications Approach for Delay Minimizing in Internet of Things. *IEEE Access, 4*, 3775–3793.

Maulin, P., & Wang, F. J. (2010). Applications, Challenges and Prospective In Emerging Body Area Networking Technologies. *IEEE Wireless Communications*, 1284–1536.

Misra, S., & Sarkar, S. (2015). Priority-based time-slot allocation in wireless body area networks during medical emergency situations: An evolutionary game-theoretic perspective. *IEEE Journal of Biomedical and Health Informatics, 19*(2), 541–548. doi:10.1109/JBHI.2014.2313374 PMID:24686307

Mohseni, P., & Najafi, K. A. (2005). 1.48-mw low-phase-noise analog frequency modulator for wireless biotelemetry. *IEEE Transactions on Biomedical Engineering, 52*(5), 938–943. doi:10.1109/TBME.2005.845369 PMID:15887544

Movassaghi, S., Abolhasan, M., Lipman, J., Smith, D., & Jamalipour, A. (2014). Wireless body area networks: A survey. *IEEE Communications Surveys and Tutorials, 16*(3), 1658–1686. doi:10.1109/SURV.2013.121313.00064

Omar, S., Adda, K., Youssef, Z., & Bernard, C. (2016). *ESR- Energy-aware and Stable routing protocol for WBAN Networks*. IEEE Publications.

Otto, C., Milenković, A., Sanders, C., & Jovanov, E. (2006). System Architecture of a Wireless Body Area Sensor Network For Ubiquitous Health Monitoring. *Journal of Mobile Multimedia, 1*(4), 307–326.

Pervez, Hussain, & Kyung. (2009). Medical Applications of Wireless Body Area Networks. *International Journal of Digital Content Technology and Its Applications, 3*(3), 185-193.

Qiu, Y., Haley, D., Chan, T., & Davis, L. (2016). Game theoretic framework for studying WBAN coexistence: 2-Player game analysis and n-player game estimation. *IEEE Australian Communications Theory Workshop*, 53-58. 10.1109/AusCTW.2016.7433609

Reddy, G. P., Reddy, P. B., & Reddy, V. K. (2013). Body area networks. *J. of Telematics and Informatics, 1*(1). Advance online publication. doi:10.12928/jti.v1i1.36-42

Riccardo, C., Flavia, M., Ramona, R., Chiara, B., & Roberto, V. (2014). A Survey on Wireless Body Area Networks: Technologies and design challenges. IEEE Communications Surveys and Tutorials, 16(3), 1635-1657.

Samaneh, M., Mehran, A., Justin, L., David, S., & Abbas, J. (2014). Wireless Body Area Networks: A Survey. IEEE Communications Surveys and Tutorials, 16(3), 1658-1686.

Seyedi, Kibret, Lai, & Faulkner. (2013). *A survey on intrabody communications for body area network applications*. Academic Press.

Tang, Q., Tummala, N., Gupta, S., & Schwiebert, L. (2005). Communication scheduling to minimize thermal effects of implanted biosensor networks in homogeneous tissue. *IEEE Transactions on Biomedical Engineering*, *52*(7), 1285–1294. doi:10.1109/TBME.2005.847527 PMID:16041992

Zou, L., Liu, B., Chen, C., & Chen, C. W. (2014). Bayesian game based power control scheme for inter-WBAN interference mitigation. *IEEE Global Communications Conference*, 240-245.

KEY TERMS AND DEFINITIONS

IWBAN: Implantable wireless body area networks.
LOS/NLOS: Line of sight/non-line of sight.
WPAN: Wireless personal area network.
WWBAN: Wearable wireless body area network.

Chapter 9
Location Information Services of Automated External Defibrillators (AEDs)

Reima Suomi

https://orcid.org/0000-0003-2169-7997

University of Turku, Finland

Eila Lindfors

University of Turku, Finland

Brita Marianne Somerkoski

University of Turku, Finland

ABSTRACT

Cardiovascular diseases are a leading death cause in the world. Cardiac arrest is one of the most usual, and very quickly fatal, especially in out-of-hospital environments. Defibrillation, aside with cardiopulmonary resuscitation, is an effective means to restart blood circulation and heart operation, even though even these forms of treatment can help just in sadly few situations. Defibrillation was invented and first demonstrated already year 1899, but first in the 2000s portable defibrillators with good automatic functions started to penetrate daily environments of people, especially in urban settings. Nowadays the starting point is that every citizen with normal human functionality should be able to use automated defibrillators. The chapter discusses how modern information and communication technology, especially mobiles services, internet, and location services based on them, could help citizens in the first crucial step in implementing their safety competence in emergency situations by using automatic defibrillators if they could only find them.

DOI: 10.4018/978-1-5225-6067-8.ch009

INTRODUCTION

Cardiovascular diseases are a leading death cause in the world. Of them, cardiac arrest is one of the most usual, and very fast fatal, especially in out-of-hospital environments, where most cardiac arrests happen. World Health Organization (WHO) gives following facts about cardiovascular diseases (CVDs) (World Health Organisation, 2020):

- CVDs are the number 1 cause of death globally: more people die annually from CVDs than from any other cause.
- An estimated 17.9 million people died from CVDs in 2016, representing 31% of all global deaths. Of these deaths, 85% are due to heart attack and stroke.
- Over three quarters of CVD deaths take place in low- and middle-income countries.
- Out of the 17 million premature deaths (under the age of 70) due to non-communicable diseases in 2015, 82% are in low- and middle-income countries, and 37% is caused by CVDs.

Cardiac arrest can hit anyone, even though risk usually grows with age. Alarmingly, the study of Ringh & al (2009) found that there was a decreasing median age (form 68 to 64 years) in their study of out-of-hospital cardiac arrest patients in Sweden. In their Japan-wide study of SCAs in years 2013-2015 (Kobayashi et al., 2020) found 4863 out-of-hospital cardiac arrest patients less than 18 years of age. As SCA hits the core of critical body functions, hearth, fast response is needed.

Defibrillation, aside with cardiopulmonary resuscitation, is an effective means to restart blood circulation and heart operation, even though even these forms of treatment can help just in sadly few situations. Not all blood circulation or heart –related traumas are treatable with automated external defibrillators. Especially, asystole, a state with flat line –pattern, telling that the hearth has no electrical activity, and also causes no blood circulation, is not shockable with an AED.

Defibrillation was invented and first demonstrated already year 1899, but first in the 2000s portable automated external defibrillators (AEDs) with good automatic functions started to penetrate daily environments of people, especially in urban settings. Nowadays the starting point is that everyone with normal human functionality should be able to use automated defibrillators, and is expected to do so. The fast and right response is symbolized in the chain of survival: finding the patient/victim as early as possible, immediately started cardiopulmonary resuscitation (CPR), immediately started defibrillation with AEDs devices, and fast advanced cardiac life support in hospital settings. AED use should start within 5 minutes from the hearth stop, and before that taken cardiopulmonary resuscitation strongly improves the changes of survival.

Despite much activity, automatic external defibrillators are still scarce, and even if they would be available, they very seldom end up to productive use. This article studies the reasons for the rather low effectiveness of the heavy AED investments. The effectiveness of the AED investments has been already widely discussed, as for example in (Ringh et al., 2009) and (Walker, Sirel, Marsden, Cobbe, & Pell, 2003). Especially, this article discusses how modern information and communication technology, especially mobiles services, Internet and location services based on them could help citizens in the first crucial step in use of automatic defibrillators, the finding of them. Even when a defibrillator is found in time, there is sadly ample evidence, that they do not end up to use, or the use cannot help the victim. However, willingness to act, and knowledge and skills to execute needed operations in using AEDs should be a part of citizens' safety competence that could be enhanced by digital mobile applications.

In most cases even in heavily urban areas professional emergency staff (EMS) is not able to arrive to the venue of the cardiac arrest fast enough (Kitamura et al., 2010; O'Keeffe, Nicholl, Turner, & Goodacre, 2011; Zakaria et al., 2014). In US, the median time from 911 call to the arrival of professional rescuers often exceeds 6 minutes, even in dense urban environments (Myerburg, Velez, Rosenberg, Fenster, & Castellanos, 2003). This reveals why bystander help is needed crucially. Still, in the US, less than 8 percent of patients with out-of-hospital cardiac arrest in public setting have an automated external defibrillator applied before EMS personnel arrive (S. C. Brooks, Hsu, Tang, Jeyakumar, & Chan, 2013; Weisfeldt et al., 2011).

The article unfolds as follows. After this introduction to the topic we discuss defibrillators, and automatic external defibrillators as a subgroup of them. Then we discuss the medical outcomes of usage of AEDs, and stress the need for fast action. Then we turn to discuss why all citizens, including laymen, should have common safety competence including knowledge, skills and a willingness to use AEDs, and what kind of reasons inhibit them from doing so. Then the concept of chain of survival is introduced, and extended to reflect possibilities and challenges in using information and communication technologies (ICT) support to find and use AEDs. In the next section we focus on the crucial chain of survival component, finding an AED, and the role of ICT-based services in this. Conclusions follow.

DEFIBRILLATORS

A defibrillator is a device that gives a high energy electric shock to the heart through the chest wall to someone who is in cardiac arrest. This high energy shock is called defibrillation, and it is an essential life saving step in the chain of survival (British Heart Foundation, 2020).

Defibrillators help in the cases of cardiac (hearth) arrhythmia. Arrhythmia means that heart beats too quickly, too slowly, or with an irregular pattern. Arrhythmia is not to be confused with hearth attack, which is the death of a segment of heart muscle caused by a loss of blood supply. AEDs are useful in the cases of ventricular fibrillation and pulseless ventricular tachycardia. They are not helping or may be even harmful in many other hearth problems.

Especially AEDs are not usable as electric shock givers in the situations of totally stopped blood circulation called in medical terms asystole. Asystole is the absence of ventricular contractions and connected to cardiac flatline, that is the state of total cessation of electrical activity from the heart, and consequently blood flow to the rest of the body. AEDs can in such cases still be used to analyze and confirm the possible (but often not probable) restart of blood circulation.

"Automated" in the notion of AED means that the device works as independently as possible. Especially it means that the AED itself decides whether an electric shock is appropriate, and gives it. Many models anyway want human to confirm and give the electric shock, already as it might be dangerous to outsiders being (by mistake) connected to the victim.

"External" means that the device is portable and not implemented to a human. Internal defibrillators are surgically implanted to the human body, and they are connected with electrodes to the human body, usually hearth muscle.

Health professionals have their own manually operated or automated defibrillators. The usually allow more decision power to the user, but often also include automatic features, if they are preferred to be used by the professional users.

Defibrillators are places on the human chest so that the two pads of the device are at the other ends of the hearth, one up on the right side and another below the hearth on the left side (as seen from the patient point of view). The pads should be in direct contact with the human skin, clothes and sometimes even hairy skin surface can be obstacles. The modern AEDs typically give two sequential shocks with power of 120-200 joules, the two shocks changing polarity during the activity. In early years of AEDs, changing polarity was not used, and the electronic energy was much higher.

In addition to doing the core defibrillation with electronic shocks, defibrillators are already helpful in analyzing the status of the hearth even if defibrillation cannot be done (non shockable rhythms), and in such way assist also the process of cardiopulmonary resuscitation (Kishimori et al., 2020).

First use of an external defibrillator on a human being was conducted in year 1947 by Claude Beck. The first portable defibrillator was invented by Frank Pantridge in Ireland in year 1965. Current developments in include web-enabled AED, also an AED that is in constant connection with the Internet. These devices offer new possibilities finding them when needed through the web, and they can also for example report themselves of their maintenance needs (Mao & Ong, 2016). Constant connection to Internet of course on the other side consumes battery recourses.

The official AED sign (Figure 1) was developed by the International Liaison Committee on Resuscitation in year 2008, and it was accepted as ISO standard 7010 E010 in year 2011. Sadly, when taking a look at Google with the keyword "AED sign", one sees hundreds of different versions of this sign. This is not of course in any way alleviating the difficulties of finding an AED in the moment of need.

Figure 1. The official AED sign (ISO standard 7010 E010)

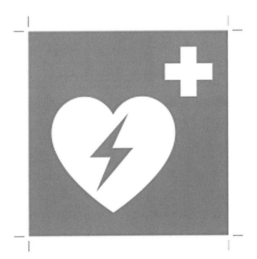

Automated external defibrillators are increasingly installed to public places. Reasons for and methods of installing vary. An usual group of AED installations is haphazard donations, where there typically is not any detailed planning for the location of the AED. Many organizations, such as insurance companies, install AEDs to their premises to show example. Cities are typically actors for planned and systematical AED acquirement and installation. In a study about Stockholm, Sweden, (Ringh et al., 2009) showed that systematic placement of AEDs to city setting are much more effective than unregulated placement.

Sun & al (2019) calculated a new positions of AEDs in Copenhagen based on real OHCA case register. They found that their reallocated AED positions would have increased AED out-of-hospital cardiac arrest (OHCA) coverage by 50 to 100 percent. Legal reasons, such as fear for liability are also a strong motivation installing AEDs (Coris, Miller, & Sahebzamani, 2005).

The current recommendation for the density of defibrillators is that they should be in places where one cardiac arrest is expected to happen every 5 years[1]. To take an example, (Folke, Lippert, & Nielsen, 2009) evaluated that in the rather urban city of Copenhagen with some 600 000 inhabitants following this standard would mean some 1100 AEDs. In the article it was counted that this resulted in the cost of $40 900 per quality-adjusted life year (QALY).

Especially it must be noted that in most cases cardiopulmonary resuscitation and defibrillation activities go hand in hand. Typical scenario is that CPR must be started and maintained, until a defibrillator is found to stabilize the hearth beat.

It is suggested by the American Heart Association (AHA) that an AED should be available within 100 meters so that it can be reached in 1,5 minutes at a brisk pace (Aufderheide et al., 2006). AED application should be started within a maximum of five minutes, and they should be accessed in a timeframe of 1-1,5 minutes (Kishimori et al., 2020). It has been assessed that every minute of delay of defibrillation start causes 9 percent decrease in neurologically intact survival (Kitamura et al., 2010).

The prices of AEDs have gone down, and their usability is good enough for a normally functional layman. Finding the defibrillator fast and effectively in the case of need is of crucial importance and improves the probability to survive out of hospital cardia arrest (Public Access Defibrillation Trial Investigators, 2004). Fortunately, the constantly increasingly more ubiquitous information and communication technology can help in the finding of the defibrillator location (Merchant & Asch, 2012), because of mobile phones and improved location-based services in them.

Results of AED Use

Out-of-hospital cardiac arrest (OHCA) Survival rates vary drastically between communities (Nichol et al., 2008). Situations, conditions and figures in different countries, environments and with different populations are different, but Figure 2 gives a broad illustration on the importance of AED use. Some 20 percent of OHCA cases happen outside home-like public inaccessible settings. According to (Becker, Eisenberg, Fahrenbruch, & Cobb, 1998) and (Pell et al., 2002) 79 to 83 percent of out-of-hospital arrests happen at home. In optimal conditions, an AED is used in some 20 percent of those cases. Survival rate is clearly improved because of the AED use, but still remains far below 10 percent. According to (Deakin, Shewry, & Gray, 2014) AEDs are successfully used in less than 2 percent of cases of out-of-hospital cardiac arrests.

Exact measurement of the improvement of survival rates is next to impossible. First, at the very moment of the hearth problems, and as much afterwards based on documentation, it is in many cases difficult if not impossible to exactly tell whether the encountered (heart-related) health problem witnessed was such one that AED could even theoretically be of use. The term shockable and non-shockable heart rhythm problems well illustrate this (Grunau et al., 2016). Fine-tuned measurement on time needed to start AED use that affects the outcome is also not easy, as exact measurement of time passing is typically not possible in the acute trauma situation.

A question of importance is also the outcome. Thresholds are many: Can the heart and blood-circulation of the victim be restarted and established? Will the patient then make it alive to the ambulance? Will

Figure 2. A broad illustration on the occurrences of out-of-hospital cardiac arrests (OHCA) and their outcomes

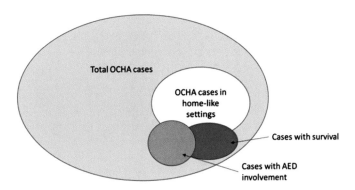

the patient arrive in life to the hospital? A typical measurement point is that of discharge from hospital, or the survival rate after 1 month (or some other period) after the discharge from the hospital. Even at those time points, the condition of the patient can vary. Typical measures are depicted in the cerebral performance categories (CPC) of (1) good cerebral performant, (2) moderate cerebral disability, (3) severe cerebral disability, (4) coma or vegetative state, and (5) death or brain death (Kishimori et al., 2020). In total, the discussion shows that saying and assessing what was a "successful" AED use case is hard to define.

AED use neither happens in isolation. As already depicted in the chain of survival, early cardiopulmonary resuscitation (CPR) is of key importance aside AED use. Rapid defibrillation performed together with CPR can improve chances of survival to more than 50% (Merchant & Asch, 2012; Public Access Defibrillation Trial Investigators, 2004; Rea et al., 2010; Weisfeldt et al., 2010). Other conditions that affect the outcome are for example the performed airway management to the patient, as well as the use of adrenaline administration to the patient (Kishimori et al., 2020). The time spent in the ambulance before arriving to the hospital surely has a deep effect on the outcomes (Dicker et al., 2019).

In Japan it was found that even in cases where there was a bystander in the case of an out-of-hospital cardiac arrest, the survival rate was 10 percent (Ambulance Service Planning Office of Fire and Disaster Management Agency of Japan, 2016). Nichol & al (2008) report better but still not good outcomes: 8,4 percent of patients of sudden cardiac arrest survive to hospital discharge. S. C. Brooks & al (2013) report that also only 8,4 percent of out-of-hospital cardiac arrest patients in North America survive to hospital discharge.

A very convincing documentation from Japan was delivered by (Kitamura et al., 2010): "Among all patients who had a bystander-witnessed arrest of cardiac origin and who had ventricular fibrillation, 14.4 percent were alive at 1 month with minimal neurologic impairment; among patients who received shocks from public-access AEDs, 31.6 percent were alive at 1 month with minimal neurologic impairment". In UK, in one sample collected by (Whitfield et al., 2005) from years 2000 to 2002, 25 percent of ventricular fibrillation patients survived to hospital discharge. The article is also a good example on what kind of data can be collected from the internal digital memories of the AEDs after use.

Readiness to Use an AED

Automated external defibrillator nonuse at a cardiac arrest emergency is a multifactorial problem with potential barriers at many points along the process pathway (S. C. Brooks et al., 2013). The trend has gone towards the conclusion and guidance that any bystander should use the AEDs in the case of cardiac arrest. In their study on Chicago airports (Caffrey, Willoughby, Pepe, & Becker, 2002) found that in 11 successfully resuscitated patients the rescuers had no training or experience in the use of automate defibrillators (albeit 3 of them had medical degrees). In their study, (Whitfield et al., 2005) conclude that the speed of response by the lay first responders in relation to AED use was similar to that reported for healthcare professionals.

Before widely recommending everyone to use AEDs, it was typical to conclude that *trained* laypersons should use them (for example see (Mao & Ong, 2016; Public Access Defibrillation Trial Investigators, 2004). The next step of increased user group would be that persons with duty (and given training) to answer to emergencies would use the devices, persons such as firemen and police officers. Medical professionals without a special education to emergency services are often also counted to this group. The best case of course is that professional emergency medical service (EMS) staff is available to do defibrillation or other tasks they assess as needed.

A key issue in AED use is the citizens' ability and willingness to use them. We refer to citizens' safety competence (Lindfors, Somerkoski, Kärki, & Kokki, 2017; Puolitaival & Lindfors, 2019), which is considered a combination of a) integrated set of attitudes b) knowledge c) skills and d) willingness to act to perform a certain task. The competence is applied in emergency situations where there is need for preparedness, and prevention and/or recognition of needs of actions in to perform a needed task in an authentic situation, e.g. the use of AED.

Automated external defibrillator nonuse at a cardiac arrest emergency is a multifactorial problem with potential barriers at many points along the process pathway (S. C. Brooks et al., 2013). The trend has gone towards the conclusion and guidance that any bystander should use the AEDs in the case of cardiac arrest. In their study on Chicago airports (Caffrey et al., 2002) found that in 11 successfully resuscitated patients the rescuers had no training or experience in the use of automate defibrillators (albeit 3 of them had medical degrees). In their study, (Whitfield et al., 2005) conclude that the speed of response by the lay first responders in relation to AED use was similar to that reported for healthcare professionals.

The AED automatically analyses the hearth situation (the word Automatic in the acronym AED), and does not recognize giving shocks if they would be dangerous or not usable, often even does not give the shock even if the user would like to do that. In principle no harm can be done with them. However, As stated earlier, "automated" in the notion of AED means the device works independently and further on, the device decides whether an electric shock is appropriate. Yet before this automated mission is accomplished, a layperson or professional who received practical AED training, is needed. The person who uses the device needs to know that AED can be used in the emergency in question. She or he has to have motivation and willingness to act (Figure 3) - to find the device and prepare it for the use. Finally, AED skills are needed. These include: to put power on AED device, to attach the pads correctly, to clear for analysis, to clear safely to deliver the shock and finally to deliver the shock. (American Hearth Association, 2016). It is documented that bystanders that have helped with AEDs in cardiac attack cases often suffer from some level of transient psychological trauma (Public Access Defibrillation Trial Investigators, 2004). It might be however that the level of trauma has nothing or very little to do with the use of the AED.

Before widely recommending everyone to use AEDs, it was typical to conclude that *trained* laypersons should use them (for example see (Mao & Ong, 2016; Public Access Defibrillation Trial Investigators, 2004). The next step of increased user group would be that persons with duty (and given training) to answer to emergencies would use the devices, persons such as firemen and police officers. Medical professionals without a special education to emergency services are often also counted to this group. The best case of course is that professional emergency medical service (EMS) staff is available to do defibrillation or other tasks they assess as needed.

An issue in itself is the possible legal liability for laymen operators of AED (or for any user if so comes). Fear of liability and legal processes is a strong demotivator to use an AED, even when it would be available (Fischer et al., 2011). Many countries and jurisdictions have implemented so-called "Good Samaritan Laws" (Pardun, 1997) to mitigate legal liability of helping bystanders (Hung, Leung, Siu, & Graham, 2019). Unfortunately, these laws vary between different countries (Mao & Ong, 2016), and for example between different states in the US, and so the helpers can never be totally assured of their legal protection. However, on most countries, leaving an emergency-situation without any actions can be considered as a negligence in the legal system.

The Extended Chain of Survival

Securing the function of the chain of survival needs a lot of supporting actions, and steps in between. Figure 3 presents one extended value chain that might lead to successful defibrillation use and restoring of vital activities for the patient. Even more detailed value chain descriptions could be easily done, but then we might lose on keeping the total picture within limits of giving a reasonable overview.

Figure 3. An extended chain of survival for out-of-hospital cardiac arrest

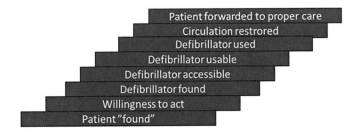

First step is to find the patient. Unfortunately, lot of cardiac arrests take place in isolated environments: home or other private property and distant and non-populated outdoor areas. No-one is to witness or get information about the cardiac arrest – the only thing that is often left is the finding of the dead person. Bardy & al (2008) found no evidence that availability of an AED would significantly improve overall survival of the victims.

The second if a cardiac attack person is found is to decide to help. For the layman who is not healthcare professional, in most countries it is not a crime not to help. Indeed, fear of harming the patient through use of defibrillators, or other means, often keeps by passers from helping. Still worse, in many environments – for example strongly in the US – the by-passers often fear legal consequences if they undertake helping actions, including use of defibrillators.

Even if will to help is there, the next crucial step is the finding of the defibrillator. As this is the key topic in this paper, this is discussed in more detail in the next section.

Even a found defibrillator might be inaccessible. It might be behind locks, or controlled by a vending machine that is out of order or too complicated to use. Defibrillators might also be protected by different strong warning signage and different kinds of alarm signals that are activated when the device is touched. All these might make the found defibrillator inaccessible, in real terms or mentally. Many studies have discussed and criticized the practice of allocating AEDs to public premises, which often are accessible only during regular office hours (Hansen et al., 2013). In their study Hansen & al found that in Copenhagen in years 1994-2011, access to AEDs in real public cardiac arrest cases was limited in 53,4 percent of cases during evening, nighttime and weekends. In some, hopefully rare, cases it might also be that public AEDS are being stolen (Public Access Defibrillation Trial Investigators, 2004), most probably for home use or to be sold on some gray market. AEDs might also fall to be victims of pure senseless vandalism.

In the next step, the AED might be in the hands of the helper. As these devices are dependent on working batteries and are complicated electrical devices needing maintenance, the next sad finding by the helper might be that the device is not usable. This condition surely gets more usual as the total amount of AEDs installed increases, and the age of the devices gets higher.

Typically, AEDs are medical devices that cannot be sold without prior acceptance of authorities. They have an expiry date and a maintenance program specified by the manufacturer. In many settings, a battery check and basic check of the devices integrity and cleanliness in expected to take place on a monthly basis (Haskell, Post, Cram, & Atkins, 2009).

A whole big issue of course is whether the device is so user-friendly that the user can operate it, even to begin. For the user, wrong language instructions of even finding the on/off button might be critical steps. Having the basic understanding on how to set the AED pads to the victim body is of course of crucial importance. Often this is clearly guided in picture form in the AED short user instructions.

The use phase is the critical. Even when the original willingness to help is there, it might be that the device never gets used because of user-related reasons. In a study about Copenhagen (Agerskov et al., 2015) found that in a period from 2011 to 2013 just in 3,8 percent of out-of-hospital cardiac arrest cases an AED was used prior to the arrival of the ambulance, even when an AED would have been reachable within 100 meters in 15,1 percent of all cases.

Doing the physical contact with the patient might just be too much for many users. One thing the "automated" refers to in the wording automated defibrillator is that the device analyzes the condition of the patient, and concludes that delivering electric shocks is not beneficial. This is of course good if and as usually the analysis is right, and is not dependent on the user. Some other kind of help should then be delivered, typically cardiopulmonary resuscitation. Other forms of help might be difficult or impossible for the non-professional helper.

Finally, it might be that the defibrillation activity is unsuccessful. Even if it is a success, might be that the further steps in the care taking chain are not successful or fast enough. These are anyway medical considerations beyond the scope of this article.

Finding a Defibrillator

At least three different roads to find an AED are usually available. If no communication-able devices like mobile phones are available, the only option is to start looking for the device in the "real" physical world. A crucial first step is a crucial initial assessment whether there is any change of finding an AED within a reasonable distance exists or not. This assessment might easily lead to totally wrong conclusions. As (Merchant & Asch, 2012) state, "perhaps the only thing worse than not knowing an AED is nearby is wasting time searching for and AED that is there not at all".

If the search is started, in successful cases there are most likely other people, even those knowing the environment well, who can be contacted for help. However, (B. Brooks et al., 2015) found that only 5 percent of people living even in high-risk cardiac arrest areas knew the location of their nearest public AED. Doing a random search without any human help might be a very frustrating exercise.

As a second road, if a mobile phone is available, calling emergency services is a natural, standard and often officially recommended way to proceed. When available, the emergency service can help in many ways: tell whether there is an AED in the near environment, send to place local helpers with AED operating skills, and if needed help orally or maybe even through visual interface in the use of the AED.

The third road might be to try to find the AED through Internet-based location services, often used through a mobile phone –based app. This might sound like a rather difficult and complicated task, but at the mobile app stores we have a lot of apps helping in finding defibrillators. Several challenges might anyway come along even with this option in the case of emergency. The first is through what service the search for the defibrillator should be conducted. Different language boundaries might inhibit the finding of the right site for locating the device. The information on the site might be outdated or otherwise false. Finally, even when the device is located, route to it might be difficult to define and/or find.

As it comes to the physical location of an AED, it must be remembered that two-dimensional coordinates of the device are often no more sufficient. In complicated built (city) environments the vertical position of the AED is of critical importance, for example if it is underground (say at a metro station) or high up (say at a sightseeing floor of a high building). Complicated multi-level street arrangements also necessitate three-dimensional information about the AED location.

A key prerequisite for finding a position of an AED is that it is registered to a publicly available register (Rucigaj, Podobnik, Gradisek, & Sostaric, 2019). It is next to impossible to assess how much AEDs are not taken to any registers. Usually AEDs that have got public financial support are registered to some registers, and the regulations in many countries demand registering for AEDs that are intended for public use. Sometimes the registers have limited access. They might just for professional use, or they might be approachable just through certain software products (for example mobile apps). In total, there is an agreement that AEDs are not properly registered in most of the countries. A new innovation to build registers of AEDs could be crowdsourcing, where citizen would be challenged to register AEDs, for example to a game-like (scavenger hunt) mobile application (Merchant & Asch, 2012).

Drone delivery of AEDs is a fresh initiative taken up. Challenges of course face even this option. Weather conditions might hinder delivery of the AED. Delivery can of course take place only to locations outdoor, and even there, complicated urban structures with multiple levels might pose a serious challenge. It is rather safe to conclude that drone delivery of AEDs could be an add-on service, but that it should not be seen as a technology to substitute AEDs permanently located to public premises

A fresh trend is that now as AEDs have become cheaper, people – especially in older age groups – buy them to their homes. AEDs are on the way to become consumer electronics – at least as basic versions.

This trend of course has its benefits and risks. A fresh innovation taken in many countries is to locate AEDs to taxis or buses (Hajari et al., 2019; Mitamura, 2008).

The general opinion is that AEDs cannot be used as weapons to kill any person (at least one in rather normal condition). The energy amount delivered by AEDs is too slow to kill anyone, and the device should not deliver any shock unless it analyses this as appropriate. Anyway, there is discussion that AED shock can deliver danger and heavy pain in the case of metal objects on the human body, such as metal jewellery or metal wires on textiles such as bras.

Mobile application stores offer possibilities for downloading apps to find the nearest defibrillator. As of 10th of April 2020 the Apple store found 11 applications with the search "defib". Most of them were AED location services, but contained also apps guiding and training in AED use. In Google Play store, department applications, the keyword "defib" returned hundreds of applications. The analysis of these applications, and trying all possible search terms in these stores is out of the scope of this article. The results anyway tell that there are plenty of applications to assist in finding and AED, but their usability and geographical coverage remains an issue to be studied later.

A very beneficial solution to the finding of AEDs could be that they would be integrated to other popular applications or location services. A kind of "silver bullet" solution would for example be that Google Maps would contain AED location information, and citizen would be aware of this and could and would like to use this information at the moment of need.

DISCUSSION

Cardiac arrest is a key cause of death in the world. It can hit anyone anywhere, even though elderly population is in the most danger. Several steps have to be mastered in order to provide successful help with defibrillators to patients. In medicine it is typical to speak of the chain of survival. It is a short version of the total truth consisting of four crucial tasks: finding the patient/victim as early as possible, immediately started cardiopulmonary resuscitation, immediately started defibrillation with AEDs or other – more professional - devices, and fast advanced cardiac life support in hospital settings.

Because of financial and other constrains, AEDs cannot be everywhere within 100 meters of 1 minute reach, as would be the recommendation. Often AEDs are typically allocated based on haphazard voluntary actions, but several cities have also taken coordinated actions to allocate AEDs to optimal locations. Studies have clearly shown that coordinated AED placement leads to better results in life saving. A key success factor is that all AEDs are registered to central, typically nation-wide, databases that are easily accessible.

There are several modes of using AEDs. On the contrary to widely spread beliefs, in most countries even laymen without any education and earlier experience are encouraged to use AEDs if need arises. An ability to use AED should be considered a part of citizen's safety competence. Laymen AED use can be improved through connections to emergency response centers, that can give guidance to the use for example through telephone connection during emergency. Better option of course would be that even the laymen have gone through some kind of related education and training, such as courses on basic life support, first aid, certified first responder, or cardiopulmonary resuscitation. The use of AED could be included in safety education as a part of safety competence development in comprehensive, vocational, higher and adult education. Additionally, voluntary courses, workshops and campaigns as part of conferences, exhibitions, trade shows and especially in social media, could be organized for citizens to enhance their ability to use AED. The next step in professionalism is that AEDs are used by special trained helpers, who anyway are not health professionals, such as guards, taxi-drivers or personnel of close-by businesses. Next step increasing professionalism is the use of AEDs by security guards, policemen and firemen (the first responder concept (Ringh et al., 2009)), if possible through the on-line support of emergency centers. The best case of course is that specialized Emergency Service Response teams use the devices, but they usually also bring their own devices with them and are not dependent on public AEDs.

Maintenance of AEDs is a big challenge. They need monthly check and maintenance, have a limited lifecycle, and are useless without a working battery delivering power.

Finding an AED is also critical. The first and decisive decision that has to be taken is whether to start to look for and AED in the case of emergency, or try to do without one. Alone this is a heavy decision, in the case of two or more helpers both activities can be undertaken simultaneously. Typical possibilities are haphazard search of the AED in real world, if possible additionally asking for guidance from local by-passers. Emergency centers can most likely tell the location of the nearest AED, if contact can be established. Then there is a possibility to try to search for an AED through different electronic services. Finding of an AED is helped if it has been fitted with international standard sign telling of its location.

CONCLUSION

Defibrillators have been around us some 50-70 years. They have surely saved millions of lives and given hundreds of millions of life-years for mankind. Yet they seem not to be an innovation that would have penetrated our life very deeply. Very few are aware of their existence, even fewer know hot to use them, still fewer would use them in real situations, and extremely few have used them. Still, over long time, many owe their lives to defibrillators and their skilled users. Studying and better understanding the user acceptance and innovation diffusion of AEDs surely remains an important research topic for many decades to come.

As any human artefact, defibrillators are not just technical or medical innovations. Their efficient usage needs a complex ecosystem, which can be erected just though commitment of key stakeholders, constant social and systemic innovation, not forgetting the core technical and medical innovations, and even some luck and favourable environmental factors.

Three central topics have come up in this analysis based on contemporary literature. First, selecting locations for AEDs is a key task, that needs careful planning in an environment where resources are not endless. Even when the installation of the AEDs in great masses could be afforded, maintaining and keeping track of the total reserve needs tremendous resources. Where to locate AEDs is a key issue now and in the future.

Second, willingness to use an AED in the case of emergency is a crucial issue. Any fear of legal consequences of (not successful) application of AED keep people from using them. It should be made universally clear that using an AED is in the case of need not just a possibility, but a duty for anyone. The automatic functions of AEDs next to totally eliminate the possibility to use them in a harmful way.

Third issue is the finding of the devices. Both real and virtual environments cause challenges. Signage of AEDs varies a lot in different places, and despite a universal standard it is not done everywhere in a standard way. Virtual world also has its challenges. There is no standard way of finding a defibrillator through digital services. Given the endless spectrum of digital devices, platforms and applications a world-wide standard search system in digital space still remains a distant dream. The fast development of various digital location services gives hope and even real developments, but variety of different installations can still cost lives in the situation of a real need.

Academic research on AEDs is rich, but mostly done by medical researchers starting from medical starting points. Computer and IS research community has allocated next to none resources to study the development and assessment of AED finding services. More research is needed to work out the fastest and most efficient strategies to find AEDs, and to understand the role of computerized, typically mobile, applications to find the AED. Additionally, further research is needed in education in considering how to educate citizens and train their ability to use digital applications in advancing their safety competence. In this case to find AEDs in time and to act in emergency where the use of AED is needed. Effective delivery and maintenance of AEDs, usability of them as well as digital applications, citizens' possibilities and ability to find and use them in emergency is a multi-scientific and multi-dimensional research and development challenge where research based innovations are needed.

REFERENCES

Agerskov, M., Nielsen, A. M., Hansen, C. M., Hansen, M. B., Lippert, F. K., Wissenberg, M., Folke, F., & Rasmussen, L. S. (2015). Public access defibrillation: Great benefit and potential but infrequently used. *Resuscitation*, *96*, 53–58. doi:10.1016/j.resuscitation.2015.07.021 PMID:26234893

Ambulance Service Planning Office of Fire and Disaster Management Agency of Japan. (2016). *Effect of first aid for cardiopulmonary arrest*. Retrieved from http://www.fdma.go.jp/neuter/topics/fieldList9_3.html

American Heart Association. (2016). *Adult CPR and AED Skills Testing Checklist*. Retrieved from https://www.google.com/url?sa=t&rct=j&q=&esrc=s&source=web&cd=19&ved=2ahUKEwjKhcTfl5DpAhVRKuwKHdA_DS0QFjASegQIARAB&url=https%3A%2F%2Fwww.cprconsultants.com%2Fwp-content%2Fuploads%2F2016%2F05%2FBLS-Adult-Skills-Checklist-2016.pdf&usg=AOvVaw1L4ObU_8YU-1h1SIlNpdEK

Aufderheide, T., Hazinski, M. F., Nichol, G., Steffens, S. S., Buroker, A., McCune, R., ... Ramirez, R. R. (2006). Community lay rescuer automated external defibrillation programs: key state legislative components and implementation strategies: a summary of a decade of experience for healthcare providers, policymakers, legislators, employers, and community leaders from the American Heart Association Emergency Cardiovascular Care Committee, Council on Clinical Cardiology, and Office of State Advocacy. *Circulation*, *113*(9), 1260–1270. doi:10.1161/CIRCULATIONAHA.106.172289 PMID:16415375

Bardy, G. H., Lee, K. L., Mark, D. B., Poole, J. E., Toff, W. D., Tonkin, A. M., ... White, R. D. (2008). Home use of automated external defibrillators for sudden cardiac arrest. *The New England Journal of Medicine*, *358*(17), 1793–1804. doi:10.1056/NEJMoa0801651 PMID:18381485

Becker, L., Eisenberg, M., Fahrenbruch, C., & Cobb, L. (1998). Public locations of cardiac arrest: Implications for public access defibrillation. *Circulation*, *97*(21), 2106–2109. doi:10.1161/01.CIR.97.21.2106 PMID:9626169

British Heart Foundation. (2020). *Defibrillators*. Retrieved from https://www.bhf.org.uk/how-you-can-help/how-to-save-a-life/defibrillators

Brooks, B., Chan, S., Lander, P., Adamson, R., Hodgetts, G. A., & Deakin, C. D. (2015). Public knowledge and confidence in the use of public access defibrillation. *Heart (British Cardiac Society), 101*(12), 967–971. doi:10.1136/heartjnl-2015-307624 PMID:25926599

Brooks, S. C., Hsu, J. H., Tang, S. K., Jeyakumar, R., & Chan, T. C. (2013). Determining risk for out-of-hospital cardiac arrest by location type in a Canadian urban setting to guide future public access defibrillator placement. *Annals of Emergency Medicine, 61*(5), 530-538. e532.

Caffrey, S. L., Willoughby, P. J., Pepe, P. E., & Becker, L. B. (2002). Public use of automated external defibrillators. *The New England Journal of Medicine, 347*(16), 1242–1247. doi:10.1056/NEJMoa020932 PMID:12393821

Coris, E. E., Miller, E., & Sahebzamani, F. (2005). Sudden cardiac death in Division I collegiate athletics: Analysis of automated external defibrillator utilization in National Collegiate Athletic Association Division I athletic programs. *Clinical Journal of Sport Medicine, 15*(2), 87–91. doi:10.1097/01.jsm.0000152715.12721.fa PMID:15782052

Deakin, C. D., Shewry, E., & Gray, H. H. (2014). Public access defibrillation remains out of reach for most victims of out-of-hospital sudden cardiac arrest. *Heart (British Cardiac Society), 100*(8), 619–623. doi:10.1136/heartjnl-2013-305030 PMID:24553390

Dicker, B., Todd, V. F., Tunnage, B., Swain, A., Smith, T., & Howie, G. (2019). Direct transport to PCI-capable hospitals after out-of-hospital cardiac arrest in New Zealand: Inequities and outcomes. *Resuscitation, 142*, 111–116. doi:10.1016/j.resuscitation.2019.06.283 PMID:31271727

Fischer, P., Krueger, J. I., Greitemeyer, T., Vogrincic, C., Kastenmüller, A., Frey, D., Heene, M., Wicher, M., & Kainbacher, M. (2011). The bystander-effect: A meta-analytic review on bystander intervention in dangerous and non-dangerous emergencies. *Psychological Bulletin, 137*(4), 517–537. doi:10.1037/a0023304 PMID:21534650

Folke, F., Lippert, F., Nielsen, S., Gislason, G. H., Hansen, M. L., Schramm, T. K., Sørensen, R., Fosbøl, E. L., Andersen, S. S., Rasmussen, S., Køber, L., & Torp-Pedersen, C. (2009). Location of Cardiac Arrest in a City Center: Strategic Placement of Automated External Defibrillators in Public Locations. *Circulation, 120*(6), 510–517. doi:10.1161/CIRCULATIONAHA.108.843755 PMID:19635969

Grunau, B., Reynolds, J. C., Scheuermeyer, F. X., Stenstrom, R., Pennington, S., Cheung, C., ... Barbic, D. (2016). Comparing the prognosis of those with initial shockable and non-shockable rhythms with increasing durations of CPR: Informing minimum durations of resuscitation. *Resuscitation, 101*, 50–56. doi:10.1016/j.resuscitation.2016.01.021 PMID:26851705

Hajari, H., Salerno, J., Weiss, L. S., Menegazzi, J. J., Karimi, H., & Salcido, D. D. (2019). Simulating Public Buses as a Mobile Platform for Deployment of Publicly Accessible Automated External Defibrillators. *Prehospital Emergency Care*, 1–7. PMID:31124734

Hansen, C. M., Wissenberg, M., Weeke, P., Ruwald, M. H., Lamberts, M., Lippert, F. K., ... Torp-Pedersen, C. (2013). Automated external defibrillators inaccessible to more than half of nearby cardiac arrests in public locations during evening, nighttime, and weekends. *Circulation, 128*(20), 2224–2231. doi:10.1161/CIRCULATIONAHA.113.003066 PMID:24036607

Haskell, S. E., Post, M., Cram, P., & Atkins, D. L. (2009). Community public access sites: Compliance with American Heart Association recommendations. *Resuscitation, 80*(8), 854–858. doi:10.1016/j. resuscitation.2009.04.033 PMID:19481852

Hung, K. K., Leung, C., Siu, A., & Graham, C. A. (2019). Good Samaritan Law and bystander cardio-pulmonary resuscitation: Cross-sectional study of 1223 first-aid learners in Hong Kong. *Hong Kong Journal of Emergency Medicine.*

Kishimori, T., Kiguchi, T., Kiyohara, K., Matsuyama, T., Shida, H., Nishiyama, C., ... Hayashida, S. (2020). Public-access automated external defibrillator pad application and favorable neurological outcome after out-of-hospital cardiac arrest in public locations: A prospective population-based propensity score-matched study. *International Journal of Cardiology, 299*, 140–146. doi:10.1016/j.ijcard.2019.07.061 PMID:31400888

Kitamura, T., Iwami, T., Kawamura, T., Nagao, K., Tanaka, H., & Hiraide, A. (2010). Nationwide public-access defibrillation in Japan. *The New England Journal of Medicine, 362*(11), 994–1004. doi:10.1056/NEJMoa0906644 PMID:20237345

Kobayashi, D., Sado, J., Kiyohara, K., Kitamura, T., Kiguchi, T., Nishiyama, C., ... Kawamura, T. (2020). Public location and survival from out-of-hospital cardiac arrest in the public-access defibrillation era in Japan. *Journal of Cardiology, 75*(1), 97–104. doi:10.1016/j.jjcc.2019.06.005 PMID:31350130

Lindfors, E., Somerkoski, B., Kärki, T., & Kokki, E. (2017). Perusopetuksen oppilaiden turvallisuuso-saamisesta. In M. Kallio, R. Juvonen, & A. Kaasinen (Eds.), Jatkuvuus ja muutos opettajankoulutuksessa (pp. 109-120). Helsinki: Suomen ainedidaktinen tutkimusseura.

Mao, R. D., & Ong, M. E. H. (2016). Public access defibrillation: Improving accessibility and outcomes. *British Medical Bulletin, 118*(1), 25–32. doi:10.1093/bmb/ldw011 PMID:27034442

Merchant, R. M., & Asch, D. A. (2012). Can you find an automated external defibrillator if a life depends on it? *Circulation: Cardiovascular Quality and Outcomes, 5*(2), 241–243. doi:10.1161/CIRCOUT-COMES.111.964825 PMID:22354936

Mitamura, H. (2008). Public access defibrillation: Advances from Japan. *Nature Clinical Practice. Cardiovascular Medicine, 5*(11), 690–692. doi:10.1038/ncpcardio1330 PMID:18779832

Myerburg, R. J., Velez, M., Rosenberg, D. G., Fenster, J., & Castellanos, A. (2003). Automatic External Defibrillators for Prevention of Out-of-Hospital Sudden Death: Effectiveness of the Automatic External Defibrillator. *Journal of Cardiovascular Electrophysiology, 14*(s9), S108–S116. doi:10.1046/j.1540-8167.14. s9.4.x PMID:12950531

Nichol, G., Thomas, E., Callaway, C. W., Hedges, J., Powell, J. L., Aufderheide, T. P., ... Dreyer, J. (2008). Regional variation in out-of-hospital cardiac arrest incidence and outcome. *Journal of the American Medical Association, 300*(12), 1423–1431. doi:10.1001/jama.300.12.1423 PMID:18812533

O'Keeffe, C., Nicholl, J., Turner, J., & Goodacre, S. (2011). Role of ambulance response times in the survival of patients with out-of-hospital cardiac arrest. *Emergency Medicine Journal, 28*(8), 703–706. doi:10.1136/emj.2009.086363 PMID:20798090

Pardun, J. T. (1997). Good Samaritan laws: A global perspective. *Loy. LA Int'l & Comp. LJ*, *20*, 591.

Pell, J. P., Sirel, J. M., Marsden, A. K., Ford, I., Walker, N. L., & Cobbe, S. M. (2002). Potential impact of public access defibrillators on survival after out of hospital cardiopulmonary arrest: Retrospective cohort study. *BMJ (Clinical Research Ed.)*, *325*(7363), 515. doi:10.1136/bmj.325.7363.515 PMID:12217989

Public Access Defibrillation Trial Investigators. (2004). Public-access defibrillation and survival after out-of-hospital cardiac arrest. *The New England Journal of Medicine*, *351*(7), 637–646. doi:10.1056/NEJMoa040566 PMID:15306665

Puolitaival, M., & Lindfors, E. (2019). Turvallisuuskasvatuksen tavoitteiden tilannekuva perusopetuksessa–dokumenttiaineistoon perustuvaa pohdintaa. In Tutkimuksesta luokkahuoneisiin (Vol. 15, pp. 119-140). Suomen ainedidaktinen tutkimusseura. Ainedidaktisia tutkimuksia.

Rea, T. D., Olsufka, M., Bemis, B., White, L., Yin, L., Becker, L., Copass, M., Eisenberg, M., & Cobb, L. (2010). A population-based investigation of public access defibrillation: Role of emergency medical services care. *Resuscitation*, *81*(2), 163–167. doi:10.1016/j.resuscitation.2009.10.025 PMID:19962225

Ringh, M., Herlitz, J., Hollenberg, J., Rosenqvist, M., & Svensson, L. (2009). Out of hospital cardiac arrest outside home in Sweden, change in characteristics, outcome and availability for public access defibrillation. *Scandinavian Journal of Trauma, Resuscitation and Emergency Medicine*, *17*(1), 18. doi:10.1186/1757-7241-17-18 PMID:19374752

Rucigaj, S., Podobnik, B., Gradisek, P., & Sostaric, M. (2019). "AED Database of Slovenia"-an analysis of operation of Slovenian national public access defibrillators registry. *Resuscitation*, *142*, e47–e48. doi:10.1016/j.resuscitation.2019.06.113

Sun, C. L., Karlsson, L., Torp-Pedersen, C., Morrison, L. J., Brooks, S. C., Folke, F., & Chan, T. C. (2019). In Silico Trial of Optimized Versus Actual Public Defibrillator Locations. *Journal of the American College of Cardiology*, *74*(12), 1557–1567. doi:10.1016/j.jacc.2019.06.075 PMID:31537265

Walker, A., Sirel, J. M., Marsden, A. K., Cobbe, S. M., & Pell, J. P. (2003). Cost effectiveness and cost utility model of public place defibrillators in improving survival after prehospital cardiopulmonary arrest. *BMJ (Clinical Research Ed.)*, *327*(7427), 1316. doi:10.1136/bmj.327.7427.1316 PMID:14656838

Weisfeldt, M. L., Everson-Stewart, S., Sitlani, C., Rea, T., Aufderheide, T. P., Atkins, D. L., ... Gray, R. (2011). Ventricular tachyarrhythmias after cardiac arrest in public versus at home. *The New England Journal of Medicine*, *364*(4), 313–321. doi:10.1056/NEJMoa1010663 PMID:21268723

Weisfeldt, M. L., Sitlani, C. M., Ornato, J. P., Rea, T., Aufderheide, T. P., Davis, D., ... Maloney, J. (2010). Survival after application of automatic external defibrillators before arrival of the emergency medical system: Evaluation in the resuscitation outcomes consortium population of 21 million. *Journal of the American College of Cardiology*, *55*(16), 1713–1720. doi:10.1016/j.jacc.2009.11.077 PMID:20394876

Whitfield, R., Colquhoun, M., Chamberlain, D., Newcombe, R., Davies, C. S., & Boyle, R. (2005). The Department of Health National Defibrillator Programme: Analysis of downloads from 250 deployments of public access defibrillators. *Resuscitation*, *64*(3), 269–277. doi:10.1016/j.resuscitation.2005.01.003 PMID:15733753

World Health Organisation. (2020). *Cardiovascular diseases (CVDs)*. Retrieved from https://www.who.int/news-room/fact-sheets/detail/cardiovascular-diseases-(cvds)

Zakaria, N. D., Ong, M. E. H., Gan, H. N., Foo, D., Doctor, N., Leong, B. S. H., ... Charles, R. (2014). Implications for public access defibrillation placement by non-traumatic out-of-hospital cardiac arrest occurrence in S ingapore. *Emergency Medicine Australasia, 26*(3), 229–236. doi:10.1111/1742-6723.12174 PMID:24712826

ENDNOTE

[1]   The guidelines are available at https://www.ilcor.org/home/

Chapter 10
M–Health and Care Coordination

Rima Gibbings
UIC, USA

Nilmini Wickramasinghe
ⓘ https://orcid.org/0000-0002-1314-8843
Swinburne University, Australia & Epworth HealthCare, Australia

ABSTRACT

Care delivery services have been traditionally dependent on direct encounters between providers and patients. With the increase in the number of aging population and the added demand for most expensive and advanced care delivery services, healthcare organizations are investing in care services that are more effective and less costly. Use of technology in healthcare systems has been a significant driver for care improvement initiatives used for controlling cost and extending care delivery services that enhance healthcare accessibility. Implementing technology in healthcare demands proper alignment between newly developed tools and care delivery system needs. In this chapter, the authors discuss the role of technology in healthcare and the value of mHealth in diverse clinical settings.

BACKGROUND

Today, most people live busy lives and are constantly travelling. One device that accompanies them where ever they go is their smart phone or mobile device. We believe that this represents an opportunity to leverage this mobile device to support superior care-co-ordination. Given the current challenges facing healthcare delivery in the US and globally, including: rapid rise of chronic conditions, aging population and longer life expectancy and the cumulative impact these have on escalating costs of healthcare delivery, robust and superior care co-ordination becomes more imperative. Such co-ordination is not feasible without the support of suitable technology.

DOI: 10.4018/978-1-5225-6067-8.ch010

HEALTH INFORMATION TECHNOLOGY

The high cost of U.S. healthcare system has been the subject of many studies and controlling it is the objective of multiple initiatives in recent years. Care delivery system structure, payment models, fragmentation in the care services, increased life expectancy; and advances in medical diagnosis and treatments have been considered as potentially contributing factors towards the cost increase (Singh & Shi, 2019) (Goyen & Debatin, 2009). Many of the health system stakeholders have eagerly participated in the design and formation of frameworks that could potentially minimize or contain cost. By some estimates advances in technology have contributed to a substantial portion of health spending increase (Goyen & Debatin, 2009). These advances include innovations in medical diagnosis and treatment procedures in addition to transformative trends that are continuously impacting healthcare information systems. Broader adoption of information systems in healthcare processes has been linked to increased patient safety and improved clinical decision-making processes (Bardhan & Thouin, 2012). Health information technology has a significant role in reducing medication errors/interactions and improving clinical communication that will ultimately reduce cost and redundancy in care processes (Laflamme, Pietraszek, & Rajadhyax, 2010). Information systems improving patient care management are developed in EMR/EHR systems and play an important role in establishing robust communication channels to support care_workflow coordination (Goyen & Debatin, 2009).

HEALTH INFORMATION TECHNOLOGY ADOPTION

Many health information systems were adopted by healthcare organizations to resolve fragmentation in the care processes and enhance the efficacy of health data processing. These systems were implemented with objectives that focused on improving the efficiency of care delivery systems, enhancing clinical monitoring tools, minimizing drug adverse reaction, and controlling or potentially eliminating redundancy in the care process by coordinating care (Chaundhry, et al., 2006). Although adopting health information technology in many care settings have been proven to improve efficiency in care delivery systems, generalizing these results has not been consistent in all settings. Several studies have determined the "human element" to be an influential factor in the process of health information technology adoption (Bruntin, Burke, Hoaglin, & Blumenthal, 2011). Research has shown that when providers are not highly satisfied with the adopted information systems, negative findings are reported as a result of this process. Healthcare organizations also reiterate on the value of staff "buy in" during the adoption process (Bruntin, Burke, Hoaglin, & Blumenthal, 2011). In addition to staff's endorsement, management's engagement in the adoption process, and managing additional workload related to newly adopted systems, multiple factors are impactful in the process of information systems' adoption. Training staff, adequate financial backing prior/during the implementation and maintenance process, and preparing healthcare organizations for possible unintended consequences of the adopted system are measures that must be taken into consideration during health system implementation process (Bruntin, Burke, Hoaglin, & Blumenthal, 2011).

EVALUATING HEALTH INFORMATION TECHNOLOGY

Evaluating health information systems is a vital step of the adoption process. The value of system evaluation is an extension of an effective adoption plan that offers a comprehensive review of all the aspects involved. To evaluate health information systems, a clear understanding of all system objectives and their goals must be outlined and compared against a set criteria (Ammenweth, Graber, Herrmann, Burkle, & Konig, 2003). A successful implementation of information systems in large organizations including healthcare organizations relies on an accurate assessment of the workflow and requirement specification gathering phase. Health information system evaluation will include assessing the methods, functions, and the technology used in the system in addition to the evaluation of the environment that hosts the system (Ammenweth, Graber, Herrmann, Burkle, & Konig, 2003). There are several methods of information system evaluation in healthcare processes. One category of these methods targets the quantitative analysis of the data lifecycle in the care system. Evaluating data generation, data management (processing, storing, communication), data analysis, and data use tasks are included in this category (Sapirie, 2000). Other categories of evaluation emphasize on the structure of the entities within the care organization itself. These evaluation models include assessing the fit between task, technology, and people and evaluating the optimal interaction between all attributes (Ammenwerth, Iller, & Mahler, 2006).

Health information systems are evaluated based on a set of assessment criteria measures that explore efficiency, quality, safety, and consistency (Ramaprasad, Syn, & Thirumalai, 2014). Evaluating health information systems that are based on complex application developments without an adequate assessment of the organizational staff (that will use the features offered by the new system), could result in unexpected results that could impact both cost and efficiency. Main users of existing (application) systems, also known as 'super users', are normally staff members with substantial knowledge of internal workflow cycles and could effectively contribute in the process of information system adoption. Clearly health information systems' evaluation and implementation both rely primarily on identifying the main goals of the organizational procedures and their strategic planning. These goals will direct the evaluation process into the formation of methodological protocols that are capable of tracking the optimal use of these systems.

IMPACT OF MHEALTH ON HEALTH CARE SYSTEMS

Geographical and spatial restrictions are influential factors in the healthcare delivery systems as they impact care accessibility and quality. Patients who live in rural areas or patients who are not able to access specialty care in a timely manner due to limited resources, could use modern technology to connect with their providers remotely. Using technology to exchange health data/information has proven its application in telemedicine and telehealth systems (Doam, et al., 2014). MHealth or m-Health is defined as the technologies of mobile computing, medical sensors, and communications used in healthcare procedures (Istepanian, Jovanov, & Zhang, 2004). MHealth could also be described as wireless technologies used in transmitting various types of health data that uses devices such as smartphones, PDAs, laptops, and tablets (Akter, D'Ambra, & Ray, 2013). MHealth is known to facilitate four main components in healthcare delivery system: supporting clinical services, supporting care practitioners, establishing helplines, and gathering data as part of the care process (Cameron, Ramaprasad, & Syn, 2017).

Using MHealth in different care settings has the potential to transform the services both on the process level and outcome level. MHealth has been reframing the care delivery system by personalizing care services/tasks, improving patient and caregiver participation in the care delivery process, improving the accessibility to preventive care services, and minimizing cost of services delivered (Malvey & Slovensky, 2014). The transformative role of mHealth in healthcare services is further established by its ability in increasing care accessibility, improving speed of care delivery processes, and reducing cost of care (Levy, 2014). Evidence demonstrates that mHealth has a positive association with improving care delivery services and enhancing care effectiveness (Akter & Ray, 2010). Populations living in low income countries are becoming more capable in accessing care services in a timely manner (Akter & Ray, 2010). MHealth technology enables patients to become better equipped in communicating with care providers and also in managing their personal care data. Adopting a comprehensive format of mHealth systems that could influence different aspects of care delivery system, could potentially result in major changes within healthcare organizations and care services. The healthcare industry, similar to other industries, has taken a cautious approach to new technology adoption and change. Managing change and facilitating systems that could be potentially disruptive to care processes require consistent commitment from industry leaders (Christensen, Bohmer, & Kenagy, 2000). Research shows that mHealth adoption has not gained the full support of practicing physicians and in some cases, it has encountered physician resistance. A substantial segment of physicians have concerns about issues resulting from patient empowerment through taking more responsibility for available care options and consequent disruptions to the traditional physician authoritative role in the care process (Malvey & Slovensky, 2014). Using fragmented mHealth applications could also significantly impact coordination in patient care (Chen, et al., 2012). Developing applications that are not fully integrated through a comprehensive care approach into relevant care systems or using applications that are commonly designed to address a limited scope of care processes could contribute to mHealth fragmentation (Malvey & Slovensky, 2014).

USE OF MHEALTH TECHNOLOGY IN CHRONIC CARE

Use of mHealth technology in healthcare could impact a wide range of elements within healthcare organizations (HCOs). MHealth technology implementation includes a set of active components that could be drivers of behavioral change in users (providers/patients). Different behavioral habits are rooted in social, environmental, and cultural determinants that in-turn could add to the complexity level of mHealth application use (Maar, et al., 2017). MHealth applications are used to improve the process of data collection, improve patient monitoring capabilities, and provide patients with timely instructions that enhance the quality of care. These applications are used in training and educating patients, enhancing overall awareness, and link providers to their patients effectively. High risk patients with low literacy have a higher chance of developing multiple mental and medical conditions which could potentially impacting their communication with care teams (Barnett, et al., 2012). Effective chronic disease care models such as collaborative care rely on health information technology (HIT) to positively impact these factors (Bauer, Thielke, Katon, Unutzer, & Arean, 2014). Patients with multiple comorbidities are considered the main users of healthcare services (Tinetti, Fried, & Boyd, 2012). In Medicare beneficiaries age 65 years or older it is estimated that 3 in 4 have multiple chronic conditions (Tinetti, Fried, & Boyd, 2012). Providing adequate and effective care to patients who have multiple chronic conditions is a considerable challenge. Multiple treatments provided simultaneously to patients could result in unintended consequences or potential harm that will negatively impact patient's health and quality of life (Tinetti, Fried, & Boyd, 2012). Determining optimal patient care outcomes is linked to identifying patient goals and preferences in addition to assessing the impact of alternative care services that are tailored to patient needs. MHealth is becoming a main component of health information technology (HIT) that enables the expansion of care services to multiple layers of patient populations. Using mHealth technology improves the patient-centeredness aspect in care services delivered. These systems focus on gathering information, communicating with care teams, and enabling stakeholders to collaborate in the management of care routines. However, certain limitations could curb or delay the adoption of mHealth applications. Patients with cognitive impairments, or mental conditions and older patients with limited accessibility to information technology and low degree of health literacy might not be well equipped to adopt such applications (Ben-Zeev, Kaiser, Christopher, Mark, & Duffecy, 2013).

USE OF CARE COORDINATION IN CHRONIC CARE

The U.S. healthcare system is facing extensive challenges in facilitating adequate and effective care for chronically-ill patients. Chronic diseases are considered physical or mental conditions such as cancer, diabetes, hypertension, stroke, heart disease, respiratory diseases, arthritis, obesity, and oral diseases (National Center for Chronic Disease Prevention and Health Promotion, 2009) that impact patients' quality of life and could potentially increase the rate of inpatient care need.

Managing chronic diseases in the U.S. consumes a substantial portion of the overall healthcare spending. According to the Centers of Disease Control (CDC), three quarters of the health expenditure in the U.S. is being spent on chronically-ill patients (Kirzinger, Munana, & Brodie, 2018). It is estimated that 96% of each dollar spent in Medicare is consumed by chronically-ill patients where this percentage is set at 83% per dollar for chronically-ill patients who utilize Medicaid services (National Association of Chronic Disease Directors Promoting Health. Preventing Disease). These measures are more significant as a quarter of the U.S. adult population is suffering from one or more chronic conditions and half of the older patients in the nation have three or more chronic conditions (Raghupathi & Raghupathi, 2018). As the number of baby boomer population rises and life expectancy of individuals increases, it is expected that the number of chronically-ill patients also will increase. Effectively managing chronic diseases has a direct link to reducing care complications and minimizing hospitalization rates which in-turn will influence healthcare cost and patients' quality of life (Raghupathi & Raghupathi, 2018). Managing chronic conditions relies on gathering data related to the at-risk population and current patients to generate appropriate care plans for chronically-ill patients (Raghupathi & Raghupathi, 2018).

Chronically-ill patients or patients who have several comorbidities require consistent medical monitoring and may require frequent interactions with different care settings. Some studies show that on average a Medicare beneficiary could visit seven physicians and four different care settings in a year (Pham, Schrag, O'Malley, Wu, & Bach, 2007). Lack of coordinated care between practitioners who are involved in the care could negatively impact the care outcome. Medicare beneficiaries on average visit two primary care practitioners and five specialty care settings in a given year while patients with multiple comorbidities could potentially visit sixteen physician practices in a single year (Bodenheimer, 2008). Each one of these settings could include a number of care providers and staff members who are directly working with a given patient's health data and coordinating care processes between all care participants involved, to exchange relevant healthcare data in a timely and effective format is a substantial undertaking. These care settings could be involved in different areas of patient care that are delivered simultaneously but could require diagnostic and treatment procedures that in some cases could be duplicated care. Furthermore, care coordination could be practiced between diverse set of providers or between patients and their care givers. Each category of coordination will additionally rely on a specific set of requirements and resources that are unique to the stakeholders involved. This type of diversity in the needs that exists in care coordination efforts could significantly increase the complexity level of optimal performance guidelines. Communication between primary care physicians and specialists must be adequate, timely, and effective to ensure the proper integration of health data sent by the target information systems (Forrest, et al., 2000). Primary care providers have a key role in coordinating their patient needs (Bodenheimer, 2008) which translates to a substantial workload that could prove challenging in the absence of appropriate health information systems.

CARE COORDINATION SYSTEMS

Improving care coordination is a key aspect of healthcare delivery systems. Fragmentation in the care delivery system could be best explained by the need for improving the decision-making processes within care systems that could potentially be improved via collaborative measures (Elhauge, 2010). Fragmentation in care could result into an incomplete understanding of how to best synchronize patient needs and preferences to available care resources. Some studies contribute the fragmented U.S. healthcare system to existing models that associate multiple payments with different services delivered to treat a medical condition or achieve an outcome (Elhauge, 2010). While there are no reward systems set to incentivize providers, who are able to reduce the volume of services by improving care coordination processes (Elhauge, 2010). Measures that evaluate care coordination have been identified partly in the form of care transition metrics that monitor a successful care continuity workflow (Chen & Ayanian, 2014). Continuity of care is an important aspect that is required in care coordination but implementing continuous care routines could not guarantee a fully coordinated care system (Chen & Ayanian, 2014). Other aspects of care coordination have been identified as patient inclusion in the process of care. Creating patient care plans that could proactively transfer accurate patient health data to all participating stakeholders have been associated with a smooth care transition between multiple practitioners while ensuring the effective management of self-care routines (Dykes, et al., 2014).

A few of the major aspects that could significantly impact the use of technology in coordinating patient care include information exchange, patient monitoring systems, patient self-management tools, and improving health communication methods (Dykes, et al., 2014.

FACILITATORS AND BARRIERS TO THE IMPLEMENTATION OF TELEHEALTH

The sudden changes in care delivery services and the higher demand that was imposed by Covid-19 across the world have introduced a long array of rapid changes in care settings. One of these changes was the accelerated adoption of telemedicine and telehealth in providing routine care checkups and patient care services. These changes were mainly recommended to minimize patient contact with providers and other clinicians in addition to reducing the spread of the virus in crowded healthcare waiting rooms. Telehealth has been used for many years as a tool that positively impacts the disproportionate access

Figure 1.

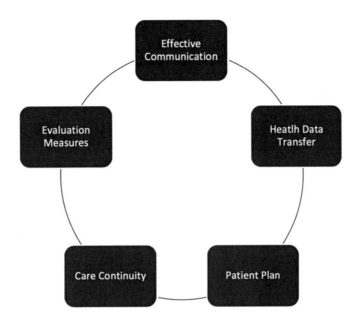

to care (Koivunen & Saranto, 2012). Unfortunately, healthcare settings have used telemedicine in very restricted settings. The main reasons for such restriction could be explained in the limited availability of coverage plan policies that include telemedicine in their care plans, and lack of technical integration between telemedicine features and provider information systems (Weigel, et al., 2020). Clinicians' familiarity and knowledge of information systems and videoconferencing will also impact the adoption process. Training nurses in school and even after they join care organizations plays a key role in the success of telehealth use and successful implementation (Koivunen & Saranto, Nursing professionals' experiences of the facilitators and barriers to teh use of telehealth applications: a systematic review of qualitative studies, 2018). Studies also show that inadequate support and lack of resource management in the process of telecare implementation is considered as a barrier in the overall adoption process (Taylor, et al., 2014).

MOBILE HEALTH IMPACT ON CARE COORDINATION

Care coordination for patients who visit multiple care settings and diverse practitioners depend upon an optimal transitioning mechanism. Improving collaboration between care team members will enhance the quality of care provided and improve the efficiency of the services delivered. This improvement is more evident in the care services required for chronically ill patients who are impacted by fragmented care. Care coordination encounters multiple challenges due to the silos created by episodic care encounters in different settings (Demiris & Kneale, 2015). Improving the coordination of care is proven to reduce the rate of hospitalizations and readmission (McWilliams, 2016).

Patient-centered medical homes (PCMHs) are care delivery models that emphasize on integration, care coordination, and patient-centeredness. Main dimensions of patient-centered care approach that enhances the connectivity of health components in the care delivery services include supportive team approach in providing care and seamless care transitioning (Bates & Bitton, 2010). Focusing on healthcare goals that are recognizable for all participants in the care routine and designing care plans to achieve these goals require a broad and robust system of data collection methods and reliable information systems that can facilitate the management of such plans (Haynes & Kim, 2016). The care plan includes data gathered during patient treatment processes, medication delivery and symptom management, nutrition and lifestyle, and physical activity that are collected from a range of diverse sources. Personal monitoring devices, EHR records, and patient portals are sources that must be integrated to form reliable care plans and goals. The goal is to enable people to live in a steady-state cloud as opposed to the acute-state cloud in terms of their health and wellness so that they can enjoy the highest possibility of quality life. This can only be done by drawing upon the mHealth care coordination framework we have outlined [figure 2].

Figure 2.

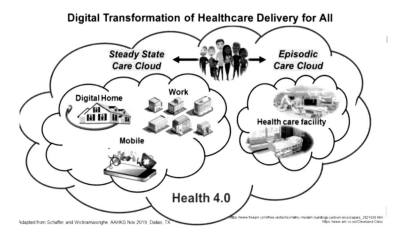

CONCLUSION

Mobile health or mHealth relies on mobile computing and data gathered by sensors. The data and information gathered and processed are used in healthcare delivery systems (Istepanian, Jovanov, & Zhang, 2004). MHealth devices are responsible for monitoring vital signs (blood pressure, blood oximetry, and physiological signals, …), tracking patient movements, and reporting on relevant physical activities. Improving care accessibility, cost-effectiveness, care personalization, and design care interventions that fit patient needs are main benefits of mHealth (Borrelli & Ritterband, 2015). Mobile health or mHealth provides multiple features for both patients and providers. These features could serve patients in the form of upcoming visits or treatment reminders and they could assist providers by gathering large sets of data through monitoring patients remotely. MHealth is used to empower care processes both in delivering patient treatments and coordinating care with other care settings (Murphy, 2016). Implementing mHealth features requires accurate evaluation and development plans. Large data sets generated by advanced mHealth devices must be appropriately integrated and analyzed to address issues that are specific to each participant in the care process (Borrelli & Ritterband, 2015)

REFERENCES

Akter, S., D'Ambra, J., & Ray, P. (2013). Development and validation of an instrument to measure user perceived service quality of mHealth. *Information & Management, 50*(4), 181–195. doi:10.1016/j. im.2013.03.001

Akter, S., & Ray, P. (2010). *mHealth - an Ultimate Platform to Serve the Unserved.* IMIA Yearbook of Medical Informatics.

Ammenwerth, E., Iller, C., & Mahler, C. (2006, January 09). IT-adoption and the interaction of task, technology and individuals: A fit framework and a case study. *BMC Medical Informatics and Decision Making, 6*(1), 3. doi:10.1186/1472-6947-6-3 PMID:16401336

Ammenweth, E., Graber, S., Herrmann, G., Burkle, T., & Konig, J. (2003). Evaluation of health information systems—Problems and challenges. *International Journal of Medical Informatics, 71*(2-3), 125–135. doi:10.1016/S1386-5056(03)00131-X PMID:14519405

Bardhan, I. R., & Thouin, M. F. (2012). *Health information technology and its impact on the quality and cost of healthcare delivery.* ScienceDirect.

Barnett, K., Mercer, S. W., Norbury, M., Watt, G., Wyke, S., & Guthrie, B. (2012). Epidemiology of multimorbidity and implications for health care, research, and medical education: A cross-sectional study. *Lancet, 380*(9836), 37–43. doi:10.1016/S0140-6736(12)60240-2 PMID:22579043

Bates, D. W., & Bitton, A. (2010). The Future Of Health Information Technology In The Patient-Centered Medical Home. *Health Affairs, 29*(4), 614–621. doi:10.1377/hlthaff.2010.0007 PMID:20368590

Bauer, A. M., Thielke, S. M., Katon, W., Unutzer, J., & Arean, P. (2014). Aligning health information technologies wiht effective service delivery models to improve chronic disease care. *Preventive Medicine, 66*, 167–172. doi:10.1016/j.ypmed.2014.06.017 PMID:24963895

Ben-Zeev, D., Kaiser, S. M., Christopher, J., Mark, B., & Duffecy, J. (2013, December). *Development and usability testing of FOCUS: A smartphone system for self-management of schizophrenia.* Academic Press.

Bodenheimer, T. (2008). Coordinating Care - A Perilous Journey through the Health Care System. *The New England Journal of Medicine, 358*(10), 1064–1071. doi:10.1056/NEJMhpr0706165 PMID:18322289

Borrelli, B., & Ritterband, L. M. (2015). Special Issue on eHealth and mHealth: Challenges and Future Directions for Assessment, Treatment, and Dissemination. *Health Psychology, 34*(Suppl), 1205–1208. doi:10.1037/hea0000323 PMID:26651461

Bruntin, M. B., Burke, M. F., Hoaglin, M. C., & Blumenthal, D. (2011). The Benefits Of Health Information Technology: A Review Of The Recent Literature Shows Predominantly Positive Results. *Health Affairs.* PMID:21383365

Cameron, J. D., Ramaprasad, A., & Syn, T. (2017). An ontology of and roadmap for mHealth research. *International Journal of Medical Informatics, 100*, 16–25. doi:10.1016/j.ijmedinf.2017.01.007 PMID:28241934

Chaundhry, B., Wang, J., Wu, S., Maglione, M., Mojica, W., Roth, E., ... Shekelle, P. G. (2006). Systematic Review: Impact of Health Information Technology on Quality, Efficiency, and Costs of Medical Care. *Annals of Internal Medicine*. PMID:16702590

Chen, C., Haddad, D., Selsky, J., Hoffman, J. E., Kravitz, R., Estrin, D. E., & Sim, I. (2012). Making Sense of Mobile Health Data: An Open Architecture to Improve Individual- and Population-Level Health. *Journal of Medical Internet Research*, *14*(4), e112. doi:10.2196/jmir.2152 PMID:22875563

Chen, L. M., & Ayanian, J. Z. (2014). Care Continuity and Care Coordination What Counts? *JAMA Internal Medicine*, *174*(5), 749–750. doi:10.1001/jamainternmed.2013.14331 PMID:24638199

Christensen, C. M., Bohmer, R. M., & Kenagy, J. (2000). Will Disruptive Innovations Cure Health Care>. *Harvard Business Review*. PMID:11143147

Demiris, G., & Kneale, L. (2015). Informatics Systems and Tools to Facilitate Patient-centered Care Coordination. *IMIA Yearbook of Medical Informatics*, 15-21.

Doam, C. R., Pruitt, S., Jacobs, J., Harris, Y., Bott, D. M., & Riley, W. L., & Oliver, A. (2014). Federal Efforts to Define and Advance Telehealth. *Work (Reading, Mass.)*.

Dykes, P. C., Samal, L., Donahue, M., Greenberg, J. O., Hurley, A. A., Hasan, O., O'Malley, T. A., Venkatesh, A. K., Volk, L. A., & Bates, D. W. (2014). A patient-centered longitudinal care plan: Vision versus reality. *Journal of the American Medical Informatics Association*, *21*(6), 1082–1090. doi:10.1136/amiajnl-2013-002454 PMID:24996874

Elhauge, E. (2010). *The Fragmentation of U.S. Health Care*. OXFORD Univeristy press. doi:10.1093/acprof:oso/9780195390131.001.0001

Forrest, C. B., Glade, G. B., Baker, A. E., Bocian, A., Van Scharader, S., & Starfield, B. (2000). Coordination of Specialty Referrals and Physician Satisfaction With Referral Care. *Archives of Pediatrics & Adolescent Medicine*, *154*(5), 499. doi:10.1001/archpedi.154.5.499 PMID:10807303

Goyen, M., & Debatin, J. F. (2009). Healthcare costs for new technologies. *European Journal of Nuclear Medicine and Molecular Imaging*, *36*(S1), 139–143. doi:10.100700259-008-0975-y PMID:19104799

Haynes, S., & Kim, K. K. (2016). A Mobile Care Coordination System for the Management of Complex Chronic Disease. *Nursing Informatics*. PMID:27332252

Istepanian, R. S., Jovanov, E., & Zhang, Y. T. (2004). Introduction to the Special Section on M-Health: Beyond Seamless Mobility and Global Wireless Health-Care Connectivity. *IEEE Transactions on Information Technology in Biomedicine*, *8*(4), 405–414. doi:10.1109/TITB.2004.840019 PMID:15615031

Kirzinger, A., Munana, C., & Brodie, M. (2018). *Public Opinion on Chronic Illness in America*. Henry J. Kaiser Foundation.

Laflamme, F. M., Pietraszek, W. E., & Rajadhyax, N. V. (2010). Reforming hospitals with IT investments. *The McKinsey Quarterly*, 27–33.

Levy, D. (2014). *Emerging mHealth: Paths for growth*. pwc.com.

Maar, M. A., Yeates, K., Perkins, N., Boesch, L., Hua-Stewart, D., Liu, P., Sleeth, J., & Tobe, S. W. (2017). A Framework for the Study of Complex mHealth Interventions in Diverse Cultural Settings. *JMIR mHealth and uHealth*, *5*(4), e47. doi:10.2196/mhealth.7044 PMID:28428165

Malvey, D., & Slovensky, D. J. (2014). mHealth Transforming Healthcare. Springer.

McWilliams, j. (2016). Cost Containment and the Tale of Care Coordination. *The New England Journal of Medicine*, 2218–2219. PMID:27959672

Murphy, J. (2016). Engaging Nurses in the Design and Adoption of mHealth Tools for Care Coordination. *Nursing Informatics*. PMID:27332334

National Association of Chronic Disease Directors Promoting Health. (n.d.). Why Public Health is Necessary to Improve Healthcare. *Preventing Disease.*

National Center for Chronic Disease Prevention and Health Promotion. (2009). *The Power of Prevention Chronic disease ... the public health challenge of the 21st cnetury.* Centers for Disease Control and Prevention.

Pham, H. H., Schrag, D., O'Malley, A., Wu, B., & Bach, P. B. (2007). Care Patterns in Medicare and Their Implications for Pay for Performance. *The New England Journal of Medicine*, *356*(11), 1130–1139. doi:10.1056/NEJMsa063979 PMID:17360991

Raghupathi, W., & Raghupathi, V. (2018). An Empirical Study of Chronic Diseases in the United States: A Visual Analytics Approach to Public Health. *International Journal of Environmental Research and Public Health*, *15*(3), 431. doi:10.3390/ijerph15030431

Ramaprasad, A., Syn, T., & Thirumalai, M. (2014). An Ontological Map for Meaningful Use of Healthcare Information Systems (MUHIS). *Proceedings of the International Conference on Health informatics*, 16-26.

Sapirie, S. (2000). *Assessing health information systems. In Design and implementation of health information systems.* World Health Organization.

Singh, D. A., & Shi, L. (2019). *Essentials of The U.S. Health Care System.* Jones & Bartlett Learning.

Tinetti, M. E., Fried, T. R., & Boyd, C. M. (2012). *Designing Health Care for the Most Common Chronic Condition - Multimorbidity.* JAMA Network. doi:10.1001/jama.2012.5265

Chapter 11
Mobile Applications for Behavioral Change:
A Systematic Literature Review

Martinson Q. Ofori
https://orcid.org/0000-0002-6581-8909
Dakota State University, USA

Omar F. El-Gayar
https://orcid.org/0000-0001-8657-8732
Dakota State University, USA

ABSTRACT

Access to the internet and the proliferation of mobile phones has resulted in a rising trend of mobile apps developed for disease self-management. This use of mobile health technology (mHealth) is viewed as an effective way to induce health behavior change. The authors conducted an evidence review of articles published in PubMed/Medline, Web of Science, and ACM Digital Library between January 2015 and January 2020 that developed and evaluated mHealth apps informed by behavior change theory. A total of 31 studies reviewed developed apps to encourage physical activity, dietary changes, diabetes, Alzheimer's disease, and others. The prevalent way of applying behavior theory to apps was through behavior change techniques (BCT) applied in 45% of the selected studies. Over 54% of the selected studies reported positive outcomes in inducing health behavior change. The results indicate that the use of behavior change theory to inform application design will result in statistically significant effects in improving health outcomes of a condition.

DOI: 10.4018/978-1-5225-6067-8.ch011

INTRODUCTION

The prevalence of chronic diseases is one of the biggest challenges to the future of healthcare. The World Health Organization (2009) (WHO) reports that the leading risk factors responsible for the cause of chronic diseases such as heart disease, cancer, and diabetes include high blood pressure (13%), tobacco use (9%) high blood glucose (6%), physical inactivity (6%), and obesity (5%). These risk factors are responsible for 44% of all global deaths (World Health Organization, 2009). Further, studies show that the prevalent mortality associated with chronic diseases correlates to non-adherence to medical regimen which has also been attributed to several factors including patient-related ones such as forgetfulness, psychosocial stress, anxieties, low motivation, and more (Currie et al., 2012; Sabaté & World Health Organization, 2003). Considering that only 50% of patients adhere to prescribed medication in developed economies and even less so in developing economies (Brown & Bussell, 2011; Sabaté & World Health Organization, 2003), it has been posited that regimen adherence should go beyond medication instructions and reflect behavioral modifications to underlying risk factors (Sabaté & World Health Organization, 2003).

To ensure these behavior changes, behavior change (BC) theory which has culminated from years of research in several disciplines, including psychology, sociology, and economics, have been used to address public health issues (Leviton, 1996). Behavior change in patients for regimen adherence is a critical component of meeting clinical goals (Klonoff, 2019). With the prevalence and high adoption rate of mobile technologies, features such as mobile applications (apps), text messaging, and electronic alarm-triggered reminders have been used for designing mobile health (mHealth) interventions. Further, it has been argued that their long-term widespread use for chronic disease self-management and effectiveness can be improved by basing their design on strong BC theory and sociotechnical design principles (El-Gayar et al., 2013).

Consequently, several studies have applied BC theory in mHealth interventions designed for self-management. The effectiveness of these interventions has been described in a wide range of reviews. However, it is often the case that reviews of this nature focus on specific conditions such as Internet-based asthma interventions (Al-Durra et al., 2015b), wearable technology for sedentary adults (Sullivan & Lachman, 2016), mobile apps for sustainable travel behavior (Sunio & Schmocker, 2017), healthy maternal behavior (Daly et al., 2018), epilepsy management (Escoffery et al., 2018), diet-tracking (Ferrara et al., 2019), or a combination of conditions (Milne-Ives et al., 2020). To evaluate a broader range health behavior change mHealth apps, Zhao et al. (2016) performed a thematic review of extant literature between 2010 and 2015. In a recent review, Han & Lee (2018) evaluated the effectiveness of mHealth apps using a broader period between 2000 and 2017. Although their study reported effectively on BCTs, the study did not report on the theories used by the applications. With the ever-changing nature of technology, and mHealth, an inherent gap exists in demonstrating the effectiveness of theory-informed apps for changing health-related behaviors.

Accordingly, and with the pervasiveness of mHealth applications, the current study aims to extend prior research by providing a systematic literature review using an updated timeframe (2015-2020) while focusing on theory and techniques in a broader context of mHealth apps targeting all manner of health-related behaviors. Specifically, this study presents a complimentary perspective that focuses on extant literature in the context of intervention efficacy based on the application of BC theories and techniques. The study reviews literature that has reported and evaluated either the use of BC theory or techniques in mHealth app design. Thus, this review aims to 1) identify and catalogue the conditions targeted by theory-informed mHealth apps, 2) identify the theories used to inform behavior change through mHealth apps, and 3) capture the presented evidence on the effectiveness of said apps.

BACKGROUND AND RELATED WORK

In the recent past, mHealth apps have been ubiquitous in chronic disease self-management but the extent to which app design is informed by behavior change theory is often unclear (Al-Durra et al., 2015a; El-Gayar et al., 2013). Consequently, mHealth apps have been found to appear as digitized versions of paper-based logbooks (El-Gayar et al., 2013). When apps are backed by research, it is often the case that popular theories are applied regardless of appropriateness or suitability (Davis et al., 2015). Michie and colleagues have attempted to support the systematic development of behavioral interventions through the creation of the hierarchically structured taxonomy of 93 behavior change techniques (BCTs) (Michie et al., 2013, 2015). Even then, extant literature shows that behavior change theory- and technique-use in app design has been applied to varying degrees of success.

For example, Zhao et al. (2016) investigated the effectiveness of achieving health behavior change through mHealth apps. Of the 6 papers (out of 23) that reported the use of theory, 3 applied the Theory of Planned Behavior while 3 used the Social Cognitive Theory. In addition, some BCTs were found to be more ubiquitous in the 12 papers that applied them: self-monitoring (12 studies), feedback provided on performance (8 studies), and tailoring messages (8 studies). The review found statistically significant effects on ensuring health behavior change. Similarly, Cho et al. (2018) found that in literature on apps developed specifically for low- and middle-income countries, only 5 studies applied behavior change theory, with the Health Belief Model being the most cited theory. Their investigation of BCTs-use identified only 7 BCTs with social support (practical) being most prevalent. However, they did not report on the effectiveness of the applications.

Han & Lee's (2018) evidence review went further back to investigate literature for the effectiveness of mHealth apps between 2000 and 2017, and found that mHealth apps positively impacted health related behaviors. Although the study did not report on the use of theory in application design, the summary characteristics of the 20 studies (including BCTs) reported on education/training (12 studies), data entry (7 studies), and feedback (5 studies) as the most prevalent. This result is echoed by Aija (2016) where a review of mHealth apps from the Google and Apple app stores found that less than 10% of possible BCTs were present in apps designed for chronic disease self-management.

Further, Milne-Ives et al. (2020), discussed apps that specifically target physical activity, diet, drug and alcohol use, and mental health and found little evidence to support the effectiveness of mobile apps for improving health outcomes in the 52 studies analyzed. Similar to other reviews, however, they found that 4 BCTs had been applied in more than half of the theory-informed interventions while out of 23 theories used in the studies, the most prevalent was the Social Cognitive Theory (8 studies) and a reference to behavior change theory in 5 papers. In another review that used an inclusive scheme coding applications as having used a BC theory or not, Fedele et al. (2017) meta-analysis on mHealth interventions designed for health behavior change in youth, also found that the use of theory to inform app design was not a moderator for effectiveness.

While the literature above covers extensively the state of the art concerning the mHealth apps-use in fostering behavior change, some limitations worth exploring still exist. In some instances, the timeframe used in some studies (Aija, 2016; Zhao et al., 2016) have become outdated due to the exponential increase in the number of available mHealth apps. In others, the focus of the study limits the generalizability of the findings (Aija, 2016; Cho et al., 2018; Fedele et al., 2017; Milne-Ives et al., 2020). Some studies (Fedele et al., 2017; Han & Lee, 2018) also investigate effectiveness of mHealth apps for behavior change appropriately but the lack of discussion on theory-use leaves a noteworthy gap in literature. Consequently, this study emphasizes the efficacy of recent theory-informed applications from extant literature by focusing on theories as applied in literature and their reported effectiveness in enforcing health behavior change based on results from randomized control trials.

METHODS

The current study follows the Preferred Reporting Items for Systematic Reviews and Meta-Analyses (PRISMA) guidelines for conducting systematic reviews (Liberati et al., 2009). PRISMA offers a standardized, and replicable approach to identifying, selecting, and critically appraising extant literature in relation to research objectives.

Data Sources and Search Strategy

We conducted a search on PubMed/Medline, Web of Science, and ACM Digital Library databases for relevant English-language peer reviewed articles, conferences, and book chapters published between January 2015 and January 2020. This study period was chosen for two reasons: 1) it complements the previous studies mentioned; 2) the number of apps published in the various app stores has increased considerably since prior studies were published. For example, Statista.com reports that there were 1.4 million apps in the Apple App Store as at January 2015. By the first quarter of 2020, however, this figure had increased to 1.85 million, plus an additional 2.56 million apps on the Google Play store. The search terms targeted mobile applications qualified with behavior change and evaluated in a randomized control trial (RCT). Table 1 details the specific search terms combination used.

Table 1. Database search criteria

Theme	Group	Keyword Combination	Relation	Tags Searched
Mobile Applications	Group 1	(smartphone OR mobile OR android OR iphone) AND (app OR application)	Group 1 AND Group 2 AND Group 3	ACM Digital Library: Anywhere Pubmed/Medline: All Fields Web of Science: Topic Search
Qualifier	Group 2	"behavior change"		
Evaluation	Group 3	(randomized AND control AND trial)		

Inclusion Criteria

With the research objectives in mind, studies were included if they constituted primarily of a mobile app based on some existing behavior change theory and consequently a clinically approved trial to evaluate the extent of behavior change associated with the use of the intervention. In order not to inadvertently rule out any publications, studies were also included if either the evaluation or intervention arm of the study was published in a separate paper not captured in our initial search.

Exclusion Criteria

We excluded all studies where the primary intervention was not a mobile app. In effect, studies that developed theoretical models or frameworks, used wearables or a primarily web-based intervention, conducted systematic reviews, comparative studies, or meta-analysis, and any other studies where the principal contribution did not include the development and subsequent evaluation of a mobile-based behavior theory-informed app was excluded.

RESULTS

As depicted in Figure 1, the literature search on three academic databases yielded 317 records, of which 272 articles remained after duplicates were removed. These records were subsequently screened based on title and abstract. In this phase, 69 articles where the primary contribution did not include a mobile app; 58 reviews, meta-analysis, and comparative studies; and 39 studies that were not mHealth focused were excluded. The remaining 106 articles underwent full text review of which 31 were accepted for qualitative synthesis. The reasons for excluding the 75 articles were related to issues such as lack of discussion on the full scope of the app and/or behavioral change elements used for intervention development (36); lack of evaluation such as trial protocols where the subsequent full RCT study had not been published yet (21); duplicate publications of the same intervention (11); and the unavailability of full text for synthesis (7).

Study Characteristics and Targeted Conditions

The articles included in this study were located mainly in developed countries with 74% of them being the subject of more than 1 paper: United States (7), Canada (4), United Kingdom (4), Australia (3), Netherlands (3), and Belgium (2). With regards to conditions targeted, a large majority of the studies (80%) were on risk factors rather than specific diseases: Dietary (10), Physical Activity (8), Smoking Cessation (5), and Alcohol Consumption (3). Apps that targeted diseases were: Diabetes (4), Alzheimer Diseases (1) and Breast Cancer prevention (1). The remaining apps focused on promotion of dental hygiene and MMR vaccination, reducing smartphone addiction and assisting patients to return to normal activities after surgery.

Regarding evaluation, 20 (65%) of the studies used a 2-arm RCT design with 2 of them employing a clustered approach while 1 other study used a cross-over approach. Additionally, 3 papers used a 2^x factorial design. Of the remaining 8 papers, 6 studies used a 3-arm RCT (1 study clustered) and the other 2 were single arm studies. The participant sample sizes for evaluation were often large sized (>100) and made up 65% (20) of the selected studies the largest being a 2-arm parallel study aimed at smoking cessation. Only 7 papers used small sample sizes (<50). Study participants were recruited in several ways several of which included internet (social media, website advertisements, or email) and phone invitations. These and other relevant details are summarized in Table 2 in the Appendix section of this paper.

Figure 1. Study selection process for systematic review

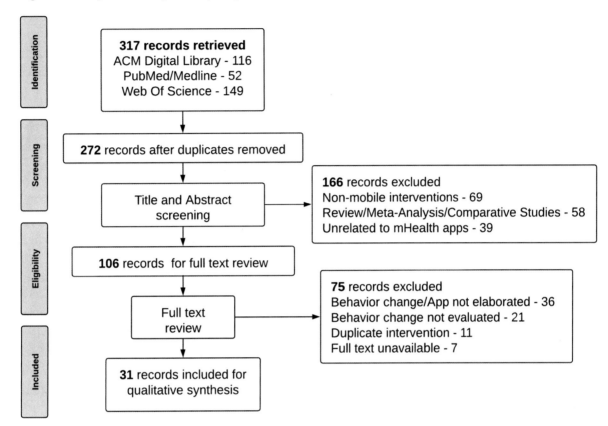

Prevalence of Behavior Change

The most prevalent method for charting behavior change in mobile apps was behavior change techniques (BCTs) (Michie et al., 2013, 2015). BCTs were applied in 14 (45%) of the selected studies. In 7 papers, they were used as a sole BC theory informing app design. A further 3 studies used them in combination with the Behavior Change Wheel (BCW), or the COM-B (Capability, Opportunity, Motivation and Behavior) model – the model that forms the hub of the BCW (Michie et al., 2011): 1 study used it with the COM-B; 1 other study combined BCTs and the BCW with UK's Medical Research Council (MRC) guidance (Craig et al., 2008), and the Multiphase Optimization Strategy (MOST) (Collins et al., 2011); and the final study applied BCTs with several other theories including the Theoretical Domains Framework (TDF) (Atkins et al., 2017), Intentional and Non-intentional Non-adherence (Lehane & McCarthy, 2007), Necessity Concerns Framework (Horne et al., 2013), Compliance and Persistence Framework (Cramer et al., 2008), and the PRIME Theory of Motivation (West, 2007) to create the BC app. Of the remaining 4 papers that used BCTs, 1 study combined it with the Action and Coping Self-Efficacy model (Schwarzer & Renner, 2000); 1 paper used it alongside the TDF; and the other 2 papers used BCTs alongside the Social Cognitive Theory and other theories to be elaborated in the ensuing sections.

Used in psychology, education, and communication, the Social Cognitive Theory (SCT) (Bandura, 1986, 2004) was also another popular theory amongst the selected articles being used in 6 papers. With its emphasis on knowledge acquisition through social contexts, it was rarely used as a sole theory for

BC app development except for 2 studies. The remaining 4 papers combined SCT with other theories: 1 study used it alongside Control Theory (CT) (Carver & Scheier, 1982); 1 other with Learning Theory (LT) (Madden, 2012) and Fogg Behavior Model (FBM) (Fogg, 2009); and in 2 papers mentioned previously, 1 paper used SCT alongside BCTs, and the other used it with CT, Theory of Planned Behavior (TPB) (Ajzen, 1985, 1991; Ajzen & Fishbein, 1980), Relapse Prevention Model (RPM) (Hendershot et al., 2011; Larimer et al., 1999), Motivational Interviewing (MI) (Elliott, 1993), as well as BTCs.

The Fogg Behavior Model (Fogg, 2009), mentioned earlier, which posits that behavior is a convergence of three elements: motivation, ability, and a prompt was used in 5 papers. The first 3 employed it as a single BC theory for app design. In the remaining 2 studies: 1 paper mentioned in the previous paragraph FB model alongside LT and SCT, and the other paper combined it with the Persuasive Systems Design Model (Oinas-Kukkonen & Harjumaa, 2009) and the Behavior Wizard Framework (Fogg & Hreha, 2010).

Other theories used in more than one of our selected studies were: the Transtheoretical Model (TTM) (Prochaska & DiClemente, 2005) which theorizes change as a progressive venture through pre-contemplating of behavior change to behavior maintenance - utilized in 2 independent papers; the TPB which, in its simplest form, states that behavior is shaped by their intentions - applied in 2 studies.

There are other theories that were only applied once in a study to influence intervention design for health behavior change. For example, 1 study used the Attitude–Social influence–self-Efficacy (ASE) (de Vries et al., 1988; Noordegraaf et al., 2012), a model which is comparable to the TPB and asserts that behavior is influenced by attitudinal beliefs, social influence, and self-efficacy beliefs. Behavioral economics principles, such as loss aversion and framing, was used by 1 author. The Mastery Hypothesis and Synergy Hypothesis, derived from theories of limited self-regulatory strength (Baumeister et al., 2007; Muraven & Baumeister, 2000) and goals system theory (Kruglanski, 1996; Kruglanski et al., 2002) respectively, were used in 1 paper. One study applied Cugelman's gamification tactics (Cugelman, 2013) in their intervention design. Further, informed by a systematic review, 1 study used a mix of techniques which included inhibition training (Verbruggen et al., 2014), mindfulness strategies (Brown et al., 2007), and location-specific goal primes (Ja, 2006). Likewise, in 1 study an intervention was created informed by prior knowledge of BC theory such as the Health Belief Model (Becker, 1974).

Effectiveness of the Intervention

Dietary

In the 10 studies that aimed to improve healthy eating using BC apps, 7 reported conclusively good results for improving health outcomes. Elbert et al. (2016) tested the efficacy of an app – informed by BCTs from extant literature and developed with the Intervention Mapping (IM) framework – which communicated textual or auditory tailored health information aimed at promoting fruit and vegetable intake over a period of 6 months. Participants reported significant effect when exposed to the audio-based intervention as compared to both the text-based intervention and the control condition. The app led to a mean increase of 3 fruits per week. However, over the same period, the result was insignificant for vegetable consumption. Mummah et al. (2016) developed a similar app using the IDEAS framework and informed by BCTs to increase vegetable consumption. In a 2-arm trial that randomized 17 participants, the app significantly increased consumption of vegetables in the intervention users.

Regarding apps that targeted weight changes using dietary interventions, Patel et al. (2016) evaluated an app that focused goal setting and self-monitoring BCTs. In their 3-arm trial that randomized participants into a 1) simultaneous weight and diet intervention; 2) sequential (weight 4 weeks) then added diet; or 3) diet only intervention over 12 weeks, it was found that all 3 apps resulted in weight loss with a high self-monitoring engagement. Similarly, van Beurden et al. (2019) found that by creating an application with components informed by theories that have been proven to manage impulsive eating, about 1 kg of weight loss could be achieved in a 1- and 3-month follow-up with medium and small effect sizes in participants. Alternatively, Brindal et al. (2018) discovered that by targeting evidence-based BCTs missing in many commercially available apps including action- and coping-planning, both a static app with face-to-face support and supportive app led to weight loss in participants over a 24-week 2-arm RCT.

Achananuparp et al. (2018) evaluated the use of an application where participants randomly lost incentives when dietary goals were not met. After controlling for other variables in a 2-arm trial, they learned that participants in the random loss incentive were significantly more likely to complete daily tasks than those in a fixed-loss incentive program. Pellegrini et al. (2015) found that by randomizing inactive adults into 3 groups: 1) *simultaneously* increase fruit and vegetable consumption, decrease leisure screen time and increase PA; 2) *sequentially* increase fruit and vegetable consumption, decrease leisure screen time and increase PA; or 3) stress management control, both interventions groups resulted in sustained improvements in fruit and vegetables, saturated fat, physical activity, and sedentary leisure screen time after 12 weeks.

Physical Activity

Across the 8 studies that reported on the development and evaluation of a PA app, 4 were exclusively PA interventions. Edney et al. (2017) reported on the development of a gamified app with social features to increase PA levels. Using the SCT, the app was evaluated in three-group, cluster-RCT where participants were assigned to one of three conditions: 1) waitlist control condition, 2) a pedometer and basic app with no BC feature, or 3) the socially-enhanced experimental condition with pedometer and BC-informed app. However, even though participants reported high engagement, the app did not lead to a significant between-group difference in moderate-to-rigorous PA after the 3-month baseline. In a secondary outcome at 9 months, participants reported nonsignificant improvements to physical health, well-being, as well as, symptoms of depression, anxiety, and stress. Korinek et al. (2018) use of SCT in their intervention to test within-person efficacy over a 14-week single-arm trial reported better results for sedentary adults. On average, the baseline step count of just under 5000 steps (reported in an initial 2-week baseline period) in participants increased by approximately 2500 steps per day after using the intervention.

Likewise, Kramer et al. (2019) and Simons et al. (2018) used BCTs in their mHealth app design but reported different outcomes. Grounding the intervention design in extant literature, Kramer et al. (2019) designed intervention components with self-monitoring prompts, planning, and incentives. After an 8-week 3-arm optimization trial where participants were randomized to receive cash, charity, or no incentive, the average baseline step count of 6,336 per day increased by about 438 steps. It was also found that participants who received cash incentives had an 8.10% probability of reaching step goals compared to the control group, with the charity group also reporting a lower 6.9% greater probability of reaching step goals compared to the control group. It must however be noted that no meaningful or statistically significant effects were found on the remaining interventions: self-monitoring prompts, action planning, and coping planning. On the other hand, Simons et al., (2018) used a 2-group cluster RCT to evaluate a PA app combined with a Fitbit activity tracker. Although participants rated the usability the app highly, there was low continuous user engagement as such, no significant intervention effects on study outcomes were reported. The outcomes were self-reported light physical activity, moderate physical activity, vigorous physical activity, MVPA, total physical activity, and steps, or self-reported occupational physical activity, active transport, household physical activity, recreational physical activity, and total physical activity.

Addiction Related

The 4 BC apps designed specifically to aid smoking cessation did not achieve the best results. For example, Baskerville et al. (2015) despite drawing on several theories to develop an evidence-based application for smoking cessation using a large sample size found no statistically significant differences between the intervention and control conditions on the key outcome measures. Tombor et al. (2016) also employed several theories in their app development for pregnant smokers. However, in a 2^5-factoial RCT, the low engagement rates led to an outcome where intervention modules did not have a statistically significant effect on smoking abstinence during pregnancy. Similarly, Herbec et al. (2019) in their 2-arm RCT found participant recruitment difficult and hence there was inconclusive evidence that their intervention could impact short term quit rates. Again, Hassandra et al. (2017) also found that intervention participants did not report superior abstinence compared to the control group.

Berman et al. (2015) designed a mobile application informed by TPB to aid university students with excessive alcohol consumption habits. Using a 3-arm RCT that randomized participants into an intervention, waitlist or control group, they found that a lower proportion of excessive drinking intervention and waitlist groups. Crane et al. (2018) also designed a similar alcohol consumption application but using the COM-B and BCTs. Participants reported insignificant - but larger - decreases in alcohol consumption in most of the intervention modules used in the 2^5-factorial trial.

The last study in this category, Foulonneau et al. (2016), developed a persuasive mobile intervention to aid smartphone addiction. A six-week single arm trial of this intervention found 15% decrease in mobile usage. Although 44% of participants reported the influence of self-monitoring on their smartphone usage, the trial itself did not permit testing of this assertion.

Diabetes, Alzheimer's, and Breast Cancer Diseases

To improve self-management among patients with type 2 diabetes (T2DM), Desveaux et al. (2016) developed a mobile application using the TTM but their 2-arm trial found no difference between glycemic controls of the intervention and control groups after testing HbA_{1c}. Kennelly et al. (2018) after developing an SCT- and CT-informed app also had relatable result in their 2-arm trial. They found that the app did not help lower the rate of gestational diabetes mellitus in overweight and obese women Goyal et al. (2017) mobile intervention, even with its high user satisfaction, also resulted in no significant improvements in primary (HbA_{1c} levels from baseline to 12 months) or secondary outcomes including self-monitoring of blood glucose and self-initiated adjustments among participants.

MacPherson et al. (2019) designed a mobile intervention using BCTs to promote exercise adherence for diabetes patients. The app was more geared towards tracking PA in adults at risk of developing T2DM, as its outcomes measure were frequency of mHealth self-monitoring and self-reported exercise in the week before and after a prompt. The study discovered a significant increase in the outcome measure 3 days after a prompt receipt in the first 6 months. This effect was however not sustained in the following 6 months.

Similarly, preventive care was the subject of Hartin et al. (2016) and Lee et al. (2017) studies respectively. Using the TTM, the former's study was designed to reduce risk of developing Alzheimer's disease in participants and found that the treatment group had favorable physiological improvements that could yield good future outcomes. The latter, in a 2-arm trial using an app informed by FBM, discovered that the Korean American population received significantly higher mammograms compared to the control group.

Others

A study by Scheerman et al. (2018) to improve oral hygiene developed a mobile app using BCTs mapped by IM. Adolescent patients who took part in the study registered a significant reduction in gingival bleeding and dental plaque in the intervention group.

Fadda et al. (2017) used gamification tactics to future behavior with regards to MMR vaccination. A 2^5-factorial RCT consisting of participants with at least 1 baby born after September 2015 discovered that increasing patient's knowledge could increase vaccination intention.

Last, den Bakker et al. (2019) study to assist patients recover faster after surgery using an app informed by the ASE model was found to be beneficial to recovery after colorectal surgery. It must however be noted that some functionalities of the intervention did not work properly and several of the participants also preferred interaction and feedback from a healthcare professional.

DISCUSSION

Principal Findings

The global ubiquity of mobile technology has created an avenue for employing mHealth solutions to improve wellness and wellbeing at an affordable rate. This has created a further need to examine the effectiveness of these solutions in relation to health behavior change and clinical outcomes. This review synthesized extant literature to identify how behavior change theory has been used in mHealth application design and examined the evidence presented to confirm the extent to which theory-informed apps can influence health. Overall, the 31 research articles identified in the current study developed various mobile applications using a variety of BC theories to improve risk factors and ensure disease self-management.

The importance of managing risk factors to reduce mortality and manage chronic diseases has been highlighted over the years by the WHO (World Health Organization, 2009). The study found a large majority of the applications pursued BC associated with improving risk factors and improving quality of life such as enhancing physical activity and diet or reducing alcohol consumption and smoking. These types of studies accounted for over 70% (22) of the selected studies, that is, without accounting for studies where the targeted health condition was in relation to oral hygiene, MMR vaccination, or even after-surgery management. Although this trend represents good news for managing highlighted risk factors, and the same applications could often be used by disease patients, more research into developing disease-specific mHealth applications may be beneficial to reducing costs and managing health.

In this study, we found that more than 30 individual BC theories were applied in the selected articles. In about 13 of these studies, it was discovered that more than one theory was applied. There was, however, no evidence that combining theories led to better clinical outcomes. In fact, one of the most critical issues pointed out in past research was the sheer number of BC theories feasible for designing and evaluating medical interventions. As mentioned earlier, an overwhelming number of interventions research is often biased towards popular theories regardless of appropriateness or suitability (Davis et al., 2015). However, this study found an uptake in the number of studies (14) that specified BCT use in designing mHealth applications even when some other BC theory was present.

In line with past research of this nature (Han & Lee, 2018; Zhao et al., 2016), the current review found an overwhelmingly positive evidence regarding the effectiveness of BC theory-use in mobile application design. This could be interpreted as the readiness of mobile apps to meet their potential to promote a culture of behavior change in patients. These findings should, however, be interpreted with caution given the distribution of the articles in this evidence review. For example, a large number of the studies that achieved positive outcomes (7/17) were those focused on dietary improvements, while most of the studies that reported statistically insignificant outcomes during intervention use were on smoking cessation (4/10). This result is also in line with Milne-Ives et al.'s (2020) review where significant evidence of behavior change were found in apps targeting physical activity and dietary change.

Evidently, several of the studies where results were negative or inconclusive also reported extraneous conditions that resulted in the interventions not working as it supposed to. Brindal et al. (2018), for example, reported positive result in both control and intervention groups due to face-to-face contact available to both groups during the trial period. Desveaux et al. (2016) and Simons et al. (2018) both suffered from low user engagement while Herbec et al. (2019) study, hoping to enlist participants through pharmacies, suffered from outright poor recruitment. Further, even when there was positive outcomes, some studies reported conditions that could also factor into the result: Scheerman et al. (2018) found a decrease in dental plaques after the 12-week follow up due to a change in brushing patterns rather than frequency or duration of brushing; compared to a prior trial; Pellegrini et al. (2015) found the evidence of positive diet and activity changes to be associated with the longer study period (12 weeks) and the existence of some minimal coach contact; and Berman et al. (2015) results suffered from possible bias as intervention and waitlist participants received an email informing them of excessive drinking habits but control group never received such an email.

Study Limitations and Implications for Future Research

Some limitations exist in this review that are worth mentioning. First, the review only targeted three health related databases and as such, some potential good publications in journals not indexed by these databases might have been excluded. Again, the reviewers' use of the search qualifier *"behavior change"* and the requirement for an explicit mention of *"randomized"*, *"control"* and *"trials"* might have resulted in similar exclusion. For example, a search in technically inclined database such as the IEEE Xplore did not return any result. Further, some potentially good interventions that may have developed commercially available application but have not been evaluated in a trial or did not fully outline how BC theory was used in their intervention, may have been excluded. Also, even though we only selected trials, we did not conduct any quality or bias assessment of the selected studies. Last, with most of the selected studies coming from developed economies and targeting the adult population, the result of the studies may not be generalizable to developing countries or younger patients.

Regardless of these limitations, this study presents several implications for future researchers. For example, the previous limitation identified the prevalence of research in high-income countries focusing on the adult population. This provides an avenue for more research in developing economies whiles researchers in high-income countries may also investigate implementing behavior change interventions that target the younger population. Studies such as these (den Bakker, Schaafsma, et al., 2019; Scheerman et al., 2018) have proved that using methods like Intervention Mapping, BCTs can be used even when some other theory(s) exist for designing intervention. Hence, we are of the view that a need exists for future studies focus on specific health conditions and report specific BCT that works for each condition when used in intervention design – even when other theories have also been applied.

CONCLUSION

Given the pervasiveness of mobile technologies for fostering health-related behavior change, the current study examined conditions targeted by theory-informed mHealth apps, the theories used to inform the app design and foster the required behavior change, and identified evidence on the effectiveness of said apps. The findings presented in the study indicated that the use of behavior change theory in application design often results in statistically significant effects in improving health outcomes of a targeted condition. This result is comparable to previous studies of similar nature (Han & Lee, 2018; Zhao et al., 2016) that has reported positive health outcomes when behavior theory is used in mHealth application design. Theoretically, the current study contributes to the body of work on mHealth interventions for behavior change by providing the current five-year retrospective on the state of the art concerning mHealth apps. The study provides a different perspective to extant literature with an emphasis on specific theories used for application design. Regardless of the good result reported in this study, for mHealth apps to remain replicable and effective, future research in this area should consider converting theory (and BCTs) from their abstract form to design principles that can inform usable patient-centered applications and subsequently foster health behavior change for all manner of conditions.

REFERENCES

Achananuparp, P., Lim, E.-P., Abhishek, V., & Yun, T. (2018). Eat & Tell: A Randomized Trial of Random-Loss Incentive to Increase Dietary Self-Tracking Compliance. *Proceedings of the 2018 International Conference on Digital Health*, 45–54. 10.1145/3194658.3194662

Agarwal, P., Mukerji, G., Desveaux, L., Ivers, N. M., Bhattacharyya, O., Hensel, J. M., Shaw, J., Bouck, Z., Jamieson, T., Onabajo, N., Cooper, M., Marani, H., Jeffs, L., & Bhatia, R. S. (2019). Mobile App for Improved Self-Management of Type 2 Diabetes: Multicenter Pragmatic Randomized Controlled Trial. *JMIR mHealth and uHealth*, 7(1), e10321. doi:10.2196/10321 PMID:30632972

Aija, L. (2016). Mobile applications for chronic disease self-management: Building a bridge for behavior change. *Frontiers in Public Health*, 4. Advance online publication. doi:10.3389/conf.FPUBH.2016.01.00103

Ajzen, I. (1985). From Intentions to Actions: A Theory of Planned Behavior. In J. Kuhl & J. Beckmann (Eds.), *Action Control: From Cognition to Behavior* (pp. 11–39). Springer., doi:10.1007/978-3-642-69746-3_2

Ajzen, I. (1991). The theory of planned behavior. *Organizational Behavior and Human Decision Processes, 50*(2), 179–211. doi:10.1016/0749-5978(91)90020-T

Ajzen, I., & Fishbein, M. (1980). *Understanding attitudes and predicting social behavior.* https://www.scienceopen.com/document?vid=c20c4174-d8dc-428d-b352-280b05eacdf7

Al-Durra, M., Torio, M.-B., & Cafazzo, J. A. (2015a). The Use of Behavior Change Theory in Internet-Based Asthma Self-Management Interventions: A Systematic Review. *Journal of Medical Internet Research, 17*(4), e89. doi:10.2196/jmir.4110 PMID:25835564

Al-Durra, M., Torio, M.-B., & Cafazzo, J. A. (2015b). The use of behavior change theory in Internet-based asthma self-management interventions: A systematic review. *Journal of Medical Internet Research, 17*(4), e89. doi:10.2196/jmir.4110 PMID:25835564

Atkins, L., Francis, J., Islam, R., O'Connor, D., Patey, A., Ivers, N., Foy, R., Duncan, E. M., Colquhoun, H., Grimshaw, J. M., Lawton, R., & Michie, S. (2017). A guide to using the Theoretical Domains Framework of behaviour change to investigate implementation problems. *Implementation Science; IS, 12*(1), 77. doi:10.118613012-017-0605-9 PMID:28637486

Bandura, A. (1986). Social foundations of thought and action: A social cognitive theory. Prentice-Hall, Inc.

Bandura, A. (2004). Health Promotion by Social Cognitive Means. *Health Education & Behavior, 31*(2), 143–164. doi:10.1177/1090198104263660 PMID:15090118

Baskerville, N. B., Struik, L. L., & Dash, D. (2018). Crush the Crave: Development and Formative Evaluation of a Smartphone App for Smoking Cessation. *JMIR mHealth and uHealth, 6*(3), e52. doi:10.2196/mhealth.9011 PMID:29500157

Baskerville, N. B., Struik, L. L., Guindon, G. E., Norman, C. D., Whittaker, R., Burns, C., Hammond, D., Dash, D., & Brown, K. S. (2018). Effect of a Mobile Phone Intervention on Quitting Smoking in a Young Adult Population of Smokers: Randomized Controlled Trial. *JMIR mHealth and uHealth, 6*(10), e10893. doi:10.2196/10893 PMID:30355563

Baskerville, N. B., Struik, L. L., Hammond, D., Guindon, G. E., Norman, C. D., Whittaker, R., Burns, C., Grindrod, K. A., & Brown, K. S. (2015). Effect of a Mobile Phone Intervention on Quitting Smoking in a Young Adult Population of Smokers: Randomized Controlled Trial Study Protocol. *Jmir Research Protocols, 4*(1). doi:10.2196/resprot.3823

Baumeister, R. F., Vohs, K. D., & Tice, D. M. (2007). The Strength Model of Self-Control. *Current Directions in Psychological Science, 16*(6), 351–355. doi:10.1111/j.1467-8721.2007.00534.x

Becker, M. H. (1974). The health belief model and personal health behavior. *Health Education Monographs, 2*(4), 324–473. doi:10.1177/109019817400200407

Berman, A. H., Andersson, C., Gajecki, M., Rosendahl, I., Sinadinovic, K., & Blankers, M. (2019). Smartphone Apps Targeting Hazardous Drinking Patterns among University Students Show Differential Subgroup Effects over 20 Weeks: Results from a Randomized, Controlled Trial. *Journal of Clinical Medicine, 8*(11), 1807. doi:10.3390/jcm8111807 PMID:31661868

Berman, A. H., Gajecki, M., Fredriksson, M., Sinadinovic, K., & Andersson, C. (2015). Mobile Phone Apps for University Students With Hazardous Alcohol Use: Study Protocol for Two Consecutive Randomized Controlled Trials. *JMIR Research Protocols, 4*(4), e139. doi:10.2196/resprot.4894 PMID:26693967

Brindal, E., Hendrie, G., Taylor, P., Freyne, J., & Noakes, M. (2016). Cohort Analysis of a 24-Week Randomized Controlled Trial to Assess the Efficacy of a Novel, Partial Meal Replacement Program Targeting Weight Loss and Risk Factor Reduction in Overweight/Obese Adults. *Nutrients, 8*(5), 265. doi:10.3390/nu8050265 PMID:27153085

Brindal, E., Hendrie, G. A., Freyne, J., & Noakes, M. (2018). Incorporating a Static Versus Supportive Mobile Phone App Into a Partial Meal Replacement Program With Face-to-Face Support: Randomized Controlled Trial. *JMIR mHealth and uHealth, 6*(4), e41. doi:10.2196/mhealth.7796 PMID:29669704

Brown, K. W., Ryan, R. M., & Creswell, J. D. (2007). Mindfulness: Theoretical Foundations and Evidence for its Salutary Effects. *Psychological Inquiry, 18*(4), 211–237. doi:10.1080/10478400701598298

Brown, M. T., & Bussell, J. K. (2011). Medication Adherence: WHO Cares? *Mayo Clinic Proceedings, 86*(4), 304–314. doi:10.4065/mcp.2010.0575 PMID:21389250

Carver, C. S., & Scheier, M. F. (1982). Control theory: A useful conceptual framework for personality–social, clinical, and health psychology. *Psychological Bulletin, 92*(1), 111–135. doi:10.1037/0033-2909.92.1.111 PMID:7134324

Cho, Y.-M., Lee, S., Islam, S. M. S., & Kim, S.-Y. (2018). Theories Applied to m-Health Interventions for Behavior Change in Low- and Middle-Income Countries: A Systematic Review. *Telemedicine Journal and e-Health, 24*(10), 727–741. doi:10.1089/tmj.2017.0249 PMID:29437546

Collins, L. M., Baker, T. B., Mermelstein, R. J., Piper, M. E., Jorenby, D. E., Smith, S. S., Christiansen, B. A., Schlam, T. R., Cook, J. W., & Fiore, M. C. (2011). The Multiphase Optimization Strategy for Engineering Effective Tobacco Use Interventions. *Annals of Behavioral Medicine : A Publication of the Society of Behavioral Medicine, 41*(2), 208–226. doi:10.100712160-010-9253-x

Craig, P., Dieppe, P., Macintyre, S., Michie, S., Nazareth, I., & Petticrew, M. (2008). Developing and evaluating complex interventions: The new Medical Research Council guidance. *BMJ (Clinical Research Ed.), 337*. Advance online publication. doi:10.1136/bmj.a1655 PMID:18824488

Cramer, J. A., Roy, A., Burrell, A., Fairchild, C. J., Fuldeore, M. J., Ollendorf, D. A., & Wong, P. K. (2008). Medication Compliance and Persistence: Terminology and Definitions. *Value in Health, 11*(1), 44–47. doi:10.1111/j.1524-4733.2007.00213.x PMID:18237359

Crane, D., Garnett, C., Michie, S., West, R., & Brown, J. (2018). A smartphone app to reduce excessive alcohol consumption: Identifying the effectiveness of intervention components in a factorial randomised control trial. *Scientific Reports, 8*(1), 4384. doi:10.103841598-018-22420-8 PMID:29531280

Cugelman, B. (2013). Gamification: What It Is and Why It Matters to Digital Health Behavior Change Developers. *JMIR Serious Games, 1*(1), e3. doi:10.2196/games.3139 PMID:25658754

Currie, C. J., Peyrot, M., Morgan, C. L., Poole, C. D., Jenkins-Jones, S., Rubin, R. R., Burton, C. M., & Evans, M. (2012). The Impact of Treatment Noncompliance on Mortality in People With Type 2 Diabetes. *Diabetes Care*, *35*(6), 1279–1284. doi:10.2337/dc11-1277 PMID:22511257

Daly, L. M., Horey, D., Middleton, P. F., Boyle, F. M., & Flenady, V. (2018). The Effect of Mobile App Interventions on Influencing Healthy Maternal Behavior and Improving Perinatal Health Outcomes: Systematic Review. *JMIR mHealth and uHealth*, *6*(8), e10012. doi:10.2196/10012 PMID:30093368

Davis, R., Campbell, R., Hildon, Z., Hobbs, L., & Michie, S. (2015). Theories of behaviour and behaviour change across the social and behavioural sciences: A scoping review. *Health Psychology Review*, *9*(3), 323–344. doi:10.1080/17437199.2014.941722 PMID:25104107

de Vries, H., Dijkstra, M., & Kuhlman, P. (1988). Self-efficacy: The third factor besides attitude and subjective norm as a predictor of behavioural intentions. *Health Education Research*, *3*(3), 273–282. doi:10.1093/her/3.3.273

den Bakker, C. M., Huirne, J. A., Schaafsma, F. G., de Geus, C., Bonjer, H. J., & Anema, J. R. (2019). Electronic Health Program to Empower Patients in Returning to Normal Activities After Colorectal Surgical Procedures: Mixed-Methods Process Evaluation Alongside a Randomized Controlled Trial. *Journal of Medical Internet Research*, *21*(1), e10674. doi:10.2196/10674 PMID:30694205

den Bakker, C. M., Schaafsma, F. G., van der Meij, E., Meijerink, W. J. H. J., van den Heuvel, B., Baan, A. H., Davids, P. H. P., Scholten, P. C., van der Meij, S., van Baal, W. M., van Dalsen, A. D., Lips, D. J., van der Steeg, J. W., Leclercq, W. K. G., Geomini, P. M. A. J., Consten, E. C. J., Koops, S. E. S., de Castro, S. M. M., van Kesteren, P. J. M., ... Anema, J. R. (2019). Electronic Health Program to Empower Patients in Returning to Normal Activities After General Surgical and Gynecological Procedures: Intervention Mapping as a Useful Method for Further Development. *Journal of Medical Internet Research*, *21*(2), e9938. doi:10.2196/jmir.9938 PMID:30724740

Desveaux, L., Agarwal, P., Shaw, J., Hensel, J. M., Mukerji, G., Onabajo, N., Marani, H., Jamieson, T., Bhattacharyya, O., Martin, D., Mamdani, M., Jeffs, L., Wodchis, W. P., Ivers, N. M., & Bhatia, R. S. (2016). A randomized wait-list control trial to evaluate the impact of a mobile application to improve self-management of individuals with type 2 diabetes: A study protocol. *BMC Medical Informatics and Decision Making*, *16*(1), 144. doi:10.118612911-016-0381-5 PMID:27842539

Edney, S., Plotnikoff, R., Vandelanotte, C., Olds, T., De Bourdeaudhuij, I., Ryan, J., & Maher, C. (2017). "Active Team" a social and gamified app-based physical activity intervention: Randomised controlled trial study protocol. *BMC Public Health*, *17*(1), 859. doi:10.118612889-017-4882-7 PMID:29096614

Edney, S., Ryan, J. C., Olds, T., Monroe, C., Fraysse, F., Vandelanotte, C., Plotnikoff, R., Curtis, R., & Maher, C. (2019). User Engagement and Attrition in an App-Based Physical Activity Intervention: Secondary Analysis of a Randomized Controlled Trial. *Journal of Medical Internet Research*, *21*(11), e14645. doi:10.2196/14645 PMID:31774402

Edney, S. M., Olds, T. S., Ryan, J. C., Vandelanotte, C., Plotnikoff, R. C., Curtis, R. G., & Maher, C. A. (2020). A Social Networking and Gamified App to Increase Physical Activity: Cluster RCT. *American Journal of Preventive Medicine*, *58*(2), e51–e62. doi:10.1016/j.amepre.2019.09.009 PMID:31959326

El-Gayar, O., Timsina, P., Nawar, N., & Eid, W. (2013). Mobile Applications for Diabetes Self-Management: Status and Potential. *Journal of Diabetes Science and Technology*, 7(1), 247–262. doi:10.1177/193229681300700130 PMID:23439183

Elbert, S. P., Dijkstra, A., & Oenema, A. (2016). A Mobile Phone App Intervention Targeting Fruit and Vegetable Consumption: The Efficacy of Textual and Auditory Tailored Health Information Tested in a Randomized Controlled Trial. *Journal of Medical Internet Research*, 18(6), e147. doi:10.2196/jmir.5056 PMID:27287823

Elliott, R. (1993). Miller, W. R. and Rollnick, S. Motivational interviewing–preparing people to change addictive behaviour. New York: Guildford Press, 1991. Pp xviii + 348. £24.95. ISBN 0–89862–566–1. *Journal of Community & Applied Social Psychology*, 3(2), 170–171. doi:10.1002/casp.2450030210

Escoffery, C., McGee, R., Bidwell, J., Sims, C., Thropp, E. K., Frazier, C., & Mynatt, E. D. (2018). A review of mobile apps for epilepsy self-management. *Epilepsy & Behavior*, 81, 62–69. doi:10.1016/j.yebeh.2017.12.010 PMID:29494935

Fadda, M., Galimberti, E., Fiordelli, M., Romano, L., Zanetti, A., & Schulz, P. J. (2017). Effectiveness of a smartphone app to increase parents' knowledge and empowerment in the MMR vaccination decision: A randomized controlled trial. *Human Vaccines & Immunotherapeutics*, 13(11), 2512–2521. doi:10.1080/21645515.2017.1360456 PMID:29125783

Fedele, D. A., Cushing, C. C., Fritz, A., Amaro, C. M., & Ortega, A. (2017). Mobile Health Interventions for Improving Health Outcomes in Youth A Meta-analysis. *JAMA Pediatrics*, 171(5), 461–469. doi:10.1001/jamapediatrics.2017.0042 PMID:28319239

Ferrara, G., Kim, J., Lin, S., Hua, J., & Seto, E. (2019). A Focused Review of Smartphone Diet-Tracking Apps: Usability, Functionality, Coherence With Behavior Change Theory, and Comparative Validity of Nutrient Intake and Energy Estimates. *JMIR mHealth and uHealth*, 7(5), e9232. doi:10.2196/mhealth.9232 PMID:31102369

Fogg, B. J. (2009). A behavior model for persuasive design. *Proceedings of the 4th International Conference on Persuasive Technology - Persuasive '09*, 1. 10.1145/1541948.1541999

Fogg, B. J., & Hreha, J. (2010). Behavior Wizard: A Method for Matching Target Behaviors with Solutions. In T. Ploug, P. Hasle, & H. Oinas-Kukkonen (Eds.), *Persuasive Technology* (Vol. 6137, pp. 117–131). Springer Berlin Heidelberg. doi:10.1007/978-3-642-13226-1_13

Foulonneau, A., Calvary, G., & Villain, E. (2016). Stop Procrastinating: TILT, Time is Life Time, a Persuasive Application. *Proceedings of the 28th Australian Conference on Computer-Human Interaction*, 508–516. 10.1145/3010915.3010947

Gajecki, M., Andersson, C., Rosendahl, I., Sinadinovic, K., Fredriksson, M., & Berman, A. H. (2017). Skills Training via Smartphone App for University Students with Excessive Alcohol Consumption: A Randomized Controlled Trial. *International Journal of Behavioral Medicine*, 24(5), 778–788. doi:10.100712529-016-9629-9 PMID:28224445

Garnett, C. (2016). *Development and evaluation of a theory- and evidence-based smartphone app to help reduce excessive alcohol consumption*. Academic Press.

Garnett, C., Crane, D., Michie, S., West, R., & Brown, J. (2016). Evaluating the effectiveness of a smart-phone app to reduce excessive alcohol consumption: Protocol for a factorial randomised control trial. *BMC Public Health, 16*(1), 536. doi:10.118612889-016-3140-8 PMID:27392430

Goyal, S., Lewis, G., Yu, C., Rotondi, M., Seto, E., & Cafazzo, J. A. (2016). Evaluation of a Behavioral Mobile Phone App Intervention for the Self-Management of Type 2 Diabetes: Randomized Controlled Trial Protocol. *JMIR Research Protocols, 5*(3), e174. doi:10.2196/resprot.5959 PMID:27542325

Goyal, S., Nunn, C. A., Rotondi, M., Couperthwaite, A. B., Reiser, S., Simone, A., Katzman, D. K., Cafazzo, J. A., & Palmert, M. R. (2017). A Mobile App for the Self-Management of Type 1 Diabetes Among Adolescents: A Randomized Controlled Trial. *JMIR mHealth and uHealth, 5*(6), e82. doi:10.2196/mhealth.7336 PMID:28630037

Han, M., & Lee, E. (2018). Effectiveness of Mobile Health Application Use to Improve Health Behavior Changes: A Systematic Review of Randomized Controlled Trials. *Healthcare Informatics Research, 24*(3), 207. doi:10.4258/hir.2018.24.3.207 PMID:30109154

Hartin, P. J., Nugent, C. D., McClean, S. I., Cleland, I., Tschanz, J. T., Clark, C. J., & Norton, M. C. (2016). The Empowering Role of Mobile Apps in Behavior Change Interventions: The Gray Matters Randomized Controlled Trial. *JMIR mHealth and uHealth, 4*(3), e93. doi:10.2196/mhealth.4878 PMID:27485822

Hassandra, M., Lintunen, T., Hagger, M. S., Heikkinen, R., Vanhala, M., & Kettunen, T. (2017). An mHealth App for Supporting Quitters to Manage Cigarette Cravings With Short Bouts of Physical Activity: A Randomized Pilot Feasibility and Acceptability Study. *JMIR mHealth and uHealth, 5*(5), e74. doi:10.2196/mhealth.6252 PMID:28550004

Hassandra, M., Lintunen, T., Kettunen, T., Vanhala, M., Toivonen, H.-M., Kinnunen, K., & Heikkinen, R. (2015). Effectiveness of a Mobile Phone App for Adults That Uses Physical Activity as a Tool to Manage Cigarette Craving After Smoking Cessation: A Study Protocol for a Randomized Controlled Trial. *JMIR Research Protocols, 4*(4), e125. doi:10.2196/resprot.4600 PMID:26494256

Hendershot, C. S., Witkiewitz, K., George, W. H., & Marlatt, G. A. (2011). Relapse prevention for addictive behaviors. *Substance Abuse Treatment, Prevention, and Policy, 6*(1), 17. doi:10.1186/1747-597X-6-17 PMID:21771314

Herbec, A., Brown, J., Shahab, L., West, R., & Raupach, T. (2019). Pragmatic randomised trial of a smartphone app (NRT2Quit) to improve effectiveness of nicotine replacement therapy in a quit attempt by improving medication adherence: Results of a prematurely terminated study. *Trials, 20*(1), 547. doi:10.118613063-019-3645-4 PMID:31477166

Horne, R., Chapman, S. C. E., Parham, R., Freemantle, N., Forbes, A., & Cooper, V. (2013). Understanding Patients' Adherence-Related Beliefs about Medicines Prescribed for Long-Term Conditions: A Meta-Analytic Review of the Necessity-Concerns Framework. *PLoS One, 8*(12), e80633. doi:10.1371/journal.pone.0080633 PMID:24312488

Ja, B. (2006). What have we been priming all these years? On the development, mechanisms, and ecology of nonconscious social behavior. *European Journal of Social Psychology, 36*(2), 147–168. doi:10.1002/ejsp.336 PMID:19844598

Kennelly, M. A., Ainscough, K., Lindsay, K., Gibney, E., Mc Carthy, M., & McAuliffe, F. M. (2016). Pregnancy, exercise and nutrition research study with smart phone app support (Pears): Study protocol of a randomized controlled trial. *Contemporary Clinical Trials, 46*, 92–99. doi:10.1016/j.cct.2015.11.018 PMID:26625980

Kennelly, M. A., Ainscough, K., Lindsay, K. L., O'Sullivan, E., Gibney, E. R., McCarthy, M., Segurado, R., DeVito, G., Maguire, O., Smith, T., Hatunic, M., & McAuliffe, F. M. (2018). Pregnancy Exercise and Nutrition With Smartphone Application Support: A Randomized Controlled Trial. *Obstetrics and Gynecology, 131*(5), 818–826. doi:10.1097/AOG.0000000000002582 PMID:29630009

Klonoff, D. C. (2019). Behavioral Theory: The Missing Ingredient for Digital Health Tools to Change Behavior and Increase Adherence. *Journal of Diabetes Science and Technology, 13*(2), 276–281. doi:10.1177/1932296818820303 PMID:30678472

Korinek, E. V., Phatak, S. S., Martin, C. A., Freigoun, M. T., Rivera, D. E., Adams, M. A., Klasnja, P., Buman, M. P., & Hekler, E. B. (2018). Adaptive step goals and rewards: A longitudinal growth model of daily steps for a smartphone-based walking intervention. *Journal of Behavioral Medicine, 41*(1), 74–86. doi:10.100710865-017-9878-3 PMID:28918547

Kramer, J.-N., Kunzler, F., Mishra, V., Presset, B., Kotz, D., Smith, S., Scholz, U., & Kowatsch, T. (2019). Investigating Intervention Components and Exploring States of Receptivity for a Smartphone App to Promote Physical Activity: Protocol of a Microrandomized Trial. *JMIR Research Protocols, 8*(1), e11540. doi:10.2196/11540 PMID:30702430

Kramer, J.-N., Künzler, F., Mishra, V., Smith, S. N., Kotz, D., Scholz, U., Fleisch, E., & Kowatsch, T. (2020). Which Components of a Smartphone Walking App Help Users to Reach Personalized Step Goals? Results From an Optimization Trial. *Annals of Behavioral Medicine*. doi:10.1093/abm/kaaa002

Kruglanski, A. W. (1996). Goals as knowledge structures. In *Linking cognition and motivation to behavior* (pp. 599–618). Guilford Press.

Kruglanski, A. W., Shah, J. Y., Fishbach, A., Friedman, R., Chun, W. Y., & Sleeth-Keppler, D. (2002). A theory of goal systems. In Advances in experimental social psychology (Vol. 34, pp. 331–378). Academic Press., doi:10.1016/S0065-2601(02)80008-9

Larimer, M. E., Palmer, R. S., & Marlatt, G. A. (1999). Relapse prevention. An overview of Marlatt's cognitive-behavioral model. *Alcohol Research & Health: The Journal of the National Institute on Alcohol Abuse and Alcoholism, 23*(2), 151–160. PMID:10890810

Lee, H., Ghebre, R., Le, C., Jang, Y. J., Sharratt, M., & Yee, D. (2017). Mobile Phone Multilevel and Multimedia Messaging Intervention for Breast Cancer Screening: Pilot Randomized Controlled Trial. *JMIR mHealth and uHealth, 5*(11), e154. doi:10.2196/mhealth.7091 PMID:29113961

Lehane, E., & McCarthy, G. (2007). Intentional and unintentional medication non-adherence: A comprehensive framework for clinical research and practice? A discussion paper. *International Journal of Nursing Studies, 44*(8), 1468–1477. doi:10.1016/j.ijnurstu.2006.07.010 PMID:16973166

Leviton, L. C. (1996). Integrating Psychology and Public Health. *The American Psychologist*, 10.

Liberati, A., Altman, D. G., Tetzlaff, J., Mulrow, C., Gøtzsche, P. C., Ioannidis, J. P., Clarke, M., Devereaux, P. J., Kleijnen, J., & Moher, D. (2009). The PRISMA statement for reporting systematic reviews and meta-analyses of studies that evaluate health care interventions: Explanation and elaboration. *PLoS Medicine, 6*(7), e1000100. doi:10.1371/journal.pmed.1000100 PMID:19621070

MacPherson, M. M., Merry, K. J., Locke, S. R., & Jung, M. E. (2019). Effects of Mobile Health Prompts on Self-Monitoring and Exercise Behaviors Following a Diabetes Prevention Program: Secondary Analysis From a Randomized Controlled Trial. *JMIR mHealth and uHealth, 7*(9), e12956. doi:10.2196/12956 PMID:31489842

Madden, G. J. (Ed.). (2012). *APA Handbook of Behavior Analysis.* American Psychological Association.

Michie, S., Richardson, M., Johnston, M., Abraham, C., Francis, J., Hardeman, W., Eccles, M. P., Cane, J., & Wood, C. E. (2013). The Behavior Change Technique Taxonomy (v1) of 93 Hierarchically Clustered Techniques: Building an International Consensus for the Reporting of Behavior Change Interventions. *Annals of Behavioral Medicine, 46*(1), 81–95. doi:10.100712160-013-9486-6 PMID:23512568

Michie, S., van Stralen, M. M., & West, R. (2011). The behaviour change wheel: A new method for characterising and designing behaviour change interventions. *Implementation Science; IS, 6*(1), 42. doi:10.1186/1748-5908-6-42 PMID:21513547

Michie, S., Wood, C. E., Johnston, M., Abraham, C., Francis, J. J., & Hardeman, W. (2015). Behaviour change techniques: The development and evaluation of a taxonomic method for reporting and describing behaviour change interventions (a suite of five studies involving consensus methods, randomised controlled trials and analysis of qualitative data). *Health Technology Assessment, 19*(99), 1–187. doi:10.3310/hta19990 PMID:26616119

Milne-Ives, M., Lam, C., De Cock, C., Van Velthoven, M. H., & Meinert, E. (2020). Mobile Apps for Health Behavior Change in Physical Activity, Diet, Drug and Alcohol Use, and Mental Health: Systematic Review. *JMIR mHealth and uHealth, 8*(3), e17046. doi:10.2196/17046 PMID:32186518

Mummah, S., Robinson, T. N., Mathur, M., Farzinkhou, S., Sutton, S., & Gardner, C. D. (2017). Effect of a mobile app intervention on vegetable consumption in overweight adults: A randomized controlled trial. *The International Journal of Behavioral Nutrition and Physical Activity, 14*(1), 125. doi:10.118612966-017-0563-2 PMID:28915825

Mummah, S. A., King, A. C., Gardner, C. D., & Sutton, S. (2016). Iterative development of Vegethon: A theory-based mobile app intervention to increase vegetable consumption. *The International Journal of Behavioral Nutrition and Physical Activity, 13*(1), 90. doi:10.118612966-016-0400-z PMID:27501724

Mummah, S. A., Mathur, M., King, A. C., Gardner, C. D., & Sutton, S. (2016). Mobile Technology for Vegetable Consumption: A Randomized Controlled Pilot Study in Overweight Adults. *JMIR mHealth and uHealth, 4*(2), e51. doi:10.2196/mhealth.5146 PMID:27193036

Muraven, M., & Baumeister, R. F. (2000). Self-Regulation and Depletion of Limited Resources: Does Self-Control Resemble a Muscle? *Psychological Bulletin, 126*(2), 247–259. doi:10.1037/0033-2909.126.2.247 PMID:10748642

Murawski, B., Plotnikoff, R. C., Rayward, A. T., Oldmeadow, C., Vandelanotte, C., Brown, W. J., & Duncan, M. J. (2019). Efficacy of an m-Health Physical Activity and Sleep Health Intervention for Adults: A Randomized Waitlist-Controlled Trial. *American Journal of Preventive Medicine*, *57*(4), 503–514. doi:10.1016/j.amepre.2019.05.009 PMID:31542128

Murawski, B., Plotnikoff, R. C., Rayward, A. T., Vandelanotte, C., Brown, W. J., & Duncan, M. J. (2018). Randomised controlled trial using a theory-based m-health intervention to improve physical activity and sleep health in adults: The Synergy Study protocol. *BMJ Open*, *8*(2), e018997. doi:10.1136/bmjopen-2017-018997 PMID:29439005

Noordegraaf, A. V., Huirne, J. A. F., Pittens, C. A., van Mechelen, W., Broerse, J. E. W., Brölmann, H. A. M., & Anema, J. R. (2012). eHealth Program to Empower Patients in Returning to Normal Activities and Work After Gynecological Surgery: Intervention Mapping as a Useful Method for Development. *Journal of Medical Internet Research*, *14*(5), e124. doi:10.2196/jmir.1915 PMID:23086834

Oinas-Kukkonen, H., & Harjumaa, M. (2009). Persuasive Systems Design: Key Issues, Process Model, and System Features. *Communications of the Association for Information Systems*, *24*. Advance online publication. doi:10.17705/1CAIS.02428

Patel, M. L., Hopkins, C. M., Brooks, T. L., & Bennett, G. G. (2019). Comparing Self-Monitoring Strategies for Weight Loss in a Smartphone App: Randomized Controlled Trial. *JMIR mHealth and uHealth*, *7*(2), e12209. doi:10.2196/12209 PMID:30816851

Patel, M. S., Asch, D. A., Rosin, R., Small, D. S., Bellamy, S. L., Heuer, J., Sproat, S., Hyson, C., Haff, N., Lee, S. M., Wesby, L., Hoffer, K., Shuttleworth, D., Taylor, D. H., Hilbert, V., Zhu, J., Yang, L., Wang, X., & Volpp, K. G. (2016). Framing Financial Incentives to Increase Physical Activity Among Overweight and Obese Adults: A Randomized, Controlled Trial. *Annals of Internal Medicine*, *164*(6), 385. doi:10.7326/M15-1635 PMID:26881417

Pellegrini, C. A., Steglitz, J., Johnston, W., Warnick, J., Adams, T., McFadden, H. G., Siddique, J., Hedeker, D., & Spring, B. (2015). Design and protocol of a randomized multiple behavior change trial: Make Better Choices 2 (MBC2). *Contemporary Clinical Trials*, *41*, 85–92. doi:10.1016/j.cct.2015.01.009 PMID:25625810

Prochaska, J. O., & DiClemente, C. C. (2005). The Transtheoretical Approach. In J. C. Norcross & M. R. Goldfried (Eds.), *Handbook of psychotherapy integration* (2nd ed.). Oxford University Press. doi:10.1093/med:psych/9780195165791.003.0007

Rabbi, M., Pfammatter, A., Zhang, M., Spring, B., & Choudhury, T. (2015). Automated personalized feedback for physical activity and dietary behavior change with mobile phones: A randomized controlled trial on adults. *JMIR mHealth and uHealth*, *3*(2), e42. doi:10.2196/mhealth.4160 PMID:25977197

Sabaté, E., & World Health Organization. (Eds.). (2003). *Adherence to long-term therapies: Evidence for action*. World Health Organization.

Sankaran, S., Dendale, P., & Coninx, K. (2019). Evaluating the Impact of the HeartHab App on Motivation, Physical Activity, Quality of Life, and Risk Factors of Coronary Artery Disease Patients: Multidisciplinary Crossover Study. *JMIR mHealth and uHealth*, *7*(4), e10874. doi:10.2196/10874 PMID:30946021

Sankaran, S., Frederix, I., Haesen, M., Dendale, P., Luyten, K., & Coninx, K. (2016). A Grounded Approach for Applying Behavior Change Techniques in Mobile Cardiac Tele-Rehabilitation. *Proceedings of the 9th ACM International Conference on PErvasive Technologies Related to Assistive Environments.* 10.1145/2910674.2910680

Scheerman, J. F. M., Meijel, B., Empelen, P., Verrips, G. H. W., Loveren, C., Twisk, J. W. R., Pakpour, A. H., Braak, M. C. T., & Kramer, G. J. C. (2020). The effect of using a mobile application ("WhiteTeeth") on improving oral hygiene: A randomized controlled trial. *International Journal of Dental Hygiene, 18*(1), 73–83. doi:10.1111/idh.12415 PMID:31291683

Scheerman, J. F. M., van Empelen, P., van Loveren, C., & van Meijel, B. (2018). A Mobile App (WhiteTeeth) to Promote Good Oral Health Behavior Among Dutch Adolescents with Fixed Orthodontic Appliances: Intervention Mapping Approach. *JMIR mHealth and uHealth, 6*(8), e163. doi:10.2196/mhealth.9626 PMID:30120085

Scheerman, J. F. M., van Meijel, B., van Empelen, P., Kramer, G. J. C., Verrips, G. H. W., Pakpour, A. H., Van den Braak, M. C. T., & van Loveren, C. (2018). Study protocol of a randomized controlled trial to test the effect of a smartphone application on oral-health behavior and oral hygiene in adolescents with fixed orthodontic appliances. *BMC Oral Health, 18*(1), 19. doi:10.118612903-018-0475-9 PMID:29415697

Schwarzer, R., & Renner, B. (2000). Social-cognitive predictors of health behavior: Action self-efficacy and coping self-efficacy. *Health Psychology: Official Journal of the Division of Health Psychology, American Psychological Association, 19*(5), 487–495. doi:10.1037/0278-6133.19.5.487 PMID:11007157

Simons, D., De Bourdeaudhuij, I., Clarys, P., De Cocker, K., Vandelanotte, C., & Deforche, B. (2018a). A Smartphone App to Promote an Active Lifestyle in Lower-Educated Working Young Adults: Development, Usability, Acceptability, and Feasibility Study. *JMIR mHealth and uHealth, 6*(2), e44. doi:10.2196/mhealth.8287 PMID:29463491

Simons, D., De Bourdeaudhuij, I., Clarys, P., De Cocker, K., Vandelanotte, C., & Deforche, B. (2018b). Effect and Process Evaluation of a Smartphone App to Promote an Active Lifestyle in Lower Educated Working Young Adults: Cluster Randomized Controlled Trial. *JMIR mHealth and uHealth, 6*(8), e10003. doi:10.2196/10003 PMID:30143477

Spring, B., Pellegrini, C., McFadden, H. G., Pfammatter, A. F., Stump, T. K., Siddique, J., King, A. C., & Hedeker, D. (2018). Multicomponent mHealth Intervention for Large, Sustained Change in Multiple Diet and Activity Risk Behaviors: The Make Better Choices 2 Randomized Controlled Trial. *Journal of Medical Internet Research, 20*(6), e10528. doi:10.2196/10528 PMID:29921561

Sullivan, A. N., & Lachman, M. E. (2016). Behavior Change with Fitness Technology in Sedentary Adults: A Review of the Evidence for Increasing Physical Activity. *Frontiers in Public Health, 4*, 289. doi:10.3389/fpubh.2016.00289 PMID:28123997

Sunio, V., & Schmocker, J.-D. (2017). Can we promote sustainable travel behavior through mobile apps? Evaluation and review of evidence. *International Journal of Sustainable Transportation, 11*(8), 553–566. doi:10.1080/15568318.2017.1300716

Tombor, I., Beard, E., Brown, J., Shahab, L., Michie, S., & West, R. (2018). Randomized factorial experiment of components of the SmokeFree Baby smartphone application to aid smoking cessation in pregnancy. *Translational Behavioral Medicine, 9*(4), 583–593. doi:10.1093/tbm/iby073 PMID:30011020

Tombor, I., Shahab, L., Brown, J., Crane, D., Michie, S., & West, R. (2016). Development of SmokeFree Baby: A smoking cessation smartphone app for pregnant smokers. *Translational Behavioral Medicine, 6*(4), 533–545. doi:10.100713142-016-0438-0 PMID:27699682

van Beurden, S. B., Smith, J. R., Lawrence, N. S., Abraham, C., & Greaves, C. J. (2019). Feasibility Randomized Controlled Trial of ImpulsePal: Smartphone App-Based Weight Management Intervention to Reduce Impulsive Eating in Overweight Adults. *JMIR Formative Research, 3*(2), e11586. doi:10.2196/11586 PMID:31038464

Verbiest, M., Borrell, S., Dalhousie, S., Tupa'i-Firestone, R., Funaki, T., Goodwin, D., Grey, J., Henry, A., Hughes, E., Humphrey, G., Jiang, Y., Jull, A., Pekepo, C., Schumacher, J., Te Morenga, L., Tunks, M., Vano, M., Whittaker, R., & Ni Mhurchu, C. (2018). A Co-Designed, Culturally-Tailored mHealth Tool to Support Healthy Lifestyles in Maori and Pasifika Communities in New Zealand: Protocol for a Cluster Randomized Controlled Trial. *JMIR Research Protocols, 7*(8), e10789. doi:10.2196/10789 PMID:30135054

Verbruggen, F., Best, M., Bowditch, W. A., Stevens, T., & McLaren, I. P. L. (2014). The inhibitory control reflex. *Neuropsychologia, 65*, 263–278. doi:10.1016/j.neuropsychologia.2014.08.014 PMID:25149820

West, R. (2007). The PRIME Theory of motivation as a possible foundation for addiction treatment. *Drug Addiction Treatment in the 21st Century: Science and Policy Issues.*

World Health Organization. (Ed.). (2009). *Global health risks: Mortality and burden of disease attributable to selected major risks.* World Health Organization.

Zhao, J., Freeman, B., & Li, M. (2016). Can Mobile Phone Apps Influence People's Health Behavior Change? An Evidence Review. *Journal of Medical Internet Research, 18*(11), e287. doi:10.2196/jmir.5692 PMID:27806926

KEY TERMS AND DEFINITIONS

App: Application.
ASE: Attitude-social influence-self-efficacy.
BC: Behavior change.
BCT: Behavior change technique.
BCW: Behavior change wheel.
BMI: Body mass index.
COM-B: Capability, opportunity, motivation, and behavior.
CT: Control theory.
FBM: Fogg behavior model.
mHealth: Mobile health.
MI: Motivational interviewing.

MMR: Measles, mumps, and rubella.
MOST: Multiphase optimization strategy.
MRC: Medical research council.
MVPA: Moderate-to-vigorous physical activity.
PA: Physical activity.
PRIMSA: Preferred reporting items for systematic reviews and meta-analyses.
RCT: Randomized control trial.
RPM: Relapse prevention model.
SCT: Social cognitive theory.
T1DM: Type 1 diabetes mellitus
T2DM: Type 2 diabetes mellitus.
TDF: Theoretical domains framework.
TPB: Theory of planned behavior.
TTM: Transtheoretical model.
WHO: World Health Organization.

APPENDIX

Table 2. Summary of selected studies

References and Study Location	Health Condition Targeted	Study Design	BC Theory	Sample Size	Primary Outcome Measure
(Achananuparp et al., 2018) - Singapore	Dietary	2-arm RCT Parallel	Loss Aversion and Framing	245	Compliance days; Compliant users
(Baskerville et al., 2015; 2018a, 2018b) - Canada	Smoking Cessation	2-arm RCT Parallel	Fogg Behavior Model	1599	Continuous self-reported abstinence
(Berman et al., 2015, 2019; Gajecki et al., 2017) - Sweden	Alcohol Consumption	3-arm RCT Parallel	Theory of Planned Behavior	330	Quantity and frequency of alcohol consumption
(Brindal et al., 2016, 2018) - Australia	Dietary	2-arm RCT Parallel	Action and Coping Self-Efficacy, Behavior Change Techniques	146	Percentage weight loss from baseline; Changes in blood pressure, fasting blood glucose, and fasting blood lipids
(Crane et al., 2018; Garnett, 2016a, 2016b) - UK	Alcohol Consumption	2^5 factorial RCT	COM-B Behavior Change Model, Behavior Change Techniques	672	Self-reported change in weekly alcohol consumption
(den Bakker et al., 2019a, 2019b) - Netherlands	Returning to normal activities after Surgery	2-arm RCT Parallel	Attitude-Social influence-self-Efficacy model	151	Reach; Dose delivered; Dose received; Fidelity; and Participants' attitudes
(Agarwal et al., 2019; Desveaux et al., 2016) - Canada	Diabetes	2-arm RCT Parallel	Transtheoretical Model of Behavior Change	223	Glucose control - HbA$_{1c}$ levels at 3 months
(Edney et al., 2017, 2019, 2020) - Australia	Physical Activity	3-arm RCT Cluster	Social Cognitive Theory	444	Physical activity from baseline to 3-month follow-up.
(Elbert et al., 2016) - Netherlands	Dietary	3-arm RCT Pretest-Posttest	Behavior Change Techniques	146	Self-reported fruit and vegetable intake at 6-month follow-up
(Fadda et al., 2017) - Italy	MMR Vaccination	2^2-factorial RCT	Cugelman's gamification tactics	184	MMR vaccination knowledge, psychological empowerment, risk perception, and preferred decisional role
(Foulonneau et al., 2016) - France	Smartphone addiction	Single arm	Fogg Behavior Model	19	N/A
(Goyal et al., 2016, 2017) Canada	Diabetes	2-arm RCT Parallel	Prior knowledge of Behavior Change Theory including Health Belief Model. Validated with Self-Care Inventory, Diabetes Family Responsibility Questionnaire and Diabetes Quality of Life for Youth Instrument	92	Change in HbA$_{1c}$ from baseline to 12 months, between the intervention and control group
(Hartin et al., 2016) - US	Alzheimer disease	2-arm RCT Parallel	Transtheoretical Model of Behavior Change	144	A set of anthropometric measures, blood-based biomarkers, objective cognitive testing, and behavior in targeted domains.
(Hassandra et al., 2015, 2017) - Finland	Smoking Cessation	2-arm RCT Parallel	Social Cognitive Theory; Theory of Planned Behavior; Control Theory; Relapse Prevention Model; Motivational Interviewing; Behavior Change Techniques	44	Self-reported 7-day point prevalence abstinence (PPA) at 7 days prior to each scheduled follow-up; Self-reported number of relapses during the last 7 days; Self-reported number of cravings during the last 7 days; Self-efficacy of being aware of experiencing cravings (AEF); self-efficacy in managing cravings (MCEF); power of control in managing cravings (CCM)
(Herbec et al., 2019) - UK	Smoking Cessation	2-arm RCT Parallel	BCW; COM-B Behavior Change Model; Behavior Change Techniques; Theoretical Domains Framework; Intentional and Non-intentional Non-adherence; Necessity Concerns Framework; Compliance and Persistence Framework; PRIME Theory of Motivation	41	Self-reported 4-week prolonged abstinence assessed at 8-week follow-up and verified by saliva cotinine levels of less than 15 ng/mL or, among participants reporting using NRT or e-cigarettes, anabasine levels of less than 1 ng/mL.
(Kennelly et al., 2016, 2018) - Ireland	Diabetes	2-arm RCT Parallel	Control Theory; Social Cognitive Theory	565	Incidence of gestational diabetes mellitus (GDM) at 28–30 weeks of gestation.
(Korinek et al., 2018) - US	Physical Activity	Single arm	Social Cognitive Theory	20	Achieving "ambitious but doable" step goals
(Kramer et al., 2019, 2020) - Switzerland	Physical Activity	3-arm RCT Parallel	Behavioral Change Techniques	274	Proportion of participant days that daily step goals were achieved
(Lee et al., 2017) - US	Breast Cancer	2-arm RCT Parallel	Fogg Behavior Model	120	Mammogram receipt
(MacPherson et al., 2019) - Canada	Diabetes	2-arm RCT Parallel	Behavior Change Techniques	69	Frequency of self-monitoring and self-reported exercise in the week before and after a prompt.
(Mummah et al., 2016a, 2016b, 2017) - US	Dietary	2-arm RCT Parallel	Behavior Change Techniques	17	Daily vegetable consumption at baseline and 12 weeks after randomization

continued on following page

Table 2. Continued

References and Study Location	Health Condition Targeted	Study Design	BC Theory	Sample Size	Primary Outcome Measure
(Murawski et al., 2018, 2019) Australia	Physical Activity and Sleep	2-arm RCT Parallel	Social Cognitive Theory, Behavioral Change Techniques	160	Self-reported minutes of moderate-to-vigorous intensity physical activity and sleep quality
(Patel et al., 2019) - US	Dietary	3-arm RCT Parallel	Behavior Change Techniques	105	Weight change at 3 months
(Pellegrini et al., 2015; Spring et al., 2018) - US	Dietary	3-arm RCT Parallel	Mastery Hypothesis, Synergy Hypothesis	212	Composite diet and activity improvement score measured for 1-week assessment periods at 3, 6, and 9 months when participants wore an accelerometer and used the assessment app to self-monitor their behaviors without receiving any feedback.
(Rabbi et al., 2015) - US	Physical Activity and Dietary	2-arm RCT Parallel	Learning Theory; Social Cognitive Theory; Fogg Behavior Model	17	Activity and dietary logs
(Sankaran et al., 2016, 2019) - Belgium	Motivation, Physical Activity, Quality of Life, Dietary, and Risk Factors for Diabetes	2-arm RCT Cross-Over	Fogg Behavior Model; Persuasive Systems Design Model; Behavior Wizard Framework	32	Usage logs; Activities registered by patients using the app, medication compliance, and evolution of various physiological parameters
(Scheerman et al., 2018a, 2018b, 2020) - Netherlands	Dental Hygiene	2-arm RCT Parallel	Behavioral Change Techniques	132	Clinical assessments and Self-administered digital questionnaires. At baseline, 6 weeks, and 12 weeks follow-up data collected before orthodontic check-up
(Simons et al., 2018a, 2018b) - Belgium	Physical Activity	2-arm RCT Cluster	Behavior Change Techniques	130	Objective measurement of physical activity, and individual interviews
(Tombor et al., 2016, 2018) - UK	Smoking Cessation	2^5-factorial RCT	UK's Medical Research Council (MRC) guidance; the Multi phase Optimization Strategy (MOST); Behavior Change Wheel (BCW); Behavior Change Techniques	565	Duration and frequency of engagement the app. Self-reported smoking abstinence up to 4 weeks from the quit date
(van Beurden et al., 2019) - UK	Dietary	2-arm RCT Parallel	Elaborated Intrusion Theory of Desire; Implementation Intentions; Associative Learning, Pavlovian conditioning, Executive response inhibition, Mindfulness, Goal priming	88	Uptake rate; Study completion rate; SD of weight loss at 3 months of follow-up.
(Verbiest et al., 2018) - New Zealand	Health-Related Behaviors	2-arm RCT Cluster	Theoretical Domains Framework; Behavior Change Techniques	83	Measure of physical activity, smoking behavior, alcohol intake, fruit and vegetable consumption behaviors at 12 weeks.

Chapter 12
Mobile Technologies in Disaster Healthcare:
Technology and Operational Aspects

Samaneh Madanian

https://orcid.org/0000-0001-6430-9611
Auckland University of Technology, New Zealand

Reem Abubakr Abbas
Auckland University of Technology, New Zealand

Tony Norris
Auckland University of Technology, New Zealand

Dave Parry
Auckland University of Technology, New Zealand

ABSTRACT

The increasing penetration of smartphones and their ability to host mobile technologies have shown valuable outcomes in disaster management; albeit, their application in disaster medicine remains limited. In this chapter, the authors explore the role of mobile technologies for clinical applications and communication and information exchange during disasters. The chapter synthesizes the literature on disaster healthcare and mobile technologies before, during, and after disasters discusses technological and operational aspects. They conclude by discussing limitations in the field and prospects for the future.

DOI: 10.4018/978-1-5225-6067-8.ch012

1. INTRODUCTION

Disasters are an inseparable part of human life disrupting the functioning of a community or a society by causing widespread human, material, economic, or environmental losses. According to the data from EM-DAT (Centre for Research on the Epidemiology of Disasters, n.d.), the numbers, severity and complexity (damage to life and property) of disasters have grown exponentially over recent decades. In 2019, 440 natural disasters were identified: these caused 24,117 deaths and affected a further 96.5 million people.

This chapter deals primarily with the human aspects of disasters and with the issues associated with the recent development and the role of mobile technologies in improving the delivery of disaster healthcare.

The chapter first describes the nature and types of disasters and introduces the concept of the disaster management cycle which provides a useful framework to illustrate the role of mobile and other e-health technologies. It proceeds by outlining the key aspects of healthcare needs in disasters and then describes in detail the current roles of mobile technologies in improving clinical care and information sharing in such events. The chapter ends with a look at the current limitations and future possibilities.

2. DISASTERS: NATURE, TYPES, AND LIFECYCLE

A disaster is a catastrophic disruption of the functioning of a community or a society overwhelming its capacity to respond.

Disasters can be natural or man-made. Environmental disasters, typified by earthquakes, volcanic eruptions, floods etc., are often short term in duration but they can cause massive destruction and loss of life leading to long-term human, material, economic and/or environmental consequences. Other catastrophes such as wars, terrorism, and pandemics are human centred in origin and frequently extend over a longer time scale than a point event but they parallel environmental disasters in their extended impact on individuals and societies. Climate change can be seen as an example of a potential disaster which has both natural and human sources.

The effects of all disaster types, especially those with a human origin, are readily magnified by globalisation, particularly by trade and travel, as is regrettably clear from epidemics such as Ebola, Zika, and the on-going and devastating COVID-19 pandemic.

Whether natural or man-made, a disaster is conveniently characterised by four phases that compromise its lifecycle: mitigation, preparedness, response and recovery (Baldini, Braun, Hess, Oliveri, & Seuschek, 2009). The first phase, mitigation, is concerned with preventing or minimising the negative impacts of disasters. The preparedness phase focuses on planning and preparing for possible disaster occurrence. The response phase, which often receives more attention than other phases, refers to the activities conducted immediately after the occurrence of the disaster to save lives and deal with damages. The fourth stage is the recovery stage which aims at restoring pre-disaster situations or improving them (Center for Disaster Philanthropy, n.d.).

These four phases are often referred to as the Disaster Management Cycle (DMC).

3. DISASTER MANAGEMENT, DISASTER MEDICINE, AND DISASTER HEALTHCARE

3.1 Disaster Management

Disaster management refers to the processes applied before, during, and after the occurrence of a disaster event (i.e. throughout the DMC) to prevent or mitigate its impacts (Nikbakhsh & Farahani, 2011).

Catastrophes such as 2004 Indian Ocean earthquake and tsunami (Telford & Cosgrave, 2007), 2005 Hurricane Katrina (Brunkard, Namulanda, & Ratard, 2008), and 2010 Haiti earthquake (Bilham, 2010) have led to a renewed interest in disaster management and its recognition as a distinct discipline. Many countries have given priority to the policy agenda in this field (Khan, Vasilescu, & Khan, 2008), and several international organisations also have taken the lead in this regard. The United Nations has introduced 'Hyogo' (United Nations, 2007) and 'Sendai' (United Nations, 2015) frameworks for a more proactive approach to disaster management and reducing disaster risks, losses and damages to communities, respectively. The World Health Organization (WHO) has also asked all countries in the world to set up hospitals with facilities for disaster relief (WHO, 2010).

In practice, the primary purposes of disaster management are logistical, e.g. dealing with damaged infrastructure, restoring services, setting up supply chains, moving victims to safety and seeing to their basic needs. Dispensing clinical treatment to those who need it is not the main role of disaster managers as has been noted after major disasters and terrorist attacks such as 9/11 (Kirsch & Hsu, 2008; Trzeciak & Rivers, 2003).

3.2 Disaster Medicine

The delivery of clinical services in a disaster is the responsibility of disaster medicine specialists trained to deliver emergency medicine under dynamic disaster conditions, which differ dramatically from normal medicine. For example, in disasters, medical resources are limited, stress levels are high, decisions have to be made rapidly with imperfect situational awareness, and training may be inadequate to maintain normal quality standards (James et al., 2010; Su et al., 2013) whilst firm guidance in international law and health policy can be lacking (Civaner, Vatansever, & Pala, 2017).

The necessary specialisms of disaster medicine span a wide spectrum that includes public health, paramedicine, and surgery; a range that demands efficient information sharing and effective communication across multiple agencies not only to clarify roles and responsibilities, but to avoid fragmentation and duplication in services (Abbas & Norris, 2018).

3.3 Challenges in Disaster Management and Disaster Medicine

Although disaster management and healthcare would seem to be natural allies in responding to disasters, these disciplines have not been able to jointly use their tools and personnel to prepare for and respond to serious events (Bissell, 2005). Post-event investigation shows frequent miscommunication and mismanagement (Russo, 2011), that lead to poor disaster responses and delayed evacuations. These deficiencies can be attributed to the different origins and priorities of the two sectors that inhibit a common understanding, and the consequent difficulties of obtaining and sharing vital information in a timely manner. Waeckerle, Lillibridge, Burkle, and Noji (1994) pointed out that disaster physicians, who have limited focus on issues beyond medical care, often need to interact with different organisations and agencies that operate under specific organisational hierarchy and operational modes. Similarly, disaster managers lack knowledge about the way the healthcare system responds to disasters (Bissell, 2005).

The above observations have led Ciottone (2006) to suggest that managers and disaster medicine specialists should join ranks to form teams of multidisciplinary responders having increased awareness of each other's roles, responsibilities, and priorities. Whatever the practicalities of this suggestion, the advances in communication and coordinated activities designed to reduce the health consequences of catastrophic events are at the heart of the integrated approach of disaster healthcare.

3.4 Disaster Healthcare

Disaster healthcare can be defined as the systematic process of using different skills and capacities – clinical, administrative, organisation, operational – to address the challenge of planning for, responding to, and recovering from the health consequences of disasters (Ardalan et al., 2009). The central goal is to provide urgent health interventions and ongoing healthcare during and after disasters (Zhong, Clark, Hou, Zang, & FitzGerald, 2014). Thus, disaster healthcare extends over all phases of the disaster cycle coordinating activities that range from preventive and resilience-building health services, through rapid response to victims' needs, to post-disaster rehabilitation programs (de Boer, 1995; Waeckerle et al., 1994).

Although early studies have acknowledged the role of information and communication technologies in transforming disaster management (Underwood, 2010; Waeckerle et al., 1994), their application in disaster medicine are still disparate and ad hoc. Using ICT to improve both disaster management and disaster medicine has the potential to bring about dramatic improvements in the efficiency, quality, access to, and cost-effectiveness of disaster healthcare (Sieben, Scott, & Palacios, 2012). Until recently, realising this potential has been a slow process but the advent of ubiquitous mobile technologies is now accelerating the acceptance of ICT and creating the conditions for massive improvements.

3.5 Challenges in Disaster Healthcare

Loss of infrastructure, lack of planning, inadequate resources, and insufficient coordination in the provision of health services during disasters (Callaway et al., 2012; Khankeh et al., 2011) are some of the factors that transfer a disaster into the healthcare environment (Hamilton, 2003).

Health response to disaster is often challenging in the first few hours of disasters due to the sheer numbers of traumatised and injured individuals. The number of injuries may overload medical facilities due to limited medical resources (Hirshberg, Holcomb, & Mattox, 2001). This stressful nature of events may consume medical staff and local responders forcing them to concentrate on medical care and delaying their awareness about the disaster situation until reports arrive at later stages. Moreover, medical personnel may be forced to deal with arriving victims without having a clue about their medical history. During such chaotic scenarios, an increase in morbidity and mortality rates can be expected.

Lack of medical history is another challenge to the provision of safe care in disasters. Disaster victims with chronic diseases may have little information about their health conditions or the dosage of medications they take (James & Walsh, 2011). Lack of crucial information adds pressure on already stressed medical staff as they try to access and collect accurate personal health information in order to prescribe the necessary treatment and medication. Inability to get hold of medical information, as is the case with evacuees, may result in increasing the risk of medical errors and threatening patient safety

(Bala, Venkatesh, Venkatraman, Bates, & Brown, 2009). Moreover, a disaster may impact the healthcare infrastructure itself adversely impacting hospitalised patients and disrupting their treatment.

Several studies have investigated the challenges associated with the delivery of healthcare in disasters (Bala et al., 2009; Chen, Gonzalez, Leung, Zhang, & Li, 2010; Lahtela, 2009; Turcu & Popa, 2009). These challenges encouraged studying disaster management and disaster medicine with a specific focus on cooperation, communication, and awareness of situations (Javed & Norris, 2012) and exploring decision-making and abilities of disaster managers (Cioca & Cioca, 2010).

A major challenge to a coordinated response to disasters is the existence of multiple often independent and territorial agencies. These agencies come from different backgrounds and have varying responsibilities that cover a wide range of aspects including infrastructure, supply chain, transport, and the well-being of the affected communities. National, international, and non-governmental organisations such as police, health, ambulance, fire and civil defence services are usually involved in the response process. Activities concerned with the delivery of healthcare are the responsibility of health professionals specialising in various medical fields including paramedicine, public health, and disaster medicine. These factors make communication and especially cross-agency communication extremely challenging particularly at times when there are high stress levels, incomplete data, and minimum time to make critical decisions.

Fortunately, developments in information and mobile technologies can greatly assist with the communication issues whilst similar advances in e-health can have major benefits in improving healthcare provision in disaster situations. The rest of the chapter focuses on the role of mobile technologies in facilitating disaster healthcare via their general role in communication and information exchange, and their more specific clinical applications.

4. APPLICATIONS OF MOBILE TECHNOLOGIES IN DISASTER HEALTHCARE

According to the International Telecommunication Union (ITU), more than 5 billion individuals are now connected to wireless networks with a majority located in low and middle-income countries (International Telecommunication Union, 2019). The driving force behind the application of mobile technologies in disaster events is the massive penetration rate of smartphones worldwide (Figure 1). According to Statista, the number of smartphone users globally has exceeded three billion with an expected increase of several hundred million in the coming years (Statista, 2020).

The widespread use of mobile phones provides an affordable platform for supporting efficient and cost-effective solutions that provide timely information. For example, in the field of humanitarian relief, the World Food Program saves about five million dollars of its annual expenses on food surveys through utilising mobile technologies including text messages, telephone interviews and online surveys (World Food Programme, 2016; Yoo, 2018).

In the context of disasters, mobile computing and social media have a huge potential for revolutionising healthcare provision (Wilson, Wang, & Sheetz, 2014). Social media platforms supported by mobile technologies have been exceptionally useful in a broad range of activities from coordinating relief activities, mapping damaged areas, identifying people in need, disseminating information and guidance, and attracting donations (Harrison, 2015).

Social media refers to a group of applications that facilitate content sharing. In disasters, gathering and interpreting information situation awareness can be enhanced through leveraging social media platforms to provide timely information and collect vast amounts of data through connecting response

Figure 1. Number of smartphone users worldwide from 2016 to 2021 (in billions)
(Statista, 2020)

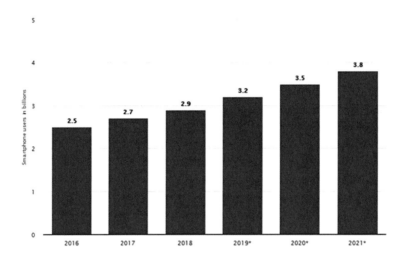

agencies and various societal sectors (Luna & Pennock, 2018). A 2016 study on the Louisiana flood revealed that connecting communities affected by disasters with external organisations through social media platforms have played a significant role in improving the accuracy of disaster-related information (Kim & Hastak, 2018a).

Data exchanged on social media can be utilised in building real-time maps and developing early warning systems (Middleton, Middleton, & Modafferi, 2014). Posts on social media platforms can be systematically studied by the authorities to identify the needs of disaster-affected communities (Yin et al., 2015). Similarly, government agencies can utilise these platforms for disseminating emergency and disaster information to the public (Kim & Hastak, 2018b). Hence, the adoption of social media technologies into disaster strategies has the potential to improve the quality of disaster response. Despite these benefits which are made possible via mobile technologies, there exists a need to verify the information exchanged over these communication channels as misinformation has the potential to increase the impacts of disasters (Luna & Pennock, 2018).

Mobile applications are being increasingly utilised in disasters; a recent example is the use of contact tracing apps in combating COVID-19. To avoid communication with high-risk contacts, these applications have been explored and in some countries utilised (Bengio et al., 2020). Built upon the idea of co-locating individuals in space and time via Bluetooth, GPS, or other technologies, contact tracing apps can identify at-risk individuals. Furthermore, mobile apps help authorities understand the spread of the virus and the degree to which communities are abiding by social distance rules (Findlay, Palma, & Milne, 2020). However, due to the fact that geospatial data can be used to identify specific individuals, contact tracing apps have come under huge scrutiny especially in democratic counties (Cho, Ippolito, & Yu, 2020). Successful use of mobile technologies depends on their uptake by their targeted audience. For example, in the case of COVID-19 contact tracing apps, download is not always mandatory (Figure 2). The Indian government argues that knowing the location and health status of individuals is a public interest (Findlay et al., 2020). Although reasonably sensible, populations worldwide may not necessarily agree with this argument and hence may simply refrain from downloading the apps or using them. This highlights the ethical and social dimensions to the uptake of mobile applications.

4.1 Communication and Information Exchange Applications

Figure 2. The uptake of contact tracing apps
(Findlay et al., 2020)

Country	App name	Mandatory?	Adoption
India	Aarogya Setu	Yes	100m downloads out of a population of 1.3bn
Norway	Smittestopp	No	1/5 of the adult population
Singapore	TraceTogether	No	25 per cent of 5.7m population
Iceland	Rakning C-19	No	40 per cent of population of 340,000

No single agency is capable of responding to the needs of disaster-affected communities without collaborating with other sectors. Accordingly, cross-agency communication is paramount for exploring possible ways of collaboration between intervening agencies. The goal of collaboration is to orchestrate the activities of different disaster stakeholders (Yang, Lee, Rao, & Touqan, 2009). It includes joint needs assessment, coordinating the provision of adequate health services, identifying affected populations and mobilising resources (IFRC, 2000). Cross-agency collaboration requires extensive investment in terms of time, resources, and funds. The different authority structures across intervening agencies guide their way of responding to emergencies and disasters and make the process of cross-agency collaboration extremely complex (Abbas, Norris, Madanian, & Parry, 2016).

Poor communication across disaster response agencies necessitates the need for education to enable these agencies to understand each other's capabilities and capacities. This, in turn, leads to the establishment of trust which is central to the flow of information across response agencies. Trust is established when agencies believe in each other's abilities, resources and skills and that they have the will to collaborate and complement each other. Agencies that trust each other share information and engage in joint problem-solving and possibly joint action. This is evident in the harmony manifested between the health sector and the rest of the government in the management of COVID-19 pandemic in New Zealand. Evidence-based decision making which was based on cross-agency trust and reliable information sharing led the New Zealand response to be praised by the World Health Organisation as 'being very systematic with a very comprehensive strategy' (TVNZ, 2020).

The main challenge in a multi-stakeholder disaster scenario is to ensure that each agency has adequate situation awareness. Endsley (1988) defines situation awareness as 'the perception of the elements in the environment within a volume of time and space, and the comprehension and the projection of their status in the near future'. Situation awareness includes having a full understanding of the situation at hand, pressing needs and required actions. However, building up such a holistic picture is a complex process (Karami, Shah, Vaezi, & Bansal, 2019). Despite credibility, a top-down approach to information exchange via official channels was found to be insufficient for achieving adequate situation awareness. Horizontal information exchange via mobile technologies proved to be exceptionally useful throughout the different phases of the disaster lifecycle.

In the mitigation stage, monitoring information can be collected and processed effectively through mobile platforms. In the preparedness stage, mobile apps can be used in disaster risk education, broadcasting early warning systems, and communicating with potential volunteers. During the response, these apps can be lifesaving as they provide a wide range of services including rapid broadcasting of critical information, indications of mass gatherings, and facilitating search and rescue operations to name a few. In the recovery stage, mobile apps can readily provide damage assessment and recovery-related information (Tan et al., 2017). The innovation of entirely mobile systems that allow rapid acquisition of data from disaster sites is made possible through mobile technologies. Technologies such as cloud computing, big data analytics, Internet of Things (IoT), and social media bring huge potential when used in conjunction with mobile technologies.

Big data, which refers to data collections that are not only very large but also highly complex and diverse (Kayyali, Knott, & Van Kuiken, 2013), enables data mining to reveal inherent patterns and associations. This technology has huge benefits like in the case of epidemiology where chronological data helps predict the onset and spread of infectious diseases such as influenza and SARS. Cloud computing enables access to information 'anywhere and anytime' and increases accessibility by using various devices such as smartphones. IoT is another technology with huge potential for improving disasters response as it enables objects to be sensed and/or controlled remotely across the existing network infrastructure. This means that objects can communicate without human intervention by embedding sensors within them; an ideal means for intervention in war and conflict zones as well as in health situations where human interaction needs to be avoided.

Social media networking via Facebook and Twitter, for example, can contribute to effective response efforts. These applications, available through smartphones and tablet, can make it possible for planners to connect with ordinary citizens and involve them in the development of strategies for disaster management (Norris et al., 2015). Social media are useful in different disaster stages. Emergency workers and volunteers use social media to find people in need, map damaged areas, organize relief efforts, disseminate news and guidance, attract donations, and help prepare for future disasters. For example, when Hurricane Sandy caused flooding in New York, the Red Cross directed some trucks and relief supplies specifically in response to tweets by victims. During the Sandy response, some 88 social media posts resulted in similar changes on the ground (Harrison, 2015). Social media can provide instant news faster than traditional news outlets or sources and can be a great wealth of information, but there is also an increasing need to verify and determine the accuracy of this information.

4.2 Clinical Applications

In disaster circumstances, mobile technologies linked to centralised information systems can provide seamless care (Brown et al., 2007; Maturana, Scott, & Palacios, 2012; Singh & Kaur, 2010). "These technologies have applications in terms of enhancing mass-casualty field care, provider safety, field incident command, resource management, informatics support, and regional Emergency Department (ED) and hospital care of disaster victims" (Chan et al., 2004, p. 1229). Recent technological advances also raise the prospect of delivering health information systems that are both portable and personalised (James & Walsh, 2011). Revolutionary mobile technologies such as telemedicine, mobile health, Electronic Health Record (EHR), social media, IoT, and big data have the potential to make a radical change in disaster healthcare.

The following sub-sections review mobile applications in the pre-, response, and post-disaster phases.

4.2.1 Pre-Disaster Applications

Well-designed disaster mitigation and preparedness plans are keys to the effectiveness of health response in disasters. Healthcare organisations should regularly assess their response plans and their readiness level. These requirements are usually provided by information systems and can now be extended and be available on mobile phones and tablets via mobile technologies. This facilitates access to information by both disaster planners and citizens.

Pre-disaster activities are designed to identify the nature and likelihood of disasters, avoid or diminish their possibility or destructive consequences, or to enable communities and response agencies to take proper actions when a disaster occurs. The objective is to ensure that proper systems, plans, procedures, and resources are in place and updated. These plans assist disaster managers, clinicians, and victims in coping with rapidly changing events. Long-term but easily adapted plans and risk reduction measures decrease the vulnerability of communities (Ahmed & Sugianto, 2009; Lettieri, Masella, & Radaelli, 2009).

Pre-disaster activities include assessing risks and taking administrative measures to prevent or reduce their impacts, zoning and building codes, vulnerability analysis, public education, development of new services and response plans, preparing resources, and training, to name a few. Mobile technologies with their ability to update information and gather feedback can assist with these activities.

Education is vital for disaster preparedness for both physicians and the public. Mobile technologies such as telemedicine and social networks are appropriate tools for this purpose. Social networks offer a way to engage with communities and bring resilience by raising public awareness about how to cope with and recover from disasters. For example, text messaging is a good method to alert target groups of health campaigns (Iwaya et al., 2013) and disseminate pre-disaster warnings. These and other mobile health technologies are particularly valuable for reaching rural communities (Eisenman et al., 2009; White, Plotnick, Kushma, & Hiltz, 2009).

To enhance community or national readiness, cloud computing and big data techniques can be utilised. These technologies can be used to assess and integrate national and local medical information and resources into a single information system. Such a system can then provide a single repository of data and information to determine disaster response capacities in a range of national and local medical environments. The system can also identify critical resources and report the whereabouts and availability of emergency medical supplies, their types and volume (Zhong et al., 2014). RFID and IoT sensors can track these resources automatically with minimal human intervention, can enhance task efficiency and accuracy, and can then share the information among all involved agencies.

To optimise future response missions, the created cloud repository can be integrated with Decision Support Systems (DSS) and EHRs. This integration offers a unified repository of patient data across all operators (AbuKhousa, Mohamed, & Al-Jaroodi, 2012) allowing customised regional services such as forecasting and tracking the progress of epidemic and pandemic diseases. Such a unified repository also would be a good platform to run different Artificial Intelligence (AI) algorithms and Machine Learning (ML) to detect any possible hidden trends.

EHRs are considered core healthcare systems. These systems improve daily healthcare delivery, as well as assist healthcare organisations to prepare better for disasters by making peoples' health backgrounds easily accessible by approved carers (Brown et al., 2007). More sophisticated mobile EHR systems linked to centralised big data repositories and supported by cloud computing and DSS are set to overcome the challenges of matching patient loads and needs with available hospital resources.

4.2.2 Disaster Response Applications

Disaster response includes actions taken during or immediately after the occurrence of a disaster to control and manage its impacts. The focus of response is on the deployment of resources and provision of emergency services to affected populations. Response services include saving lives, providing relative welfare, giving aid and assistance, and preventing or reducing the spread of the crisis impacts. These activities are conducted according to plans that aim at minimising the disaster's impacts on people, properties and environment (Ahmed & Sugianto, 2007; Altay & Green, 2006; Baldini et al., 2009).

Evacuation, sheltering, search and rescue, emergency relief, and damage control are crucial activities following the occurrence of a disaster. Often, the circumstances under which these activities are carried out change rapidly causing more pressure on response teams. Disaster response is a time-critical phase that demands access to reliable information in order to deliver life-saving services. In such scenarios, mobile technologies can facilitate the allocation of resources, assist with triage, and provide critical data on patients' medications, allergies, and pre-existing conditions.

Despite the imperative of disaster education and disaster medicine training for medical personnel (Ducharme, 2013; James et al., 2010), a great number of health practitioners do not receive this training (Walsh et al., 2012). To tackle these knowledge gaps, mobile health systems and telemedicine can be used to overcome this deficiency by supporting clinicians in the field (Blaya, Fraser, & Holt, 2010). In addition to alleviating time and space barriers, telehealth provides convenient access to expert advice (Sutjiredjeki et al., 2009).

To support disaster response teams and help affected communities, central authorities and decision makers need to communicate different types of information such as the number of casualties and the required and available medical resources. For example, IoT, RFID and sensor networks facilitate these tasks by automatically collecting and transmitting precise and real-time data to responders and other decision makers thereby helping them to make informed decisions (Petersen, Baccelli, Wählisch, Schmidt, & Schiller, 2015). As these technologies have embedded memory, they have the ability to collect and store data without relying on the network infrastructure. Collected data can be later uploaded when the broken connection is re-established.

RFID and IoT technologies can be utilised in identifying, mobilising, and dispatching disaster victims, rescue personnel, and medical resources (Chan, Killeen, Griswold, & Lenert, 2004; Shamdani & Nicolai, 2012), thus addressing issues of misidentification of patients and medications (Lahtela, 2009). This has a significant impact on patient safety in the context of disaster response. Paper triage which has several proven limitations (Fry & Lenert, 2005; Lenert, Palmer, Chan, & Rao, 2005) including inefficient information retrieval and poor saving mechanisms can be replaced by IoT and RFID technologies. When integrated with mobile health, these technologies can benefit providers' handoffs during triage (Callaway et al., 2012; Kyriacou, Pattichis, & Pattichis, 2009).

To overcome the issue of data silos, because of IoT and RFID, cloud services can be used to integrate and exchange fragmented data from disparate sources. The data then can rapidly be shared across multiple organisations in different geographical areas (AbuKhousa et al., 2012).

During disasters, medical staff deal with casualties who may include unconscious individuals, infant and children, or victims who cannot effectively communicate to give information about their medical status or their previous medical history (James & Walsh, 2011). In these situations, the ability to access patients' medical history and personal information can improve the quality of provided care as well as support the continuity of care.

Disaster response activities are prone to human errors. However, DSS(s) can assist with rapid and accurate decisions under conditions of uncertainty. These systems are efficient tools for coordinating operations and assisting the making of crucial decisions regarding task assignments (Thompson, Altay, Green III, & Lapetina, 2006). Moreover, DSS can facilitate the tasks of hospital-based providers by helping to make decisions regarding rapid transport of victims to the appropriate facility (Rüter, 2006), matching the number of inbound patients with availability i.e. number and type of hospital beds (Bradt, Abraham, & Franks, 2003), as well as prioritising victims for treatment (Fajardo & Oppus, 2010).

4.2.3 Post-Disaster Applications

Recovery refers to long-term activities performed after disasters to support systems, bring order to the disaster-stricken areas, restore the situation to normal, and stabilise or even improve the levels of normal condition (Ahmed & Sugianto, 2007; Lettieri et al., 2009). This stabilisation phase may last for quite a long time. Recovery includes reconstruction, rehabilitation, and performance assessment.

Monitoring the health condition of disaster-affected populations during recovery is of great importance albeit extremely challenging given the need to restore capacities and capabilities to pre-disaster levels. The ability of mobile systems to expedite information exchange eases pressure on healthcare systems and allows the monitoring process to proceed alongside the provision of normal health services.

Continuous monitoring of disaster casualties and people with long-term chronic diseases and mental patients can be supported by IoT technologies in the post-disaster phase (Tun, Madanian, & Mirza, 2020). Equipping patients with IoT devices or sensors reduces the necessity of hospitalisation since patients' vital signs can be monitored continuously in real-time and with minimum human intervention regardless of the geographical location of physicians and patients. This provides care for the patient while reducing the strain on the healthcare system. EHRs can be integrated with IoT sensors to incorporate monitored data into the patient's medical record thus facilitating future delivery of care if any emergency arises. EHRs can utilise mobile technologies to educate patients on public health (Brown et al., 2007) and promote health self-management (Archer, Fevrier-Thomas, Lokker, McKibbon, & Straus, 2011). Instead of physical consultation, patients can receive tele-consultation, tele-diagnosis, or tele-education in a preferred location and at a convenient time (Sutjiredjeki et al., 2009). These services have the potential to provide better healthcare when there is a lack of specialists or experts in disaster-stricken areas. Tele-health services are increasingly being used to reduce disruption in care (Vo, Brooks, Bourdeau, Farr, & Raimer, 2010) and to alleviate time and space barriers between healthcare providers and their patients (Sutjiredjeki et al., 2009).

5. DISCUSSION

In disasters, healthcare routine procedures are disrupted, and healthcare needs to shift quickly from routine activities and procedures and adjust to a status of great uncertainty. In such chaotic situations, decisions need to be taken in a short time and under stressful conditions that often include a shortage of medical resources including health personnel.

Information and communication technologies can significantly enhance the provision of disaster healthcare. Among these technologies, mobile applications play a central role in information gathering and exchange and communication due to ubiquity and ease of use. Interestingly, several mobile technologies such as EHRs and telemedicine can be applied in various DMC phases for both clinical and non-clinical purposes. In different phases of DMC, mobile devices (such as tablets) are becoming so powerful that they can support and link to different databases, enabling medical personnel and governments to get informed decisions. Furthermore, ubiquity and communication features of these devices support greater involvement and care for communities in rural areas or disadvantaged communities such as refugees, people with disabilities and mental health patients. Tablets and mobile phones facilitate the acquisition of up-to-date information from the authorities or seek mental health support. Non-clinical uses of mobile applications through social media, for instance, can facilitate communication and data sharing with outside-disaster sites for support purposes.

Integrating different technologies, where possible, often augment their impact. EHR and telemedicine integration provides a robust system that enables continuity of care in disaster recovery, regardless of patients' and physicians' geographical locations. Madanian and Parry (2019) propose a framework that integrates IoT, cloud computing, and big data to assist authorities in managing disasters. The framework suggests the use of IoT sensors in collecting disaster data which is then integrated and shared in a cloud repository that uses big data algorithms to detect and identify hidden trends. The output of such integration may provide healthcare risk analysis and forecasts that assist with disaster preparedness, response, and recovery. The outcome of integrating technologies may extend over all stages of the DMC. This can be seen in countries were information and communication technologies, including mobile technologies, were recently utilised to alleviate the COVID-19 crisis. Remote patient monitoring, providing test-results electronically, case management, contact tracing are some of the outcomes of integrating technologies.

During the lockdown period of COVID-19, mobile apps proved indispensable. While the golden rule during lockdown was to be socially distant, the recommendation was to make sure communities were still socially connected. This was made possible using mobile applications. People used mobile apps to communicate with the elderly to ensure that their mental health does not get negatively impacted by being kept distant from family members and friends. Families were allowed to communicate with their loved ones who were critically ill as nurses and critical care providers used iPads and mobile phones to avoid mental stress of their patients and their families.

A technological approach to information that assumes technology can solve all problems is known as *technocratic utopianism*. According to Davenport, Eccles, and Prusak (2009), '*no technology has yet convinced an unwilling manager to share information*'. Hence, information exchange as well as successful uptake of mobile applications should consider human factors especially in disaster situations where stress levels are high and the time to make critical decisions is scarce. Disaster responders often miss the opportunity to seek information from a reliable source due to lack of understanding about the nature of information owned by various agencies. To facilitate cross-agency information sharing in disasters, response agencies need to have trust in each other's abilities, resources and skills (IFRC, 2000). Such confidence requires the establishment of successful working relationships during peace time. Relationship building can be established formally or informally. Formally, disaster response agencies need to systematically encourage cross-agency information sharing. Education and training are essential means for the successful implementation of mobile technologies which rely primarily on efficient information sharing (Kotabe, Sakano, Sebayashi, & Komukai, 2014). An approach that aims at fostering understanding and information requirements of various disaster response agencies is crucial for ensuring appropriate development of mobile technologies.

6. CONCLUSION AND FUTURE WORK

Mobile technologies and their applications have the potential to bring several opportunities to disaster healthcare. In this chapter, the application of these technologies in the different phases of the disaster lifecycle are presented. To fully utilise these technologies human and operational aspects need to be considered.

A survey of clinical and communication applications identifies key factors that need to be recognised to exploit opportunities offered by information and communication technologies including the systematic and integrated approach to disaster healthcare across all stages of the disaster cycle. Integrated healthcare demands an interdisciplinary approach to information sharing in disasters. A golden opportunity lies in the establishment of the new discipline of disaster eHealth (DEH).

DEH can be seen as a discipline that lies at the intersection between disaster management, disaster medicine, and e-health. It refers to 'the application of information and e-health technologies in a disaster situation to restore and maintain the health of individuals to their pre-disaster levels' (Norris et al., 2015). The aims of DEH is to establish effective communication between disaster managers and disaster healthcare professionals through effective utilisation of e-health technologies. This integration of human capacities, medicine and technology has the potential to identify relevant information requirements of both sectors thus improving the quality of healthcare delivery in disasters. To appropriately and adequately identify information requirements, disaster stakeholders including emergency managers, disaster medicine specialists, the general public, victims, indigenous peoples, people with disabilities and refugees should be consulted.

Software development of mobile applications requires a needs-based approach rather than a technology approach. This refers to having a good understanding of what the audience users require in a given application. This is significantly important for usability aspects with regards to the needs of people with specific needs including the elderly and people with disabilities. For these applications proper requirement analysis and extra attention to interface and usability design are extremely important for the uptake of these technologies. These criteria are also important for disaster response applications as users may be working in austere environments that require them to wear gloves, for example. These considerations could be determinant to the acceptance and adoption of mobile applications by the public in general and disaster medicine specialists in specific.

Dependency on the network infrastructure or energy sources to power mobile devices is one of the barriers that may hinder their use in DMC. Although some technologies such as IoT and RFID have embedded power sources, the majority of mobile technologies are infrastructure-dependant. Solutions include using satellite communications or solar power as alternative energy sources. However, there exists a need to explore ways of providing access to mobile technologies when the infrastructure is damaged. Moreover, factors that impact successful implementation and uptake of mobile technologies require further research.

ACKNOWLEDGMENT

Part of this book chapter has been published as a PhD thesis.

Madanian, S. (2019). *Disaster e-Health Scope and the Role of RFID for Healthcare Purposes* (Doctoral thesis, Auckland University of Technology, Auckland, New Zealand). Retrieved from http://hdl.handle.net/10292/12813

REFERENCES

Abbas, R., & Norris, A. C. (2018). *Inter-agency communication and information exchange in disaster healthcare.* Paper presented at the 15th Information Systems for Crisis Response and Management, Rochester, NY. http://idl.iscram.org/files/reemabbas/2018/2160_ReemAbbas+TonyNorris2018.pdf

Abbas, R., Norris, T., Madanian, S., & Parry, D. (2016). *Disaster e-health and interagency communication in disaster healthcare: A suggested road map.* Paper presented at the Health Informatics New Zealand (HiNZ), Auckland, New Zealand. https://www.researchgate.net/publication/311404397_Disaster_E-Health_and_Interagency_Communication_in_Disaster_Healthcare_A_Suggested_Road_Map

AbuKhousa, E., Mohamed, N., & Al-Jaroodi, J. (2012). e-Health cloud: Opportunities and challenges. *Future Internet, 4*(3), 621–645. doi:10.3390/fi4030621

Ahmed, A., & Sugianto, L. F. (2007). *A 3-tier architecture for the adoption of RFID in emergency management.* Paper presented at the Proceedings of the International Conference on Business and Information 2007, Tokyo, Japan.

Ahmed, A., & Sugianto, L. F. (2009). RFID in emergency management. In J. Symonds, J. Ayoade, & D. Parry (Eds.), *Auto-identification and ubiquitous computing applications* (pp. 137–155). IGI Global. doi:10.4018/978-1-60566-298-5.ch008

Altay, N., & Green, W. G. III. (2006). OR/MS research in disaster operations management. *European Journal of Operational Research, 175*(1), 475–493. doi:10.1016/j.ejor.2005.05.016

Archer, N., Fevrier-Thomas, U., Lokker, C., McKibbon, K. A., & Straus, S. E. (2011). Personal health records: A scoping review. *Journal of the American Medical Informatics Association, 18*(4), 515–522. doi:10.1136/amiajnl-2011-000105 PMID:21672914

Ardalan, A., Masoomi, G., Goya, M., Ghaffari, M., Miadfar, J., Arvar, M., . . . Aghazadeh, M. (2009). Disaster health management: Iran's progress and challenges. *Iranian Journal of Public Health, 38*(1), 93-97. Retrieved from http://ijph.tums.ac.ir/index.php/ijph/article/view/2860

Bala, H., Venkatesh, V., Venkatraman, S., Bates, J., & Brown, S. H. (2009). Disaster response in health care: A design extension for enterprise data warehouse. *Communications of the ACM, 52*(1), 136–140. doi:10.1145/1435417.1435448

Baldini, G., Braun, M., Hess, E., Oliveri, F., & Seuschek, H. (2009). *The use of secure RFID to support the resolution of emergency crises.* Paper presented at the 43rd Annual 2009 International Carnahan Conference on Security Technology, Zurich, Switzerland. 10.1109/CCST.2009.5335517

Bengio, Y., Janda, R., Yu, Y. W., Ippolito, D., Jarvie, M., Pilat, D., Struck, B., Krastev, S., & Sharma, A. (2020). The need for privacy with public digital contact tracing during the COVID-19 pandemic. *The Lancet Digital Health, 2*(7), e342–e344. doi:10.1016/S2589-7500(20)30133-3 PMID:32835192

Bilham, R. (2010). Lessons from the Haiti earthquake. *Nature*, *463*(7283), 878–879. doi:10.1038/463878a PMID:20164905

Bissell, R. A. (2005). Public health and medicine in emergency management. In D. McEntire (Ed.), *Disciplines, Disasters, and Emergency Management*. FEMA, Emergency Management Institute.

Blaya, J. A., Fraser, H. S. F., & Holt, B. (2010). E-health technologies show promise in developing countries. *Health Affairs*, *29*(2), 244–251. doi:10.1377/hlthaff.2009.0894 PMID:20348068

Bradt, D. A., Abraham, K., & Franks, R. (2003). A strategic plan for disaster medicine in Australasia. *Emergency Medicine*, *15*(3), 271–282. doi:10.1046/j.1442-2026.2003.00445.x PMID:12786649

Brown, S. H., Fischetti, L. F., Graham, G., Bates, J., Lancaster, A. E., McDaniel, D., Gillon, J., Darbe, M., & Kolodner, R. M. (2007). Use of electronic health records in disaster response: The experience of Department of Veterans Affairs after Hurricane Katrina. *American Journal of Public Health*, *97*(Supplement_1), S136–S141. doi:10.2105/AJPH.2006.104943 PMID:17413082

Brunkard, J., Namulanda, G., & Ratard, R. (2008). Hurricane Katrina deaths, Louisiana, 2005. *Disaster Medicine and Public Health Preparedness*, *2*(4), 215–223. doi:10.1097/DMP.0b013e31818aaf55 PMID:18756175

Callaway, D. W., Peabody, C. R., Hoffman, A., Cote, E., Moulton, S., Baez, A. A., & Nathanson, L. (2012). Disaster mobile health technology: Lessons from Haiti. *Prehospital and Disaster Medicine*, *27*(02), 148–152. doi:10.1017/S1049023X12000441 PMID:22588429

Center for Disaster Philanthropy. (n.d.). *The disaster life cycle*. Retrieved from https://disasterphilanthropy.org/issue-insight/the-disaster-life-cycle/

Centre for Research on the Epidemiology of Disasters. (n.d.). *The international disaster database*. Retrieved from http://www.emdat.be/

Chan, T. C., Killeen, J., Griswold, W., & Lenert, L. (2004). Information technology and emergency medical care during disasters. *Academic Emergency Medicine*, *11*(11), 1229–1236. doi:10.1197/j.aem.2004.08.018 PMID:15528589

Chen, M., Gonzalez, S., Leung, V., Zhang, Q., & Li, M. (2010). A 2G-RFID-based e-healthcare system. *Wireless Communications, IEEE*, *17*(1), 37–43. doi:10.1109/MWC.2010.5416348

Cho, H., Ippolito, D., & Yu, Y. W. (2020). *Contact tracing mobile apps for COVID-19: Privacy considerations and related trade-offs*. Retrieved from https://arxiv.org/abs/2003.11511?utm_source=feedburner&utm_medium=feed&utm_campaign=Feed%253A+arxiv%252FQSXk+%2528ExcitingAds%2521+cs+updates+on+arXiv.org%2529

Cioca, M., & Cioca, L. I. (2010). Decision support systems used in disaster management. In C. S. Jao (Ed.), *Decision Support Systems*. INTECH. doi:10.5772/39452

Ciottone, G. R. (2006). *Disaster medicine*. Mosbey Elsevier.

Civaner, M. M., Vatansever, K., & Pala, K. (2017). Ethical problems in an era where disasters have become a part of daily life: A qualitative study of healthcare workers in Turkey. *PLoS One, 12*(3), e0174162. Advance online publication. doi:10.1371/journal.pone.0174162 PMID:28319151

Davenport, T., Eccles, R., & Prusak, L. (2009). Information politics. In D. A. Klein (Ed.), *The Strategic Management of Intellectual Capital*. Butterworth-Heinemann.

de Boer, J. (1995). An introduction to disaster medicine in Europe. *The Journal of Emergency Medicine, 13*(2), 211–216. doi:10.1016/0736-4679(94)00147-2 PMID:7775793

Ducharme, J. (2013). Best practices in emergency medicine: What we have to consider if we wish to get it right. *Clinical Governance: An International Journal, 18*(4), 315–324. doi:10.1108/CGIJ-04-2012-0013

Eisenman, D. P., Glik, D., Gonzalez, L., Maranon, R., Zhou, Q., Tseng, C. H., & Asch, S. M. (2009). Improving Latino disaster preparedness using social networks. *American Journal of Preventive Medicine, 37*(6), 512–517. doi:10.1016/j.amepre.2009.07.022 PMID:19944917

Endsley, M. R. (1988). Design and evaluation for situation awareness enhancement. *Proceedings of the Human Factors Society Annual Meeting, 32*(2), 97-101. 10.1177/154193128803200221

Fajardo, J. T. B., & Oppus, C. M. (2010). A mobile disaster management system using the android technology. *WSEAS Transactions on Communications, 9*(6), 343–353.

Findlay, S., Palma, S., & Milne, R. (2020). *Coronavirus contact-tracing apps struggle to make an impact*. Retrieved from https://www.ft.com/content/21e438a6-32f2-43b9-b843-61b819a427aa

Fry, E. A., & Lenert, L. A. (2005). *MASCAL: RFID tracking of patients, staff and equipment to enhance hospital response to mass casualty events*. Paper presented at the AMIA Annual Symposium Proceedings, Washington, DC.

Hamilton, J. (2003). An internet-based bar code tracking system: Coordination of confusion at mass casualty incidents. *Disaster Management & Response, 1*(1), 25–28. doi:10.1016/S1540-2487(03)70007-8 PMID:12688307

Harrison, L. (2015). *Social media: indispensable during disasters*. Retrieved from https://www.medscape.com/viewarticle/847183

Hirshberg, A., Holcomb, J. B., & Mattox, K. L. (2001). Hospital trauma care in multiple-casualty incidents: Acritical view. *Annals of Emergency Medicine, 37*(6), 647–652. doi:10.1067/mem.2001.115650 PMID:11385336

IFRC. (2000). *Disaster preparedness training programme: Improving coordination*. Retrieved from https://www.ifrc.org/Global/Impcoor.pdf

International Telecommunication Union. (2019). *The State of Broadband: Broadband as a Foundation for Sustainable Development*. Retrieved from https://www.itu.int/dms_pub/itu-s/opb/pol/S-POL-BROADBAND.20-2019-PDF-E.pdf

Iwaya, L. H., Gomes, M. A., Simplício, M. A., Carvalho, T. C., Dominicini, C. K., Sakuragui, R. R., Rebelo, M. S., Gutierrez, M. A., Näslund, M., & Håkansson, P. (2013). Mobile health in emerging countries: A survey of research initiatives in Brazil. *International Journal of Medical Informatics, 82*(5), 283–298. doi:10.1016/j.ijmedinf.2013.01.003 PMID:23410658

James, J. J., Benjamin, G. C., Burkle, F. M. Jr, Gebbie, K. M., Kelen, G., & Subbarao, I. (2010). Disaster medicine and public health preparedness: A discipline for all health professionals. *Disaster Medicine and Public Health Preparedness, 4*(02), 102–107. doi:10.1001/dmp.v4n2.hed10005 PMID:20526129

James, J. J., & Walsh, L. (2011). E-health in preparedness and response. *Disaster Medicine and Public Health Preparedness, 5*(04), 257–258. doi:10.1001/dmp.2011.84 PMID:22146662

Javed, Y., & Norris, T. (2012). Measuring shared and team situation awareness of emergency decision makers. *International Journal of Information Systems for Crisis Response and Management, 4*(4), 1–15. doi:10.4018/jiscrm.2012100101

Karami, A., Shah, V., Vaezi, R., & Bansal, A. (2019). Twitter speaks: A case of national disaster situational awareness. *Journal of Information Science, 46*(3), 313–324. doi:10.1177/0165551519828620

Kayyali, B., Knott, D., & Van Kuiken, S. (2013). The big-data revolution in US health care: Accelerating value and innovation. *McKinsey & Company, 2*(8), 1-13.

Khan, H., Vasilescu, L. G., & Khan, A. (2008). Disaster management cycle-a theoretical approach. *Journal of Management and Marketing, 6*(1), 43–50. http://www.mnmk.ro/documents/2008/2008-6.pdf

Khankeh, H. R., Khorasani-Zavareh, D., Johanson, E., Mohammadi, R., Ahmadi, F., & Mohammadi, R. (2011). Disaster health-related challenges and requirements: A grounded theory study in Iran. *Prehospital and Disaster Medicine, 26*(3), 151–158. doi:10.1017/S1049023X11006200 PMID:21929828

Kim, J., & Hastak, M. (2018a). Online human behaviors on social media during disaster responses. *The Journal of the NPS Center for Homeland Defense and Security, 14*, 7–8. https://www.hsaj.org/articles/14135

Kim, J., & Hastak, M. (2018b). Social network analysis: Characteristics of online social networks after a disaster. *International Journal of Information Management, 38*(1), 86–96. doi:10.1016/j.ijinfomgt.2017.08.003

Kirsch, T. D., & Hsu, E. B. (2008). Disaster medicine: What's the reality? *Disaster Medicine and Public Health Preparedness, 2*(1), 11–12. doi:10.1097/DMP.0b013e31816564ca PMID:18388650

Kotabe, S., Sakano, T., Sebayashi, K., & Komukai, T. (2014). Rapidly deployable phone service to counter catastrophic loss of telecommunication facilities. *NTT Technical Review, 12*(3), 1–11.

Kyriacou, E. C., Pattichis, C. S., & Pattichis, M. S. (2009). *An overview of recent health care support systems for eEmergency and mHealth applications.* Paper presented at the Annual International Conference of the IEEE in Engineering in Medicine and Biology Society, Minneapolis, MN. 10.1109/IEMBS.2009.5333913

Lahtela, A. (2009). *A short overview of the RFID technology in healthcare.* Paper presented at the 4th International Conference on Systems and Networks Communications, Porto, Portugal. 10.1109/ICSNC.2009.77

Lenert, L. A., Palmer, D. A., Chan, T. C., & Rao, R. (2005). An intelligent 802.11 triage tag for medical response to disasters. *AMIA Aannual Symposium Proceedings*.

Lettieri, E., Masella, C., & Radaelli, G. (2009). Disaster management: Findings from a systematic review. *Disaster Prevention and Management: An International Journal*, *18*(2), 117–136. doi:10.1108/09653560910953207

Luna, S., & Pennock, M. J. (2018). Social media applications and emergency management: A literature review and research agenda. *International Journal of Disaster Risk Reduction*, *28*, 565–577. doi:10.1016/j.ijdrr.2018.01.006

Madanian, S., & Parry, D. (2019). IoT, cloud computing and big data: Integrated framework for healthcare in disasters. *Studies in Health Technology and Informatics*, *264*, 998–1002. doi:10.3233hti190374 PMID:31438074

Maturana, C., Scott, R. E., & Palacios, M. (2012). e-Health and the haddon matrix: Identifying where and how e-health can assist in disaster managment. In M. J. F. Lievens (Ed.), Global Telemedicine and eHealth Updates: Knowledge Resources (Vol. 5, pp. 373-377). Grimbergen, Belgium: International Society for Telemedicine & eHealth (ISfTeH).

Middleton, S. E., Middleton, L., & Modafferi, S. (2014). Real-time crisis mapping of natural disasters using social media. *IEEE Intelligent Systems*, *29*(2), 9–17. doi:10.1109/MIS.2013.126

Nikbakhsh, E., & Farahani, R. Z. (2011). Humanitarian logistics planning in disaster relief operations. *Logistics Operations and Management: Concepts and Models, 291*.

Norris, A. C., Martinez, S., Labaka, L., Madanian, S., Gonzalez, J. J., & Parry, D. (2015). *Disaster e-Health: A new paradigm for collaborative healthcare in disasters*. Paper presented at the The 12th International Conference on Information Systems for Crisis Response and Management, Kristiansand, Norway. http://idl.iscram.org/files/acnorris/2015/1252_ACNorris_etal2015.pdf

Petersen, H., Baccelli, E., Wählisch, M., Schmidt, T. C., & Schiller, J. (2015). The role of the Internet of Things in network resilience. In R. Giaffreda, D. Cagáňová, Y. Li, R. Riggio, & A. Voisard (Eds.), *Internet of Things. IoT Infrastructures* (pp. 283–296). Springer International Publishing. doi:10.1007/978-3-319-19743-2_39

Russo, C. (2011). *Emergency communication remains a challenge ten years after 9/11*. Retrieved from http://www.homelandsecuritynewswire.com/emergency-communication-remains-challenge-ten-years-after-911

Rüter, A. (2006). *Disaster medicine-performance indicators, information support and documentation: A study of an evaluation tool*. Linköping University. Retrieved from http://swepub.kb.se/bib/swepub:oai:DiVA.org:liu-7990?tab2=abs&language=

Shamdani, A., & Nicolai, B. (2012). *Applications of RFID in incident management*. Paper presented at the The 7th International Multi-Conference on Computing in the Global Information Technology, Venice, Italy.

Sieben, C., Scott, R. E., & Palacios, M. (2012). e-Health and disaster management cycle. In M. Jordanova & F. Lievens (Eds.), Global Telemed eHealth Updates: Knowl Resources (pp. 368-372). Academic Press.

Singh, B., & Kaur, M. (2010). IT applications in healthcare. *Proceedings of the International Conference and Workshop on Emerging Trends in Technology.* 10.1145/1741906.1741940

Statista. (2020). *Number of smartphone users worldwide from 2016 to 2021.* Retrieved from https://www.statista.com/statistics/330695/number-of-smartphone-users-worldwide/

Su, T., Han, X., Chen, F., Du, Y., Zhang, H., Yin, J., Tan, X., Chang, W., Ding, Y., Han, Y., & Cao, G. (2013). Knowledge levels and training needs of disaster medicine among health professionals, medical students, and local residents in Shanghai, China. *PLoS One, 8*(6), e67041. doi:10.1371/journal.pone.0067041 PMID:23826190

Sutjiredjeki, E., Soegijoko, S., Mengko, T. L. R., Tjondronegoro, S., Astami, K., & Muhammad, H. U. (2009). *Application of a mobile telemedicine system with multi communication links for disaster reliefs in indonesia.* Paper presented at the World Congress on Medical Physics and Biomedical Engineering, Munich, Germany. 10.1007/978-3-642-03904-1_96

Tan, M. L., Prasanna, R., Stock, K., Hudson-Doyle, E., Leonard, G., & Johnston, D. (2017). Mobile applications in crisis informatics literature: A systematic review. *International Journal of Disaster Risk Reduction, 24*, 297–311. doi:10.1016/j.ijdrr.2017.06.009

Telford, J., & Cosgrave, J. (2007). The international humanitarian system and the 2004 Indian Ocean earthquake and tsunamis. *Disasters, 31*(1), 1–28. doi:10.1111/j.1467-7717.2007.00337.x PMID:17367371

Thompson, S., Altay, N., Green, W. G. III, & Lapetina, J. (2006). Improving disaster response efforts with decision support systems. *International Journal of Emergency Management, 3*(4), 250–263. doi:10.1504/IJEM.2006.011295

Trzeciak, S., & Rivers, E. P. (2003). Emergency department overcrowding in the United States: An emerging threat to patient safety and public health. *Emergency Medicine Journal, 20*(5), 402–405. doi:10.1136/emj.20.5.402 PMID:12954674

Tun, S. Y. Y., Madanian, S., & Mirza, F. (2020). Internet of things (IoT) applications for elderly care: A reflective review. *Aging Clinical and Experimental Research.* Advance online publication. doi:10.100740520-020-01545-9 PMID:32277435

Turcu, C., & Popa, V. (2009). *An RFID-based system for emergency health care services.* Paper presented at the International Conference on Advanced Information Networking and Applications Workshops, Bradford, UK. 10.1109/WAINA.2009.107

TVNZ. (2020). *World Health Organisation praises New Zealand for its 'very systematic' response to Covid-19 pandemic.* Retrieved from https://www.tvnz.co.nz/one-news/new-zealand/world-health-organisation-praises-new-zealand-its-very-systematic-response-covid-19-pandemic

Underwood, S. (2010). Improving disaster management. *Communications of the ACM, 53*(2), 18–20. doi:10.1145/1646353.1646362

United Nations. (2007). *Hyogo framework for action 2005-2015: Building the resilience of nations and communities to disasters*. Retrieved from https://www.unisdr.org/files/1037_hyogoframeworkforaction english.pdf

United Nations. (2015). *Sendai framework for disaster risk reduction 2015-2030*. Retrieved from https://www.unisdr.org/files/43291_sendaiframeworkfordrren.pdf

Vo, A. H., Brooks, G. B., Bourdeau, M., Farr, R., & Raimer, B. G. (2010). University of Texas Medical Branch telemedicine disaster response and recovery: Lessons learned from hurricane Ike. *Telemedicine Journal and e-Health*, *16*(5), 627–633. doi:10.1089/tmj.2009.0162 PMID:20575732

Waeckerle, J. F., Lillibridge, S. R., Burkle, F. M. Jr, & Noji, E. K. (1994). Disaster medicine: Challenges for today. *Annals of Emergency Medicine*, *23*(4), 715–718. doi:10.1016/S0196-0644(94)70304-3 PMID:8161037

Walsh, L., Subbarao, I., Gebbie, K., Schor, K. W., Lyznicki, J., Strauss-Riggs, K., ... James, J. J. (2012). Core competencies for disaster medicine and public health. *Disaster Medicine and Public Health Preparedness*, *6*(1), 44–52. doi:10.1001/dmp.2012.4 PMID:22490936

White, C., Plotnick, L., Kushma, J., Hiltz, S. R., & Turoff, M. (2009). An online social network for emergency management. *International Journal of Emergency Management*, *6*(3), 369–382. doi:10.1504/IJEM.2009.031572

WHO. (2010). *Hospitals must be protected during natural disasters*. Retrieved from https://www.who.int/news-room/detail/11-12-2010-hospitals-must-be-protected-during-natural-disasters

Wilson, E. V., Wang, W., & Sheetz, S. D. (2014). Underpinning a guiding theory of patient-centered e-health. communications of the association for information systems. *Communications of the Association for Information Systems*, *34*. Advance online publication. doi:10.17705/1CAIS.03416

World Food Programme. (2016). *Mobile vulnerability analysis and mapping (mVAM)*. Retrieved from https://www.wfp.org/publications/2016-mobile-vulnerability-analysis-mapping-mvam

Yang, J., Lee, J., Rao, A., & Touqan, N. (2009). Interorganizational communications in disaster management. In V. Weerakkody, M. Janssen, & Y. Dwivedi (Eds.), *Handbook of Research on ICT-Enabled Transformational Government: A Global Perspective* (pp. 240–257). IGI Global. doi:10.4018/978-1-60566-390-6.ch013

Yin, J., Karimi, S., Lampert, A., Cameron, M., Robinson, B., & Power, R. (2015). *Using social media to enhance emergency situation awareness*. Paper presented at the 24th International Joint Conference on Artificial Intelligence, Buenos Aires, Argentina.

Yoo, T. (2018). *4 ways technology can help us respond to disasters*. Retrieved from https://www.weforum.org/agenda/2018/01/4-ways-technology-can-play-a-critical-role-in-disaster-response/

Zhong, S., Clark, M., Hou, X.-Y., Zang, Y., & FitzGerald, G. (2014). Progress and challenges of disaster health management in China: A scoping review. *Global Health Action*, *7*(1), 24986. doi:10.3402/gha.v7.24986 PMID:25215910

Chapter 13
Modern Healthcare With Wearable Sensors and Wireless Technology

Anitha Mary
Karunya University, India

Jegan R.
ⓘD https://orcid.org/0000-0001-6115-3455
Karunya Institute of Technology and Sciences, India

Suganthi Evangeline
Karunya Institute of Technology and Sciences, India

ABSTRACT

In today's world, people are most concerned about their health and safe living especially bed ridden people needing extensive care and assistance. A strict routine has to be followed by the patients after operation. Wearable sensors play an important role in monitoring physiological signals for the patient at home. With wireless technology, these physiological parameters can be monitored continuously. Also, the medical staffs and doctors are given immediate warning and causality services can be provided as early as possible. This chapter addresses the importance of wireless technology in healthcare sector.

1. PATIENT FALL MONITORING SYSTEM

Elderly people are subjected to encounter fall frequently. It is the most significant cause of injury. These ultimately leads to the cause of many disabling fractures that could eventually leads to death and left with complications (NIS Senior Health 2013), such as infection or pneumonia. If proper treatment is not provided then it leads to the consequences of serious conditions. By reducing the delay in assisting and treatment such consequences can be minimized (Frank et.al., 2012). The unexpected human fall is detected by the 3-axis MEMS accelerometer. The principle behind this work is to detect the changes in

DOI: 10.4018/978-1-5225-6067-8.ch013

the human position and the motion using an analogue sensor, which tracks the acceleration change in three orthogonal directions. When the fall is detected, the exact fall location with the latitude and longitude values are provided to the end user using wireless technology such as Global Positioning System (GPS) (Lord et.al., 2006).

1.1 Methodology

Figure 1. Block diagram for patient fall monitoring system

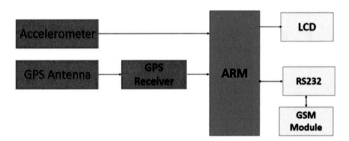

The prototype developed shown in Figure 1 consists of a set of biomedical sensor attached to the body of the person whose health condition is to be monitored. In this work, three axis accelerometer are used to detect the fall of the person. These sensors are connected to LPC2148 Advanced RISC Machine (ARM) micro controller. The microcontroller receives the signals from the sensors and processes the data and checks for the condition of the person. If the condition is normal then the microcontroller keeps on repeating the same process of receiving the data from the sensors and monitoring the position of the person. Whenever the condition steps out the normal range it checks for two or more values, if still the same condition prevails microcontroller sends alert messages to the care takers and concerned health care professionals about the unusual health condition of the person. Once doctor receives message and immediate response can be provided to the affected person. The SMS is sent in response to the person in need of help through the GSM modem which receives message and medicine name is displayed on LCD connected to controller through port pins.

1.2 ARM LPC2148 Microcontroller

NXP Semiconductors (formerly Philips Semiconductors) designed a 32 bit microcontroller grouped under LPC series. It has the CPU with emulation and debugging support and also with In-circuit programming features which supports 32 kB to 512 kB high speed flash memory. The microcontroller used in the prototype is with 128 bit wide memory interface with pipelined architecture which enables faster code execution. There is an alternative instruction set to ARM 32 bit is Thumb 16 bit which is ideal for critical code size applications that reduces code by more than 30% with minimal performance penalty (NXP Semiconductors 2011).

Each microcontroller unit consists of the processor core which is the heart of the core, memories includes static RAM (SRAM) memory, flash memory. In some higher applications cache memory is also used for storage purposed. It also support serial communications interfaces ranging from a Universal Serial Bus (USB) 2.0 Full-speed device, multiple Universal Asynchronous Receiver and Transmitter (UART),

Serial Peripheral Interface (SPI), Synchronous serial port (SSP) to Inter Integrated Circuit (I2C) and on-chip SRAM of 8 kB up to 40 kB. These added interface enables the ARM based products well suited for the applications in networking and also in imaging. Advanced ARM machined are providing both with large buffer size and high processing power. All ARM based microcontrollers are provided with 32-bit timers, 10-bit ADC/DAC, Real Time Clock (RTC). With the help of 45 fast GPIO lines with external interrupt pins, makes the ARM based controller suitable for industrial control and medical systems.

1.3 ADXL 335 Tri Axial Accelerometer

ADXL335 is a 3-axis accelerometer provided with signal conditioned voltage outputs. It is known for the compactness and it consumes less power. It is used to measure the acceleration with the full-scale range of ± 3 g. It can be used to measure both static and dynamic acceleration such as tilt-sensing, acceleration resulting from motion, shock, or vibration (Analog devices 2009). It contains a poly-silicon

Figure 2. ADXL335 accelerometer sensor

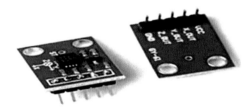

Figure 3. Sensor interfacing with LPC2148 using PROTEUS Simulation Environment

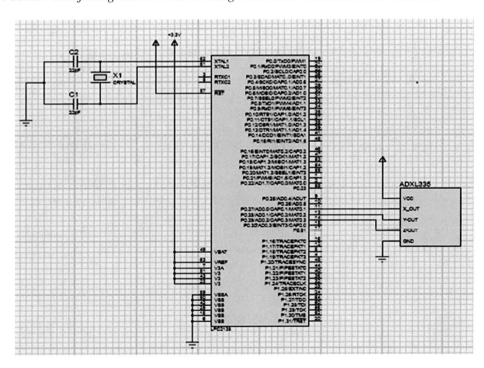

surface-micro machined sensor and signal conditioning circuitry which enable to implement open-loop acceleration measurement architecture. The changes of acceleration in 3 axes are monitored continuously and the output signals are directly proportional to acceleration. When the changes in acceleration is exceeding the threshold values, it is considered as fall. Figure 2 shows the ADLX335 accelerometer sensor and Figure 3 Sensor Interfacing with LPC2148 using PROTEUS Simulation Environment.

1.4 Global Positioning System

The Global Positioning System (GPS) is capable of giving the location and time information irrespective of climatic conditions anywhere on the earth. It is possible with the help of the signals it receives from the unobstructed line of sight from three or more GPS satellites. The system can be employed and it can used in defence, social and commercial applications. The communication pattern used by GPS is serial mode in which the location of the person is sent to the concerned care taker. According to National Marine Electronics Association (NMEA) standards, these serial data are send (US Environmental Protection agency 2015).

The first six bytes of the data received from GPS module is decoded using online decoder and it is further compared with the pre-stored string and if matched then only the data is further accounted. If not, the process is repeated again due to error in the message reception. The GPS is used to find the latitude and longitude of the person's location. These data are received by the processing unit through MAX 232 serial I/O module and displayed on LCD or transmits required data to mobile phones through GSM.

1.5 Global System for Mobile Communications (GSM)

European Telecommunications Standards Institute (ETSI) developed GSM (Global System for Mobile Communications) standard which defines the protocols for second-generation (2G) digital cellular networks. The GSM modems are most frequently used to provide mobile internet connectivity, many of them can also be used for sending and receiving SMS and MMS messages (European Standard 2001). Computers use AT commands to control modems. The various merits of using AT commands such as it is used to send SMS from SIM300 GSM module, delete a SMS from inbox, receive an incoming call, dialling a new number from SIM300, hanging up a call. GSM modems also support an extended set of AT commands.

1.6 Interfacing ADXL335 Accelerometer Sensor With LPC2148 Microcontroller

The ARM7 LPC2148 uses three channels of ADC for reading X, Y and Z axis from ADXL335. The output of the accelerometer is sent to the ADC channel resulting in the digitized form of 10 bit representation. The digital output of ADC is converted into voltage by a formula

$$Output(V) = Output(digital) * \frac{33}{1023} \tag{1}$$

The Co-ordinates values are displayed on LCD and also it is sent to the mobile phones of the care taker/ relatives of the fallen person using GSM as Short message Service (SMS).The location of the human fall is determined using GPS.

1.7 Calibration

In LPC2148 has 10 bit ADC

$$Step\ size = \frac{V_{ref}}{2^{10}} \tag{2}$$

where,

V_{ref} – used to detect step size

$$D_{OUT} = \frac{V_{input}}{Step\ size} \tag{3}$$

where,

D_{OUT} – Decimal output digital data

V_{input} – Analog input voltage

Table 1 summarises the zero bias values and its equivalent voltage levels given to analog to digital converting unit and Table 2 summarizes the calculated digital value for various g ranges. The experiment by interfacing tri axis accelerometer with ARM microcontroller is conducted by varying its axis position in order to find the threshold value. The threshold values for different types of fall has been recorded and tabulated in Table 3.

Table 1. Zero bias level of X, Y, and Z axis

Zero g BIAS LEVEL(RATIOMETRIC)	CONDITIONS	MIN	TYP	MAX	UNIT
X_{OUT} , Y_{OUT}	3V	1.35	1.5	1.65	V
Z_{OUT}	3V	1.2	1.5	1.8	V
Offset vs Temperature			±1		mg/°c

Table 2. Calibration of ADXL335

	RANGE(g)	VOLTAGE	ADC RANGE	ADC VALUE
	0	1.35		1A3
	1.2	1.62		1F6
	1.5	2.02		273
ADXL335	1.8	2.43	0-3.3V	2F2
	2	2.70		346
	2.2	2.97		399
	2.4	3.04		3ED

Table 3. Threshold value for ADXL335

POSITION	X-AXIS	Y-AXIS	Z-AXIS
NORMAL	0.319	1.274	1.650
FORWARD FALL	0.322	1.687	1.970
BACKWARD FALL	0.319	1.487	1.380
LEFT SIDE FALL	0.312	1.690	1.650
RIGHT SIDE FALL	0.325	1.512	1.85

By comparing all the values, we have set the threshold values as

X=0.322V, Y=1.320V, Z=1.700V

1.8 Interfacing GPS and GSM With LPC2148

Figure 4 shows how to interface GPS and GSM to LPC2148 microcontroller. GSM and GPS is connected ARM7 LPC2148 through UART0. In the place of COM2 in Figure 4 either GPS or GSM can be connected. Text message may be sent through the modem by interfacing only three signals viz., TX, RX and GND. GPS connection requires only TX and GND .The transmitter of GPS is connected to the receiver of UART0. GPS transmits the latitude and longitude and the data is received shown in Figure 5. Then GSM modem sends SMS message which contains the latitude and longitude value in text mode.

Figure 4. Circuit diagram to interface GPS and GSM with LPC2148

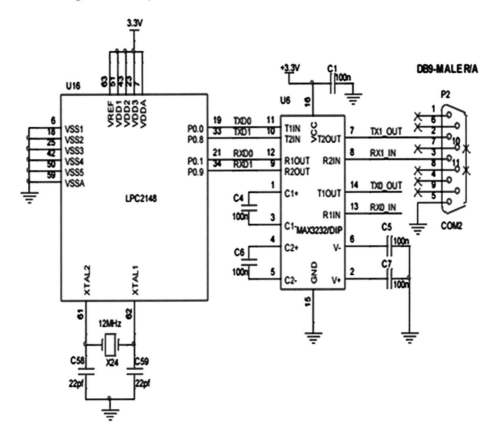

Figure 5. Alert messages for fall detection

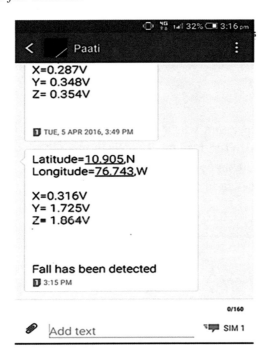

2. MONITORING OF PATIENT BODY TEMPERATURE

The most predominant symptom of any infection of foreign objects is the rise of temperature. It is one of the main indication which is used to detect any symptoms related to stress which ultimately leads to severe health conditions like stroke, heart attack. The measurement of body temperature is extremely useful for determining their physiological conditions as well as for other things such as activity classification or even harvesting energy from body heat (Aminian et.al., 2013). The main aim of the work is to monitor the temperature of human and update in cloud. This work will create a great impact to analyse the person's body temperature over a period of time. This system will enable the physicians to come to a conclusion of diagnostics and also they will be virtually connected with the patients. On the other hand it is of wearable kind and it is possible to take it anywhere, anytime (Subhas Chandra Mukhopadhyay 2015).

2.1 Methodology

In order to measure the body temperature of an individual, the wearable device is connected to the person's wrist or any other comfortable part in which the thermistor is in contact with the body such that the temperature would be monitored and sent to the micro controller and from the microcontroller to the server through the IOT (The temperature is monitored on the website as shown in Figure 6. The doctor gets an access to the patient's temperature and ensures the requirements are given accordingly as per the schedule (Aruna Devi et.al., 2016).

Figure 6. Block diagram of the system

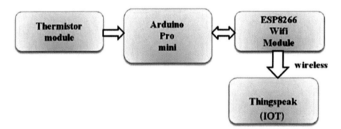

To build the wearable temperature sensor module, the components are used such as thermistor, arduino pro mini and ESP8266 Wi-Fi module. The Wi-Fi module is connected to internet. When the thermistor detect the temperature and send the data to thingspeak and it save the value for future use. The interfacing diagram is shown in Figure 7.

Figure 7. Circuit diagram for interfacing Wi-Fi module with microcontroller

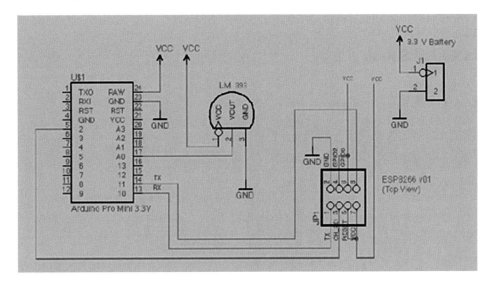

2.2 ESP8266 Wifi Module

It is a low cost Wi-Fi module with full TCP/IP (Transmission Control Protocol/Internet Protocol) stack and CPU (Central Processing Unit) which allows TCP/IP communication possible between microcontrollers to a Wi-Fi network using Hayes-style commands. The flash memory capacity is 1 Mb. It is low cost and can be useful for many Wi-Fi applications (Ada-fruit 2015).

2.3 ATmega328 Microcontroller

The Arduino microcontroller board is based on the ATmega328 architecture. It has Harvard architecture with memory capability of 32K flash memory, 2K SRAM data memory and 1024 bytes of EEPROM. Additional features includes 32 8- bit general purpose registers, 3 timer/counters, 6 channel 10-bit ADC, 14 digital input/output pins, 6 analogue inputs. The operating voltage is between 1.8-5.5 volts (Atmel 2016).

2.4 LM393-Thermitor Module

The thermistor module is used to detect the temperature change and it works like dual differential comparator. It has advantages like it has low operating voltage, consumes less power and compactness are the primary specifications in circuit design for portable consumer products (On semiconductor 2016).

2.5 Software Module- Thingspeak

Thingspeak is an open source Internet of Things (IOT) application uses HTTP protocol over Internet. It is mainly used to update the measured sensor values at regular interval of time. It has the features of collecting and sharing data from private channels. It involves MATLAB support for analysis and visualisations. It also responsible for creating alerts, event scheduling, apps integration and also it has wide community support (Kyriazis, D. et al. 2013).

2.6 Experimental Set-up

Figure 8. Experimental setup for patient body temperature measurement system

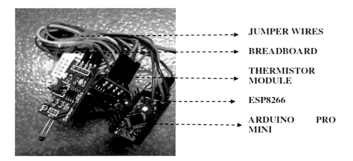

Figure 8 shows the Experimental setup for patient body temperature measurement system. ESP8266 is configured using AT commands by setting to preferred mode for communication. The thermistor sense the temperature and sends to microcontroller, it is responsible of converting into 3 different parameter i.e. Kelvin, Fahrenheit, Celsius. The measured temperature values are send to IOT by initially creating a webserver. It is done by connecting ESP8266 and then type the IP address in the webpage the output will be displayed. To access the data from internet the slight change is to be done in configuration. ESP8266 is configured by checking its TCP/IP with username and password, now this module is configured and connected to internet.

2.7 Results and Discussion

The wearable temperature monitoring experiment set up has been verified and results are sent to cloud. The concerned person can able to get the result anywhere using intranet and internet. The temperature values are expressed both in Celsius and also in Fahrenheit. Figure 9 shows the Intranet results of body temperature and it is shown in both kelvin and Frahenheit and Figure 10 shows the temperature measurement in Thingspeak.

Figure 9. Intranet results of body temperature

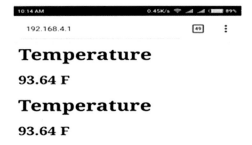

Figure 10. Body temperature shown in Thingspeak

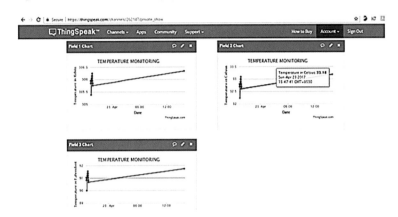

3. VITAL PARAMETER MEASUREMENT USING PPG SIGNAL

3.1 Significance of Remote Patient Monitoring

Remote Patient Monitoring (RPM) allows the continuous remote monitoring of bio signals for elderly peoples, patients having seizures, cardiac diseases, with high blood pressure, high blood sugar etc., without disturbing their personal life. It helps in 24*7 monitoring of patients which helps the physicians for better diagnostics. It allows the patients to be monitored outside clinical setting, even allowing them at their own home. RPM helps in providing better monitoring for antenatal care and even post-operative monitoring. Wireless transmission of the bio-monitoring signals was performed by means of the Bluetooth technology and other technologies(Chen et.al., 2012), developed for cable replacement when connecting devices still maintain a high level of security. However, the wire connection between the recording sites and the processing unit may disturb subject's daily activities (Vaidehi et.al., 2013). In order to have a continuous data acquisition and monitoring without any disturbances we use Radio Frequency (RF) connectivity based wireless transmission of PPG data (Perkins et.al., 2009). Through these data values we could calculate the Heart rate, Respiratory rate and can measure various other parameters (Klingeberg and Schilling 2012, carlos et.al., 2013, hadjidj et.al., 2013).

3.2 Importance of PPG Signal

The word plethysmograph is a combination of two ancient Greek words 'plethysmos' which means increase (Shelley 2007) and 'graph' which is the word for write (Alnaeb et.al., 2007), and is an instrument mainly used to determine and register the variations in blood volume or blood flow in the body which occur with each heartbeat. Various types of plethysmograph exist, and each of them measures the changes in blood volume in a different manner with a specific transducer and has certain applications (Cheang et.al., 2003). It uses a probe which contains a light source and a detector to detect cardio-vascular pulse wave that propagates through the body. The PPG signal reflects the blood movement in the vessel, which goes from the heart to the fingertips and toes through the blood vessels in a wave-like motion (Tokutaka 2009). It is an optical measurement technique that uses an invisible infrared light sent into the tissue and the amount of the backscattered light corresponds with the variation of the blood volume (Alnaeb et.al.,

185

2007). Hertzman was the first to find a relationship between the intensity of backscattered light and blood volume in 1938 (Hertzman 1938). The low-cost and simplicity of this optical based technology could offer significant benefits to healthcare (e.g. in primary care where non-invasive, accurate and simple-to-use diagnostic techniques are desirable). Further development of PPG could place this methodology among other tools used in the management of vascular disease (Elgendi et.al., 2012).

3.3 Principle Behind PPG Sensor

Figure 11. PPG sensor

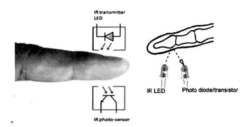

The photoplethysmogram sensor consist of an infrared light source (typically a photodiode emitting light at a wavelength of around 900 nm) and a photo detector (phototransistor) as shown in Figure 11. The light source is used to illuminate the tissue (e.g. skin) and a photo detector is used to measure the small variations in light intensity associated with changes in the blood vessels volume. It gives a voltage signal, which is proportional to the amount of blood present in the blood vessels. This type of sensors gives only a relative measurement of the blood volumetric changes and it cannot quantify the amount of blood (Tamura 2014).

Figure 12. PPG pulse waveform

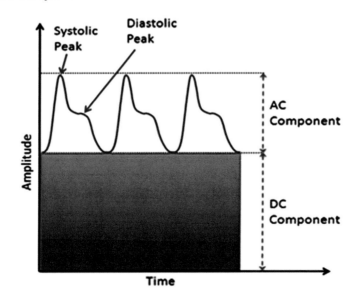

Most illuminated constituents, such as bone, muscle, venous blood, and various other cellular structures, absorb a constant amount of light, since their volumes and densities do not change over short periods of time. The volume of the arterial blood, however, is modulated by the beating of the heart. Each time the heart contracts, an additional bolus of blood are forced through the arterial pathways. With this variation in arterial volume comes a proportional variation in light absorption that can be measured by an optical sensor (Sandeep et.al.,2014). An increase in arterial blood volume causes a corresponding decrease in the amount of light that reaches the photo detector. The amount of light absorbed by the tissues contains two significant aspects, as shown in Figure 12. The first is the constant absorbance, or DC component, influenced by the nonvascular tissues and residual arterial and venous blood volumes. The second is a modulated absorbance, or AC component, caused by the variations in arterial blood volume. Together, they affect the amount of light that illuminates the photo detector to produce a pulsatile waveform (Rajasekaran et.al., 2016, Rajasekararn 2018)

3.4 Heart Rate Measurement Using PPG Signal With Wireless Technology

Figure 13. Block diagram for heart rate measurement system using PPG sensor

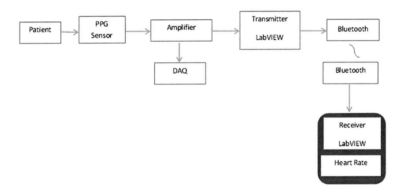

Figure 13 shows the Block diagram of heart rate measurement system using PPG Signal. The PPG from the patient is obtained using the sensors. The electrode gel is used for obtaining better contact between the electrode and the patient. The Bio-Kit physionet is used as a power supply for the Bio-Kit PPG amplifier. The Bio-Kit PPG amplifier is connected to Data Acquisition (DAQ) device. The ports in the DAQ are made to acquire the signal using the connectors and it is sent to the system. LabVIEW software is used for displaying and processing of PPG. LabVIEW program is given such that the detection of Heart rate from PPG is obtained and it is made to display whether the patient is normal or abnormal. The measured Heart rate can sent to the other system using Bluetooth module. The Bluetooth module transmits the patient Heart rate with the patient name, ward name and also displays whether the patient is abnormal i.e. Tachycardia or Bradycardia. Using Bluetooth module the physician can receive the message in the other computer displaying if the condition is abnormal (Rajasekaran et.al., 2015)

3.5 Experimental Setup

Figure 14. Experimental setup for heart rate measurement using PPG signal with Bluetooth technology

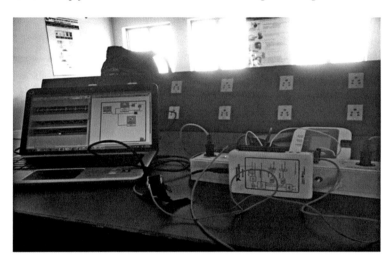

The PPG signal is obtained using PPG sensor. The obtained PPG is made to process using the Lab-VIEW software. The Heart rate is obtained and the detection of the abnormal signals like Bradycardia and Tachycardia are found. The signal obtains the Heart rate based on the threshold peak detector in the PPG signal. The result is obtained from LabVIEW is by setting an alarm for the abnormal signal based on Heart rate. The heart rate from PPG is transmitted through the Bluetooth module. Thus the patient's data is transmitted and received using Bluetooth module. Using LabVIEW makes the user to understand visually also, with the help of LabVIEW the person at the client can also visualize the same information as that of server as shown in Figure 15. The PPG data available in the server side can reach out client and its front panel is shown in Figure 16

Figure 15. Front panel of server

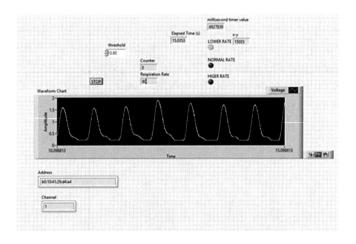

Figure 16. Front panel of client

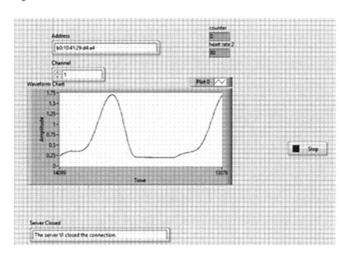

4. OXYGEN SATURATION MEASUREMENT USING PPG SIGNAL

Measuring to an arterial pressure waveform complete with dichroitic oxygen saturation level is an important part in monitoring patient's health condition. This is commonly monitored by a pulse oximeter, which has been widely adopted around the world as a standard measure during anesthesia, neonatal care and post-operative recovery. Measuring oxygen level continuously is very important for aged people, pregnant women and in many other critical situations. Modern pulse oximeter devices aim to measure the arterial oxygen saturation of the blood (SaO2). This measurement is denoted as SpO2. The aim of modern device manufacturers is to achieve the best correlation between the measured SpO2 and the actual SaO2 during the normal range of operating conditions (Addison 2004). The photo plethysmogram (PPG) signal bears a strong resemblance notch. The pulse oximeter works in either transmittance or reflectance mode by shining two wavelengths of light, red and infrared, through an appropriate part of the body and collecting the reflected or transmitted light via a photodetector. The red (660nm) and the IR PPG (940nm) signals are detected by the photodiode and its output is converted to voltage by a trans-impedance amplifying circuit, and is given to the Data Acquisition System after appropriate amplification. The acquired analogue signals are taken into the LabVIEW platform which hosts SpO2 on a real time basis. During systole, the heart pumps out the blood therefore, the arteries contain more blood than during diastole. This causes existence of more light absorbing components (Hb and HbO2) to exist in blood during systole. Due to the pulsatile nature of blood, the output of the photo detector contains an AC component. It also contains a large DC component caused by constant light absorption of venous blood, tissue, bone etc. However, signal manipulation is easier when the output of the photo detector is transformed to voltage. Therefore the ratio R is calculated in terms of voltage, not intensity. The photo detector produces a current signal which is proportional to the light intensity transmitted through finger from LEDs. The current signal produced by the photodiode can be converted to voltage signal at the output node of the trans-impedance amplifier. Photodiodes are used for light detection, conversion, and measurement.

4.2 SpO₂ Calculation

Figure 17. Block diagram for SpO2 measurement

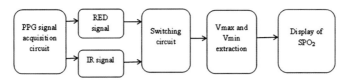

Figure 17 explains the SpO2 Calculation. The signals are first fed to the SpO2 program which calculates the saturation of oxygen in blood. First the maximum and minimum peaks of the PPG signal were found. Using these values SpO2 was calculated. The normal range of PPG signal is 0.5 to 5 Hz. So the high frequency noise can be removed by using a low pass filter with cut off frequency 5 Hz. For calculation of SpO2, the Vmax and Vmin components of both red and IR signals are extracted

5. HEART RATE MEASUREMENT USING ECG SIGNAL

5.1 Monitoring of ECG Signal Over Wireless Transmission

Figure 18. System architecture of remote monitoring

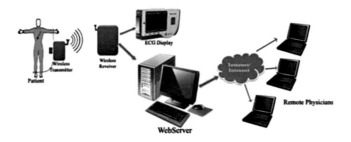

The system shown in Figure 18 makes use of a standard ECG amplifier to acquire the ECG signal from patient. This acquired analogue signal converted to digital and is transmitted wirelessly in licensed health-care spectrum to the nearby fixed receiver. The receiver will reproduce the same analogue waveform from the transmitter and is given to the ECG display. The wireless transceiver is enough powerful for transmitting the signal to nearby monitoring room and allows monitoring without disturbing the patient For RPM, at the receiver end, a PC based web server is installed which can publish the received signal on a webpage which allows the real-time monitoring of patient through Internet/Intranet. Thus RPM can be used to monitor a patient even outside the clinical settings. It allows the patients to be with their loved ones at their own homes while being monitored.

Electrocardiogram (ECG) is used to measure the heart's electrical conduction system. It picks up electrical impulses generated by the polarization and depolarization of cardiac tissue and translates into a waveform. ECG is a trans- thoracic interpretation of the electrical activity of the heart over a period of time, as detected by electrodes attached to the surface of the skin and recorded by a device external to the body. The recording produced by this non-invasive procedure is termed an electrocardiogram. The waveform is then used to measure the rate and regularity of heartbeats, as well as the size and position of the chambers, the presence of any damage to the heart, and the effects of drugs or devices used to regulate the heart, such as a pacemaker (Page et.al.,2014). Figure 19 shows the Block diagram of heart rate measurement using ECG signal. The ECG from the patient is obtained using the electrodes. The electrodes are of three lead and the ring type of electrode is used. The electrode gel is used for obtaining better contact between the electrode and the patient. LabVIEW program is given such that the detection of Heart rate from ECG is obtained and it is made to display whether the patient is normal or abnormal. The obtained Heart rate is sent to the physician mobile using Bluetooth module. The conditions for Heart Arrhythmia is that, if the Heart rate is above 150bpm then it is Tachycardia, if the Heart rate is less than 60bpm it is Bradycardia and if the Heart rate is above 150bpm it is Atrial Flutter.

Figure 19. Block diagram of heart rate measurement using ECG signal

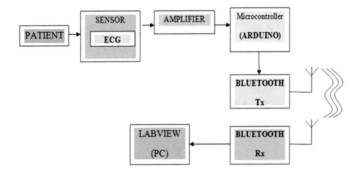

Figure 20. Experimental setup for heart rate measurement system

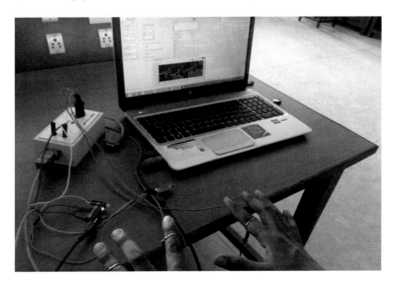

Figure 20 shows the Experimental Setup for heart rate measurement system. By using the LabVIEW, ECG signal is acquired and processed by placing ring electrodes on the finger and monitored continuously to detect abnormal alterations in the heart rate at an early stage.

5.2 Results and Discussion

The signal acquisition is done by real time signal from patient using the electrodes and it is implemented using LabVIEW. The acquired signal is then made to analyze the signals and distinguish whether the obtained signal is a normal signal or Tachycardic or Brady cardiac signal. If the signal that is obtained is an abnormal signal, then an alarm is set to indicate the patient with abnormal ECG. The type of ECG is obtained using the abnormality in heart rate. The ECG heart rate detection is done by detecting the baseline drift estimation to eliminate the signal from noise. The heart rate is detected using the R-R peaks from the Baseline Drift Elimination signal. The output is shown in the Figure 21.

Figure 21. Output showing the front panel using LabVIEW

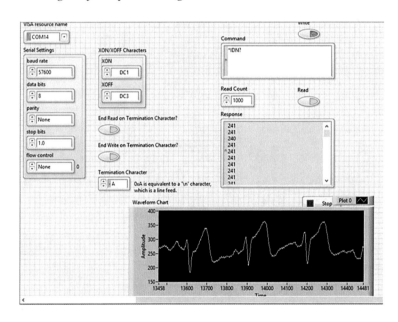

The real time signal is read in LabVIEW and the detection of heart rate and the abnormality in the heart rate is obtained. The signal is processed and the abnormal signal is detected and an alarm is shown in the front panel of LabVIEW. The filtered ECG signal is is displayed. The output of the signal either normal or abnormal is displayed using light emitting diodes in LabVIEW. The block diagram and the front panel is shown in Figure 22. The heart rate calculation is done from the given ECG signal.

Wireless heart rate detection is important because it can be wirelessly connected to the other system, hence communication is possible. Here the ECG monitoring system is based on labview. The client captures the ECG from the Bluetooth connection.

We have built a prototype using parts of the case from a commercial blood pressure monitor for the wrist. All necessary sensors are placed inside (acceleration and pressure) or at the outside (temperature)

Figure 22. Block diagram showing the type of signal with an alarm

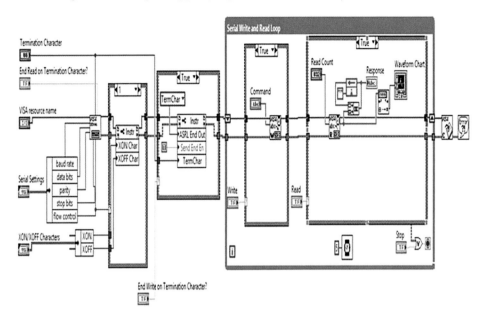

of the case except for the ECG electrodes which are placed at the chest and are connected by cables. The device is powered by system itself. It currently transmits every sample of the sensor raw data wirelessly to the stationary computer where the data will be stored and processed with a common time base. Our prototype only collects and forwards the data and does not perform any calculations for data compression or analysis yet.

6. CONCLUSION

With wireless technology, these physiological parameters can be monitored continuously and also immediate warning and causality services can be given to the medical staffs and doctors are given as early as possible. Patient fall detection and body temperature are done with wireless technology. The wireless communication of PPG signal, in order to get database anywhere within the hospital was presented in this chapter. This is especially helpful in monitoring the postoperative patient, though a separate person to watch them is not necessary. The doctor can view the patient details anywhere within the hospital. Also it is a continuous monitoring of the PPG signal for a long time, which shows the results of Heart Rate and SpO2. With ECG Signal, the heart rate measurement was done.

REFERENCES

Alnaeb, M., Alobaid, N., Seifalian, A., Mikhailidis, D., & Hamilton, G. (2007). Optical Techniques in the Assessment of Peripheral Arterial Disease. *Current Vascular Pharmacology*, 5(1), 53–59. doi:10.2174/157016107779317242 PMID:17266613

Aminian, M., & Naji, H. R. (2013). A Hospital Healthcare Monitoring System Using Wireless Sensor Networks. *J Health Med Inform, 4*(121). doi:10.4172/2157-7420.1000121

Analog devices Small, Low Power, 3-Axis ±3g Accelerometer. (2009). https://www.sparkfun.com/datasheets/Components/SMD/adxl335.pdf

Banka & Mary. (2014). Remote Monitoring of Heart Rate, Blood pressure and temperature of a person. *International Journal of Emerging Technology in Computer Science and Electronics, 8*(1).

8bit AVR Microcontrollers. (2016). http://www.atmel.com/Images/Atmel-42735-8-bit-AVR-Microcontroller-ATmega328-328P_Datasheet.pdf

Cheang, P., & Smith, P. (2003). *An overview of non-contact photoplethysmography*. Electronic Systems and Control Division Research, Dept Electron and Elect Eng.

Devi, Winster, & Sasikumar. (2016). Patient health monitoring system (PHMS) using IoT devices. *International Journal of Computer Science & Engineering Technology, 7*(3).

Elgendi, M. (2012, February). On the analysis of fingertip photoplethysmogram signals [Review]. *Current Cardiology Reviews, 8*(1), 14–25. doi:10.2174/157340312801215782 PMID:22845812

Frank, W. (2012, April). Lack of exercise is a major cause of chronic diseases. *Comprehensive Physiology, 2*(2), 1143–1211. PMID:23798298

Global System for Mobile communication (GSM). (2001). *Requirements for GSM operation on railways, European Standard (Telecommunications series)*. http://www.etsi.org/deliver/etsi_en/301500_301599/301515/01.00.00_20/en_301515v010000c.pdf

Introduction to GPS - US Environmental protection agency. (2015). https://www.epa.gov/sites/production/files/2015-10/documents/global_positioning_system110_af.r4.pdf

Kyriazis, D. (2013). Sustainable smart city IoT applications: Heat and electricity management & Eco-conscious cruise control for public transportation. *World of Wireless, Mobile and Multimedia Networks (WoWMoM), 2013 IEEE 14th International Symposium and Workshops on*, 1–5.

LM393. LM393E, LM293, LM2903, LM2903E, LM2903V, NCV2903 On semiconductor. (2016). https://www.onsemi.com/pub/Collateral/LM393-D.PDF

Lord, S. R., Menz, H. B., & Sherrington, C. (2006). Home environment risk factors for falls in older people and the efðcacy of home modiðcations. *Age and Ageing, 35*(Suppl 2), ii55–ii59. doi:10.1093/ageing/afl088 PMID:16926207

LPC2148 Microcontroller. (2011). https://www.nxp.com/docs/en/data-sheet/LPC2141_42_44_46_48.pdf?

Mary. (2014). Modelling and control of MIMO Gasifier system during coal quality variations. *International Journal of Modelling. Identification and Control, 22*(4), 131–139.

Mary & Sivakumar. (2012). A Reduced Order Transfer Function Models for Alstom Gasifier using Genetic Algorithm. *International Journal of Computer Applications, 46*(5), 1-6.

Mukhopadhyay. (2015). *Wearable Sensors for Human Activity Monitoring. IEEE Sensors Journal, 15(3)*.

Nihseniorhealth: About falls. (n.d.). Available online: http://nihseniorhealth.gov/falls/aboutfalls/01.html

Rajasekaran, K. (2016). *Smart technologies for Non-invasive Biomedical Sensors to measure physiological parameters. In Handbook of Research on Healthcare Administration and Management.* IGI Global Publication.

Rajasekaran, K. (2016). *Smart technologies for Non- invasive Biomedical Sensors to measure physiological parameters. In Handbook of Research on Healthcare Administration and Management.* IGI Global Publication.

Rajasekaran, Rekh, & Mary. (2015). *Non-Invasive Hemoglobin Measurement: A Great Blessing to the Rural Community.* Academic Press.

Shelley, K. (2007). Photoplethysmography: Beyond the Calculation of Arterial Oxygen Saturation and Heart Rate. *Anesthesia and Analgesia*, 105. PMID:18048895

Ubbink, T. (2004). Toe Blood Pressure Measurements in Patients Suspected of Leg Ischaemia: A New Laser Doppler Device Compared with Photoplethysmography. *European Journal of Vascular and Endovascular Surgery*, 27(6), 629–634. doi:10.1016/j.ejvs.2004.01.031 PMID:15121114

Unno, N., Inuzuka, K., Mitsuoka, H., Ishimaru, K., Sagara, D., & Konno, H. (2006). Automated Bedside Measurement of Penile Blood Flow Using Pulse-Volume Plethysmography. *Surgery Today*, 36(3), 257–261. doi:10.100700595-005-3139-8 PMID:16493536

Watson. (2014). A novel time–frequency-based 3D Lissajous figure method and its application to the determination of oxygen saturation from the photoplethysmogram. *Measurement Science & Technology*.

Chapter 14
Non-Invasive Active Acousto-Thermometer

Oleg Victorovich Sytnik

A. Ya. Usikov Institute for Radiophysics and Electronics of the National Academy of Science of Ukraine, Ukraine

ABSTRACT

The problem of detecting and identifying the heat transfer processes in living tissues using a noninvasive ultrasound technique is discussed. An optimal method, which is optimal in terms of maximum of likelihood, is proposed to detect the temperature variations within internal layers of the living tissue. The properties of signals returned from different tissues are examined. The ultrasound velocity for different temperatures and the salt composition of a specimen under study is estimated. Results of the algorithm simulation are given.

INTRODUCTION

Remote monitoring of the temperature in different types of a medium is a topical issue both in engineering, biology, and medicine (Dmitriev, 1987). Specifically, when treating cancer diseases through hyperthermia, in diagnosing internal inflammatory processes, etc. the application of contact methods results in the hazardous injury of vitals (Pasechnik, 1991). Therefore the immediate goal of to-day us to develop special technical tools that would provide the non-invasive monitoring of the temperature in the living organism areas under study.

To obtain some reliable information on the internal layers of living tissues, technical facilities are needed to radiate, receive and extract information from echo signals. To this end both active (Sytnik, 2002) and passive (Pasechnik, 1991) systems can be employed. The operation of passive systems is based upon the reception and processing of object self-radiations.

However, the passive accoustothermometry techniques allow making an integral estimate of the temperature along the observation beam. Yet if the temperature profile is to be restored, it is necessary to scan an area under study from different points and to solve a set of integral equations. As a results, one cannot obtain on-line information. At the same time the accuracy of measurements is largely depth-

DOI: 10.4018/978-1-5225-6067-8.ch014

dependent. As shown in (Anosov, 1995), an acceptable accuracy is attained at a depth of no more than 3 to 5 cm, which, in many instances, is insufficient. Moreover, bone and fatty tissues can lead to dramatic distortion of a temperature spatial profile. To obtain reasonable accuracies signal storing should take quite a long time, which is found to be comparable to the typical period of time during which the thermodynamic processes occur in living tissues.

The above shortenings can be avoided if one falls back upon an idea of determining the degree to which the local areas of the living tissue are heated. This idea is based upon the measurement of the temporal or phase delay of an ultrasound signal as it passes through a heated region (Dmitriev, 1987),(Sytnik, 2002). In the general case the delay is governed by the rate at which the ultrasound propagates in tissues. This rate, in its turn, is dependent upon the tissue temperature and the blood salt composition. If the aforementioned composition is considered to show no dramatic change on being heated, then the phase shift between the signal that has passed through the tissues prior to and after heating will result from the temperature gradient. In other words, the power of the ultrasound signal transmitted into a human organism should be brought up to a level so that a signal returned from the remotest point of a signal propagation path could not only exceed the self-radiation of tissues and the receiver noise more than once, but also keep the tissues from being appreciably heated. In this instance, the typical targets are the boundaries of transition between fatty, muscular, bone and tumor-affected tissue, blood vessel walls, etc. The variation in the position of these targets along the same path upon heating will enable the temperature gradient profile to be restored.

PHYSICAL PRINCIPLES OF THE PROPOSED TECHNIQUE

A plot of the sound wave velocity as a function of temperature $c(T)$ for homogeneous media (say, water) and for different sounding signal frequencies using the data drawn from the reference (Hutte,1934), is presented on Figure 1.

As far as medical applications are concerned, hyperthermia in particular, the temperature interval between 39^0 and 45^0 C is of certain interest. The experimental studies indicated that the derivative of sound velocity with respect to $dc\,/\,dT^0C$ over this particular temperature interval is insignificant (Figure 2), and for the carrier frequency of sounding signal $f = 0,88 f = 0,88$ MHz yields an increment of a complete returned-signal phase $\Delta\Psi$ on the order of 0,1 of phase degree (or 1,8*10^{-3} rad) by a temperature degree according to the Celsius scale.

In terms of obtaining a high accuracy of measurement and ensuring the simplicity of hardware realization it would be more expedient to estimate the sound velocity from the variations in the phase difference between a reference coherent signal and the signals echoed from typical inter-layer inhomogeneities rather than the echo-signal delay time. Specifically, upon recording the time interval within which the echo signal are being sampled and comparing the phase difference between the fluctuations in these samples one can easily notice the variations in signal propagation on those propagation paths where both a rise in temperature and a relevant change in the sound propagation are observed to occur. As the sounding signal frequency increases, the requirements for the equipment sensitivity tend to be less stringent. This tendency is clearly apparent from the experimental data (see Figure 3), where the curves are given as $f = 1,76$ MHz and $f = 3,0$ MHz.

Figure 1. The temperature-dependent sound propagation velocity in water

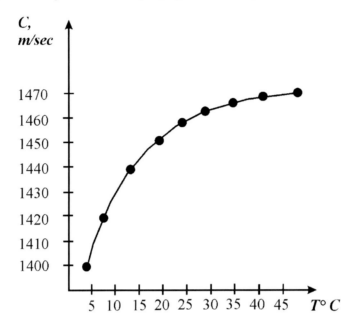

The sound propagation velocity as a function of the salt content in water is shown in Figure 4, whereas the derivative of the sound velocity with respect to salt concentration (solid line) and the corresponding full phase incursion, $\Delta\Psi$, at a constant temperature of 15^0 C (dotted line) are shown in Figure 5.

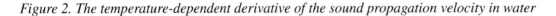

Figure 2. The temperature-dependent derivative of the sound propagation velocity in water

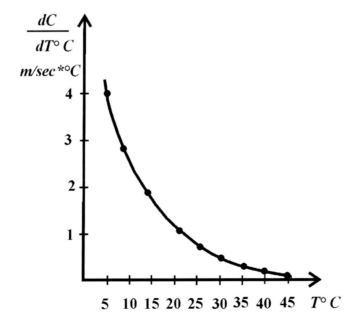

Figure 3. The increment of the complete signal phase as a function of temperature

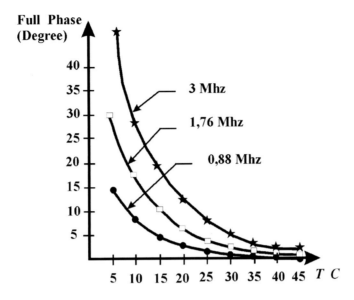

In conducting experiments the typical size of a homogeneous area was chosen to be as $\Delta h = 1$ cm. The sound propagation in tissues was considerably impacted not only by temperature conditions but also by the salt content of liquids and apparently by the degree to which the tissues got saturated.

Figure 4. The sound propagation velocity as a function of the salt content in water

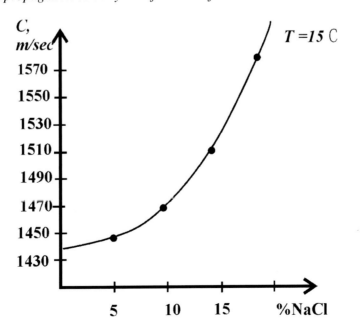

Figure 5. The increment of the full signal phase as a function of the salt content in water at a constant temperature

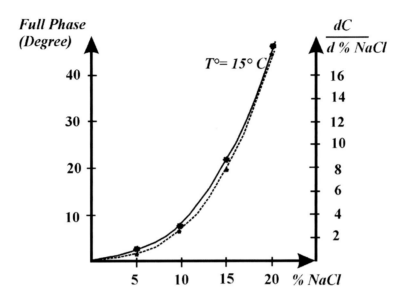

REQUIREMENTS FOR HARDWARE/SOFTWARE FACILITIES OF AN ACOUSTOTHERMOMETER

Proceeding from the analysis of experimental data cited above, when an active ultrasound locator was used to measure the temperature gradients in tissues, as they were heated up by an external source it was necessary that the related equipment meet the following requirements:

1. In order to attain the accuracy of measurement of temperature range between $39^0...45^0$ C and the typical size $\Delta h = 1$ cm of the tissue inhomogeneity one needs to obtain the sensitivity in terms of measuring the phase difference $\Delta \Psi$ for:

Table 1. Phase sensitivity for different ultrasound frequencies

Frequencies of Sounding Signal	Phase Sensitivity
$f = 0,88$ MHz	$\Delta \Psi = 0,06$ deg. (or $1,1*10^{-3}$ rad);
$f = 1,76$ MHz	$\Delta \Psi = 0,12$ deg. (or $2,1*10^{-3}$ rad);
$f = 3,0$ MHz	$\Delta \Psi = 0,2$ deg. (or $3,5*10^{-3}$ rad);

2. A short-term phase instability of a reference oscillator should be, at least, an order of magnitude lower than the above values. Specifically, the standard short-term instability of the quartz-controlled reference oscillator, which is reduced to 1 sec, is equal to 10^{-6}, i.e., at $f = 1,76$ MHz $\Delta f = 1,76$

Hz per second for the interval, $\Delta h = 1$ cm, and $C \approx 1500$ m/sec, phase incursion $\Delta \Psi = 4,2 \cdot 10^{-3}$ deg/sec. Therefore, in order to ensure the prescribed accuracy of ΔT measurement, the phase noise of the reference oscillator can be ignored.

3. In the course of processing a signal integration interval in view of the fact that a returned signal is influence by a pulse rate, breathing and involuntary movements of a human being.

To obtain absolute values of temperature one should know the behavior of the plotted curve $c\left(T\right)$ in specific tissues. As indicated in (Dmitriev, 1987), a growing pattern of the curve $c\left(T\right)$ is not typical for all types of tissues. Therefore an additional calibration of the device is required when conducting absolute measurements along each sounding beam.

The parameters of an ultrasound meter are selected from the same considerations as those of any radar facility. That is to say, the sounding pulse duration and the pulse recurrence rate are chosen in terms of requirements for resolution and a maximum sounding depth respectively. The temperature variation sensitivity will be determined by the properties of a medium and dependent upon the absolute temperature value. The experimental data given in (Anosov, 1995) indicate that a prominent increase in heating of, say, a fatty tissue by about 1^0 C is noted at ultrasound signal energy flux densities of ~ 500 W/cm² and with a pulse length, $\tau_{pulse} = 50$ msec.

Therefore, in order to obviate the influence of the measuring system on tissues the radiated pulse power should not be over 10 W. At the same time the sounding pulse duration resulting from the requirement for depth resolution should not be in excess of 2,4 msec. This suggests that it is essential to allow for the effect of noise (the intrinsic noise of equipment and the noise caused by tissue radiation) upon the resultant accuracy of measurement. In addition, an instantaneous echo-signal response is unfit for use in the measuring algorithm, because the signal is impacted by biological factors such as a pulse rate, breathing, etc. It is just for this reason that the signal is to be statistically preprocessed.

STATISTICAL PROCESSING OF ACOUSTOTHERMOMETER SIGNALS

On analog output of locator is a mixture of $x\left(t\right)$ of desired harmonic signal $S\left(t\right)$ (having known frequency ω_0 and unknown amplitude a and phase ϕ) and noise $n\left(t\right)$:

$$x\left(t\right) = S\left(t, \theta_1, \theta_2\right) + n\left(t\right) \tag{1}$$

where

$$S\left(t, \theta_1, \theta_2\right) = a\cos\left(\omega_0 t - \phi\right) = a\cos\left(\phi\right)\cos\left(\omega_0 t\right) + a\sin\left(\phi\right)\sin\left(\omega_0 t\right);$$

$\left[-T; T\right]$ is the interval of signal $S\left(\bullet\right)$ existence, i.e., $t \in \left[-T; T\right]$, or

$$\left|t\right| \leq T; \quad \theta_1 = a\cos\left(\phi\right); \quad \theta_2 = a\sin\left(\phi\right); \quad n\left(t\right)$$

is the normal Gaussian noise with zero mathematical expectation and spectral density, N_0.

The problem, ought to be solved, is to evaluate the unknown parameters of a deterministic summand from the maximum likelihood criterion (Levin, 1975). Upon solving this problem the minimal r.m.s. estimation errors will be written as

$$\sigma_{\hat{a}}^2 = N_0 \, / \, 2T \tag{2}$$

$$\sigma_{\hat{\phi}}^2 = N_0 \, / \, \left(2Ta^2\right) \tag{3}$$

The statistical estimates (2), (3) may be thought of as optimal ones if the interference stationary conditions is met. However, with a tissue being heated up by an external source, not only does the sound propagation velocity vary within them, but also the changes in the self-radiation intensity occur. Therefore prior to evaluating the signal phase incursions along the sound propagation path it is necessary to perform the preliminary corrective filtering of the acoustothermometer receiver output signal. It is exactly for this purpose that a dynamic Kalman filter is qurte a suitable device (Kalman, 1961), (Sotskov, 1985), (Shelukhin, 1984), (Brammer, 1982).

Now equation (1) can be re-writing in the following form:

$$x\left(t\right) = a\left(t\right)\cos\left(\omega t\right) + n\left(t\right) \tag{4}$$

where $n\left(t\right)$ is the normal Gaussian noise with zero mathematical expectation and variance of σ_n^2.

The trend of function $a\left(t\right)$ can be described by the differential equation:

$$\frac{da\left(t\right)}{dt} = Fa\left(t\right) + v\left(t\right) \tag{5}$$

where $F = const$ defines the amplitude variation dynamics under the change in temperature of a specific layer; $v\left(t\right)$ is the excitation noise, i.e., the Gaussian noise with variance σ_v^2 and a zero main value. The observation factor for the model (4) will have this form (Kravchenko, 2003):

$$H\left(t\right) = \cos\left(\omega_0 t\right) \tag{6}$$

The transmission constant of the Kalman dynamic filter can be found from the Ricatti differential equation with a given equation of state (5) and an observation factor (6) (Kalman, 1961), (Sotskov, 1985), (Shelukhin, 1984), (Brammer, 1982):

$$K\left(t\right) = \frac{\sigma_s^2}{2\sigma_n^2}\cos\left(\omega_0 t\right) \tag{7}$$

where $\sigma_s^2 = E\left\{\varepsilon_t^2\right\}$ is the variance of the signal amplitude estimate.

Thus, the signal filtering to obtain smoothed estimates is reduced to this form:

$$\frac{da(t)}{dt} + \left(F + \frac{\sigma_s^2}{2\sigma_n^2}\right)a(t) = \frac{\sigma_s^2}{\sigma_n^2}x(t)\cos(\omega_0 t) \tag{8}$$

Equation (8) indicates that in this particular case the Kalman filter consists of a synchronous detector, an inertial section (of the low-pass filter with variable parameters) and an amplifier having the gain as given in (Kalman, 1961).

As discussed in (Kravchenko, 2003), (Kravchenko, 2009), the minimum of the r.m.s. filtering error is achieved when the Kravchenko-Rvachev atomic functions $fup_N(t)$, are employed as an integrating link, these functions being represented in the analytical form (Kravchenko, 2003):

$$v(t) = \frac{1}{2\pi}\int_{-\infty}^{\infty}\left[\frac{\cos(ut)\cdot\sin\left(\frac{u}{2}\right)}{\frac{u}{2}}\right]^{N+1}du \tag{9}$$

The Kravchenko weighting function appears as $fup_N(t) = up(2t)\cdot v(t)$, where the function $up(t)$ has the following Fourier transform-based representation:

$$up(t) = \frac{1}{2\pi}\int_{-\infty}^{\infty}e^{jut}\prod_{k=1}^{\infty}\frac{\sin\left(u\cdot 2^{-k}\right)}{u\cdot 2^{-k}}du \tag{10}$$

When synthesizing the integrating section of the Kalman filter, the application of functions (9) appears to be premising owing to their unique properties. Specifically, function $fup_N(t)$ for each N is even, positive having an upper bound

$$\sup\left\{fup_N(t)\right\} = \left[-(N+2)/2, (N+2)/2\right]$$

encompassing the unit area: $\int_{-1}^{1}fup_N(t)dt = 1$. The derivative of function $fup_N(t)$ has a direct coupling with

$$fup_{N-1}(t): fup_N'(t) = fup_{N-1}(t+0,5) - fup_{N-1}(t-0,5).$$

Besides, function $fup_N(t)$ can be calculated from recurrent relations

$$fup_N\left(t\right) = 2^{-N}\sum_{k=0}^{N-1}C_{N-1}kfup_{N-1}\left(2t - k + \left(N - 1\right)/2\right).$$

Besides, there are some more properties of function $fup_N\left(t\right)$ which are detailed in (Kravchenko, 2003).

It should be noted that the fluctuation component level in the dynamic trend of a signal decreases by 6 to 8 dB when the Kalman filter with an integrating section is applied in terms of functions $fup_N\left(t\right)$ relative to an ordinary low-pass filter.

IMPLEMENTATION OF ACOUSTOTHERMOMETER SIGNALS PROCESSING ALGORITHM

The diagram (Figure 6) schematically shows radiated acoustic pulses (grey rectangles) and continue returned signal from human body as a time function (The time intervals in Figure 6 are given in µs). Here the heating region stands out as being shaded, and the typical targets, which were experimentally chosen, are schematically displayed according to the standard dimensions of tumors.

Figure 6. The diagram of a returned signal in time

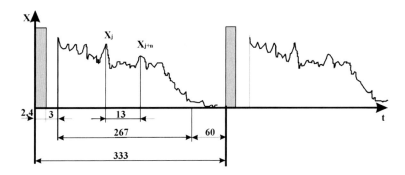

The amplitude and phase estimates of a tissue-radiated signal are obtained and smoothed via the Kalman filter and are subsequently used in a two-channel device. The phase channel serves to calculate the increments of the head region temperature according to the following relations (Anosov, 1995):

$$\left.\begin{aligned} G_{j,n}^{l} &= \frac{1}{b}\frac{c_0^2\Delta\bar{\Psi}_{j,n}}{\omega_0 z + c_0\Delta\bar{\Psi}_{j,n}} \\ \Delta T_j &= \mathrm{mod}\left\{G_{j,n}^{l} - G_{j,n}^{l-1}\right\} \end{aligned}\right\} \tag{11}$$

where $b = \Delta c / \Delta T$ is the constant of calibration, which is determined by comparing with in-situ measurements on the body surface; c_0 is the ultrasound wave velocity in a tissue prior to heating; ω_0 is the circular carrier frequency of a sonar; z is the distance to the point at which temperature measurements are performed; $\overline{\Psi}_{j,n}$ - is the mean value of the signal phase difference between the typical reflectors j and $(j + n)$ reflectors inside and beyond the heating region; l - is the time at which measurements were taken; $G^l_{j,n}$ - is the intermediate temperature-dimensional coefficient; ΔT_j - is the increment of growth in acousto-brightness temperature at the j -th point.

In order to obtain the profile of acousto-brightness temperatures it is necessary to do scanning by a chosen strobe pulse along the entire propagation path and to calculate the value of ΔT using formulas (11). As seen from Figure 6, this strobe pulse is equal to 13 µsec.

The full representation of a signal processing algorithm in the phase channel is shown in Figure 7. Figure 8 presents an algorithm for signal processing in the amplitude channel. The information provided by the signal from the amplitude channel is unused for temperature calculations. However, it allows the structural changes in the tissues under study to be monitored and it is likewise helpful in accurately choosing the typical targets along the ultrasound wave propagation path.

EXPERIMENTAL STUDIES INTO ACOUSTOTHERMOMETER OPERATIONS

The experimental studies on the ultrasound wave acoustothermometer were carried out in a vessel containing a salt water solution (1% solution of table salt). The walls and the bottom of the vessel were coated with a sound-absorbing material that excludes the sound interference. The ultrasound point reflecting baffles were used as typical targets. These reflectors are matched to the sonar's resolution bin (elements), which was came to 2 mm for a specimen under study. The distance between the baffles (reflectors) was 1 cm. The initial value of the sound velocity $C_0 = 1500$ m/sec whereas the constant value $b = 2$. Figure 9 shows the experimental temperature-dependent phase difference $\Delta \Psi$ under slow cooling of the solution for two distances d between the sound reflecting baffles.

As seen from Figure 9, one can observe the method in question to be highly sensitive to temperature variations (see curve 1, $d = 5$ cm) over the temperature interval between 39^0 and 44^0 C, which is of considerable interest for medical applications. This enables one to measure the time-dependent temperature gradient in a single linear resolution element (2 mm along the signal propagation direction) with an error of no more than $0,1^0$ C. Curve 2 indicated the same dependence, but at $d = 7,2$ cm.

It is apparent from the analysis of experimental data that if one strives to keep the measurement error within $0,1^0$ C it is essential that the effect of hardware errors and destabilizing factors should not go beyond a series of allowable limits. More specifically it concerns:

1. The errors resulting from a fluctuation component, which combine the errors caused by a) the equipment inherent noise; b) acoustic noise of an object under study and c) discretization noise $\sigma^2 = N_0 / (2n\tau a^2)$, where N_0 is the noise spectral density; n is the number of pulses being stored; τ is the pulse duration; a is the signal amplitude. With $\tau = 2,4$ µsec; $F = 3$ kHz, an interval of storage of 0,5 sec and for the required accuracy in measuring signal phase difference, the power *S/N* ratio must be no less than 35 dB;

Figure 7. A signal processing algorithm in the phase channel

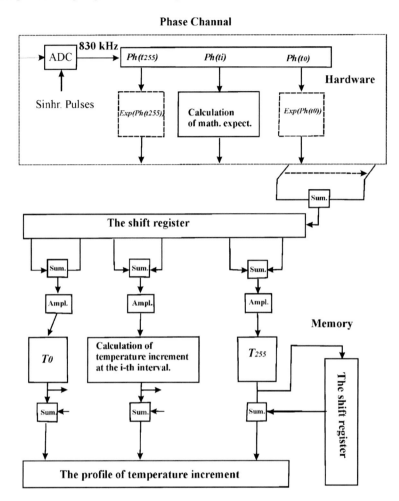

2. Phase noise of a reference oscillator; for the typical instability of the sensors reference oscillator at a carrier frequency of 1,76 MHz; the typical linear dimension of 1 cm and the propagation speed of 1500 m/sec, the r.m.s. value of the phase error is equal to $4,2 \cdot 10^{-3}$ deg/sec;

3. The errors resulting from absorption and scattering of signals on the way of ultrasound wave propagation can be estimated from the absorption factor value; itis experimentally found (Sytnik, 2002) that the signal absorption factor in a muscle tissue amounts to a value on the order of 0,2 cm^{-1} whereas the factor of reflection from boundaries equals to a value on the order of 10^{-6} . Therefore the errors resulting from absorption of a signal and its scattering can be disregarded;

4. The contribution of quantization noise to a resultant error is due to an analog-to-digital converter finite word length; the quantization noise restricts the maximum attainable signal-to-noise ratio and, consequently, the maximum achievable accuracy in calculating the phase difference of received signals; with 8-bit ADC the maximum attainable *S/N* ratio is equal to 21 dB, whereas for 16-bit ADCs this ratio is 45 dB, respectively. This leads to a restriction of accuracy in measuring temperature gradient to 1 K and 0,1 K, respectively;

Figure 8. An amplitude channel processing algorithm

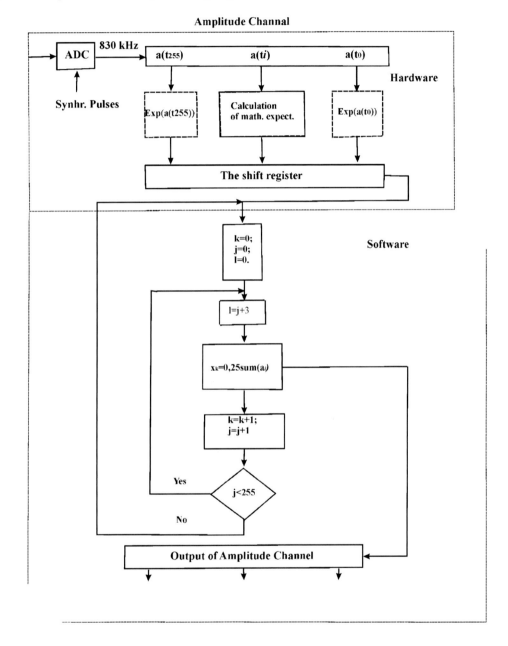

5. The pulse waveform effect upon a resultant error can be ignored. Since the measurement procedure is based upon the principle of determining the phase difference between signal samples according to carrier oscillations, the change in the pulse waveform has an impact upon the magnitude of radiated oscillation energy and, consequently, upon the *S/N* ratio at the receiver input. If 90 dB radiation power reserve is provided in the sonar arrangement, then this impact is insignificant;

6. The errors resulting from the tumor location depth relative to the surface are associated with a decrease in the *S/N* ratio by about 9 dB per each 10 cm for a single signal passage. Hence, an error

Figure 9. Temperature-dependent variations in phase differences with the solution getting slowly cooled off

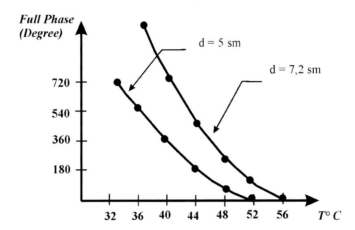

in estimating the temperature gradient cannot exceed 1 K at a distance of 20 cm when an initial *S/N* ratio is 60 dB. Yet with an initial 90 dB S/N ratio the estimated error will not be over 0.1 K;

7. Systematic errors that are caused by accuracy in specifying the constants C_0 and $b = \Delta C / \Delta T$ are determined using the initial calibration by a phantom, and here these error do not make an impact upon relative measurement errors.

CONCLUSION

To sum up what has been stated above, it would be important to call readers attention to the following points. The noninvasive technique for measuring temperature gradients in living biological tissues, aggressive media, certain fields of technology and other applications has been proposed. In contrast to the well-known technique (Dmitriev, 1987), (Pasechnik, 1991), (Anosov, 1995), the matter of the above-mentioned method lies in the fact that the pulsed sounding signal is radiated into a medium under study. Next is receiving of a reflected signal and phase-pulsed processing of received signal. The main advantages of the proposed technique over passive non-contact methods are as follows 1) sounding is performed at a dramatically greater depth by an order of magnitude greater; 2) the measurement error is weakly depth-dependent and a possibility to obtain the temperature gradient profile in one measurement cycle.

Special procedures are worked out to describe, and to correct as well as algorithms for statistical processing of measurement data on sounding signals in the course of sounding the living tissues by ultrasound waves.

As theoretical and experimental approaches to studying problems in question suggested, a high sensitivity of the method to time-varying temperature changes is observed over a temperature interval between 39^0 and 44^0 C. This allows one to measure the temperature gradient in a single resolution element with an error of up to $0,1^0$ C.

A software/hardware integrated system for gathering and handling the data on the temperatures of inner layers in a medium under investigation is developed. In addition, the requirements for technical facilities are set with the goal of obtaining specified measurement errors. The measurement error that is experimentally attained during the measurements at a depth of 7,2 cm for an average inhomogeneity of some 1 cm in diameter is not more than $0,1^0$ C. This indicates that an accuracy of the known passive method (Pasechnik, 1991) is almost by an under of magnitude greater.

It is shown that since an increasing behavior of the temperature-dependent sound wave velocity function is not observable for all types of tissues, an additional calculation of the device must be performed when making absolute measurements along each sounding bean on the surface of a specimen under study using the contact methods. The lines along which the evolution of technique described above is expected to proceed have been substantiated.

An opportunity is shown to synthesize a model for ultrasound wave propagation in a layered-inhomogeneous medium and scanning of a piezoelectric transducer over the surface of an object along with cooperative processing of returned signals received at different angles.

REFERENCES

Dmitriev, V. N., Solntseva, L. V., & Gavrilov, L. R. (1987). An acoustic method for determining the temperature of locally heated biological tissues [in Russian]. *Meditsinskaya Radiologiya, 1,* 82–86.

Pasechnik, V. I. (1991). Acoustic tomography of biological object [in Russian]. *Radiotekhnika, 8,* 65–72.

Klochko, G. I., Logvinenko, A. I., & Sytnik, O. V. (2002). A signal processing algorithm for remote acoustic temperature meter [in Russian]. *Radiotekhnika, 2,* 18–25.

Anosov, A. A., Isrefilov, M. G., & Pasechnik, V. I. (1995). Accuracy of solving an inverse problem of acoustothermography in non-correlation reception [in Russian]. *Radiotekhnika, 9,* 49–57.

Hutte. (1934), *Mannual (Handbook)*. Mashinistroenie. (in Russian)

Levin, B. R. (1975). *Theoretical foundations of statistical radio engineering.* Sov. Radio. (in Russian)

Kalman, R. Ye., & Bewsy, R. S. (1961). Now results in linear filtering and prediction theory, *Proc. of the American Society of mechanical engineers. Ser. D., 83*(1), 123–141.

Sotskov, B. M., & Shcherbakov, V. Yu. (1985). Theory and technology of Kalman filtering in the presence of interfering parameters [in Russian]. *Zarubezhnaya Radioelektronika, 2,* 3–29.

Shelukhin, O. I., & Alyabiev, S. P. (1984). Preliminary filtering in a Kalman filter under the a priori uncertainty conditions [in Russian]. *Radiotekhnika, 8,* 53–57.

Brammer, K., & Ziefling, G. (1982). *Kalman-Bewsy filter.* Nauka. (in Russian)

Kravchenko, V. F. (2003). *Lectures on the theory of atomic functions an some of their application.* Radiotechnika. (in Russian)

Kravchenko, V. F., Labun'ko, O. S., & Lerer, A. M. (2009). *Calculation methods in present-day radiophysics.* Fizmatlit. (in Russian)

KEY TERMS AND DEFINITIONS

Acousto-Brightness Temperature: Is gradient amplitude of reflected acoustic signal.

Hyperthermia: A method of treating cancer (malignant tumors), in which the patient's body, parts thereof, or individual organs are exposed to high temperatures (above 39 ° C, to 44-45 ° C).

Increment of the Total Phase of the Signal: Is the phase change of the signal due to the propagation delay of the signal to the target and back, expressed in radians (or degrees).

Kalman Filter: Is dynamic adaptive filter the amplifier factor of which calculated from the Riccati differential equation using statistical information of signal and noise.

S/N Ratio: Is a ratio of acoustic signal power to dispersion of noise.

Sound Velocity: Is a velocity of ultrasound wave front in homogeneous tissue.

Ultrasound Wave Acoustothermometer: Is a device which radiate ultrasound waves to living tissue and calculate the temperature gradient as a function of time using information from reflected signal.

Chapter 15
Sport and Wellness Technology to Promote Physical Activity of Teenagers:
An Intervention Study

Eeva Kettunen
University of Jyvaskyla, Finland

Markus Makkonen
https://orcid.org/0000-0002-1553-211X
University of Jyvaskyla, Finland

Tuomas Kari
University of Jyvaskyla, Finland

Will Critchley
University of Jyvaskyla, Finland

ABSTRACT

Life-long physical activity patterns are established during teenage years, so promoting physical activity is important. Sport and wellness technology has potential for promoting physical activity. Yet, research concerning its use among teenage populations is sparse. This intervention study investigated whether using a sport and wellness technology application could affect teenagers' physical activity intention, its antecedents, and the effects of these antecedents on intention. The study uses the theory of planned behavior (TPB) combined with self-efficacy as a theoretical model. The results showed no statistically significant difference between the intervention and control group in terms of the means and variances of the four constructs (attitude, subjective norm, self-efficacy, and intention) in the theoretical model. However, there was a statistically significant difference in the effect of self-efficacy on intention in the intervention group. Using sport and wellness technology in physical activity interventions among teenagers has potential and further research is warranted.

DOI: 10.4018/978-1-5225-6067-8.ch015

INTRODUCTION

According to the World Health Organization, over 80% of the world's adolescent population is not physically active enough. What makes the situation even worse is the steadily decreasing trend of physical activity and the increasing trend of sedentary behavior of this population (Brodersen et al., 2007; World Health Organization, 2018; Knell et al., 2019). Today's teenagers live in an environment that offers them an increasing number of options for sedentary leisure activities as well as an increasing number of barriers to physical activity.

Health related behavioral patterns concerning, for example, physical activity, sleep, and nutrition are being established during the teenage years, and these learned patterns are usually maintained throughout life (Kumar et al., 2015). Thus, promoting healthy behaviors, such as physical activity, during the teenage years has an important impact on the overall life quality of a person. Enabling exercise participation and promoting physical activity has the ability to foster personal competence and improvement. This, in turn, will help teenagers to achieve personal goals regarding their physical activity intentions and is important for the formation and maintenance of long-term health behaviors (Hagger et al., 2001). Research has also shown that physical activity during this age can boost academic achievement (Kari et al., 2017) and have far-reaching consequences for life-long educational (Kari et al., 2017) and labor-market outcomes (Kari et al., 2016).

Today, technology plays a major role in teenagers' lives because many of them are constantly online and use various applications and devices on a daily basis. It is reasonable to also consider using technology in health and physical activity promotion and interventions. For example, the role of sport and wellness technology devices and applications in health promotion could be highlighted more. Typically, sport and wellness technology applications and devices, such as wearable devices, have been designed for adults who are already physically active and want to maintain their active lifestyle or improve their performance level (Carrino et al., 2014). Teenagers associate the need of wearable sport and wellness technology devices with serious goals and a strong aim for achieving them (Carrion et al., 2015).

There is a gap in research related to teenagers and their use of internet, mobile applications, and wearable fitness devices for health-related purposes (Wartella et al., 2016). There are few wearables created especially for teenagers, and they have mainly focused on game related elements and connectivity (Carrion et al., 2015). Understanding the effects sport and wellness technology has on teenagers is relevant for sport technology companies in being able to create products and services that not only attract this target group but are also effective and useful.

The use of interactive technology might increase the appeal of physical activity promotion interventions (Direito et al., 2015). However, there is a lack of empirical evidence supporting the effectiveness of these targeted health behavior interventions and research on how sport and wellness technology can stimulate health behavior change in younger populations (Masteller et al., 2017). When designing intervention programs, understanding what motivates young people to participate in physical activity is essential (Dos Santos et al., 2016). The focus should be on strategies that include psychosocial issues, sport competence, and physical self-worth (Masteller et al., 2017).

This paper reports the findings from a five-week-long intervention study that was conducted in order to increase the knowledge about sport and wellness technology and its effects on the physical activity of teenagers. More specifically, drawing from IS and exercise psychology perspectives, the aim was to find out whether the use of a sport and wellness technology application could affect the physical activity intentions of teenagers, its antecedents, as well as the effects of these antecedents on intention by using the theory of planned behavior (TPB) combined with the concept of self-efficacy as a theoretical framework. This study, which followed a mixed methods approach, included 64 teenagers divided into an intervention group and a control group, of which the intervention group was provided with a sport and wellness technology application for the five-week intervention period.

The paper is structured as follows. After this introductory section, the theoretical background is presented, followed by sections on methodology, results, discussion and conclusions. Finally, the limitations and future research are discussed.

BACKGROUND AND THEORETICAL MODEL

The theoretical model of the study is based on the Theory of Planned Behavior (TPB) by Ajzen (1985, 1991), which is an extension of the Theory of Reasoned Action (TRA) (Fishbein et al., 1975; Ajzen & Fishbein, 1980). According to the TPB, an individual's stated intention to perform a certain behavior in a given time and context is a proximal predictor of behavior. This intention is a function of a person's attitude, subjective norm, and perceived behavioral control (PBC). Attitude is based on an individual's perceptions of the intended behavior and his/her evaluation of the behavior outcome. Subjective norm refers to a person's estimate of the extent that other important people to them would like the person to engage in that behavior. PBC refers to a person's perception of his/her abilities and the limiting facilitating factors related to the intended behavior, such as barriers to access. The TPB differs from the TRA by including PBC as a behavioral antecedent. The TPB has often been used in studies about behavioral intentions (Hagger et al., 2001), such as in physical activity related studies with adults (Godin, 1994; Hausenblas et al., 1997) and young people (Hagger et al., 2001; Plotnikoff et al., 2011; Craig et al., 1996). According to these studies, attitude and PBC tend to be the most important antecedents of physical activity intention. However, in the case of young people, the importance of subjective norm is higher (Hagger et al., 2001).

Alfred Bandura (1986) introduced the concept of self-efficacy, which refers to a person's beliefs in his/her capabilities of performing a specific task. Self-efficacy is not about the person's skills but rather a person's judgments regarding what they can do with these skills. People with high levels of self-efficacy are more likely to perceive difficult tasks as challenges and, therefore, perform better, whereas people with low levels of self-efficacy might avoid doing tasks which they perceive being difficult. Self-efficacy also relates to motivation. If a task is perceived as too difficult or too easy compared to one's own skills, motivation to continue can decrease. Conversely, tasks that are perceived as moderately difficult and challenging can produce the experience of achievement, thus bringing satisfaction (Bandura, 1998). Self-efficacy can also influence health-related behavior, including physical activity and exercise (Bandura, 1991).

According to Bandura (1986), there are four different sources of information affecting the person's self-efficacy: performance accomplishments, vicarious experience, verbal persuasion, and physiological states. Performance accomplishments are based on mastery experiences, and they are the most powerful source of self-efficacy. Vicarious experiences mean experiences received through observing other people. Verbal persuasion means comments and feedback heard from other people. Finally, physiological states refers to the perceived emotional arousal, such as stress, experienced in a specific situation.

The construct of self-efficacy is part of Bandura's social cognitive theory (Bandura, 1986), which emphasizes that the reactions, actions, and social behavior of an individual are influenced by actions they have observed from others. The social cognitive theory highlights the role of observational learning and social experience learning in personality development. It has often been used as a framework theory for studies focusing on motivation and physical activity. The theory of self-efficacy has been one of the most widely used theories when studying self-confidence in the field of health promotion (Kroll et al., 2007) and physical activity and sports (Feltz & Lirgg, 2001). Self-efficacy has also been demonstrated to have high influence in the adoption of physical activity (McAuley & Blissmer, 2000). The influence appears especially during the phase when the physical activity has not yet become habitual (Bandura, 1986). Self-efficacy has also been associated with the long-term maintenance of physical activity (McAuley et al., 2011). People with a high level of self-efficacy tend to participate more frequently, persist longer, and also exert more effort, thus enhancing their performance (Bandura, 1986), for example in regards to exercising and physical activity. Thus, self-efficacy plays an important role in everyday life when aiming to become more physically active and improve fitness.

The concept of self-efficacy was integrated to the TPB in 1991 (Ajzen, 1991). Self-efficacy has been closely associated with PBC, explaining the internal perceptions regarding personal abilities but leaving out the limiting facilitating factors. Dividing PBC into two parts, internal and external, has been recommended (Terry & O'Leary, 1995), proposing that self-efficacy reflects the internal aspects of control, such as the abilities to perform physical activity, and that PBC refers to the external aspects of control, such as the barriers for performing physical activity. Another conceptualization of PBC is presented by Fishbein and Ajzen (Fishbein & Ajzen, 2010) who divide it into two dimensions referred to as capacity and autonomy. Of these, capacity refers to the perception that one can, is able to, or is capable of performing the behavior and thus is comparable to self-efficacy. In contrast, autonomy refers to the perceived degree of control over performing the behavior. However, in some studies, the terms PBC and self-efficacy have been used interchangeably (Fishbein & Cappella, 2006).

This study is based on the theoretical model of Hagger et al. (2001), which used the TPB, combined with the concept of self-efficacy, to explain the exercise intentions of teenagers. However, the present study deviates from the theoretical model of Hagger et al. (2001) by concentrating only on self-efficacy and omitting PBC due to the aforementioned considerable conceptual overlap of these two constructs. In contrast to Hagger et al. (2001), the present study was also conducted study as an intervention study instead of a cross-sectional survey study. The theoretical model of the present study, in which intention (INT) is explained by attitude (ATT), subjective norm (SN), and self-efficacy (SE), is illustrated in Figure 1. The importance of attitude and self-efficacy related to exercise intentions is also highlighted in a study by Fishbein & Cappella (2006). Furthermore, intention and self-efficacy have been found to be the two strongest predictors regarding physical activity behavior of teenagers (Foley et al., 2008).

METHODOLOGY

Study Design and Data Collection

This study followed a mixed methods approach. The study was done in Finland and included 64 teenage participants of whom 34 were girls and 30 were boys. The age group was between 13 to 15 years old. The participants were divided into two groups. The intervention group consisted of 34 participants (18 girls, 16 boys) and the control group consisted of 30 participants (16 girls, 14 boys). The participants were recruited from three local junior high schools with the help of schoolteachers. The intervention group

Figure 1. Theoretical model of the study

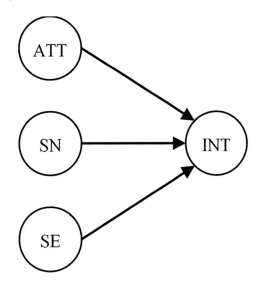

participants were recruited from two schools and the control group participants from a third school, in order for the groups to not know about the existence of the other group. All the students who expressed their interest were selected to the study regardless of their physical activity background. In Finland, the physical activity recommendation for teenagers (ages 12–18) is 1–1.5 hours per day (Husu et al., 2011). In the introduction phase, both groups were told the topic of the study was related to physical activity and exercise motivation. All the participants provided a signed consent form from their parents. The data was collected during winter 2017–2018 in two phases. In the beginning and end of the five-week intervention, the participants filled out a questionnaire about their perceptions regarding their own exercising and physical activity. These questionnaires provided data for the quantitative part of the study. The questionnaire used in the study was the same originally used by Hagger et al. (2001). To ensure the participants' level of understanding, the questionnaire was translated into Finnish. The translation was tested using academic representatives and representatives of the target group's demographic. In addition to the quantitative questionnaires, all participants filled out another questionnaire consisting of qualitative questions. The aim of the questionnaire was to find out in more detail the background of the participants related to physical activity and exercising, what kind of previous experience they had related to using sports and wellness technology, and how they perceived the role of technology in regards to exercise motivation.

Like the theoretical model, the measurement of the model constructs was based on the prior study by Hagger et al. (2001). In accordance with it, intention, attitude, and self-efficacy were each measured by using a reflective measurement model with three indicators. In contrast, subjective norm was measured by only one indicator, which is "quite common and consistent with TPB" (Courneya & Friedenreich, 1999, p. 116) although it obviously makes it impossible to statistically control the potential measurement error. The seven indicators that were measuring intention, attitude, and subjective norm were originally adapted from the reasoned action approach (Fishbein & Ajzen, 2010), whereas the three indicators that were measuring self-efficacy were developed in the study by Hagger et al. (2001) and applied from it. All the indicator wordings are reported in Table 1. The measurement scale of subjective norm and intention was a seven-point Likert scale, whereas the measurement scale of attitude was a seven-point semantic differential scale. In turn, the measurement scale of self-efficacy was a 10-point confidence scale ranging from 0% to 100%.

Table 1. Indicator wordings

Item	Wording
INT1	I intend to participate in physical activities that make me out of breath at least three times during my free time in the next week.
INT2	I plan to participate in physical activities that make me out of breath at least three times during my free time in the next week.
INT3	I will participate in physical activities that make me out of breath at least three times during my free time in the next week.
ATT1	Doing physical activities that make me out of breath at least three times in a week is bad vs. good.
ATT2	Doing physical activities that make me out of breath at least three times in a week is boring vs. exiting.
ATT3	Doing physical activities that make me out of breath at least three times in a week is unpleasant vs. fun.
SN	Most people important to me think I should do physical activities that make me out of breath at least three times in a week.
SE1	How confident are you in doing physical activities that make you out of breath at least three times in the next week when you are going out with your friends?
SE2	How confident are you in doing physical activities that make you out of breath at least three times in the next week when the weather is bad?
SE3	How confident are you in doing physical activities that make you out of breath at least three times in the next week when you have homework to do?

After the first round of questionnaires were finished, all the participants in the intervention group downloaded and installed a free sport and wellness technology application which they were asked to use for the next five weeks in a way most suitable for them. The aim of the study was not to intentionally try to increase the level of physical activity of the target group but rather to see whether using a sport and wellness technology application has an impact on their exercise intention from an exercise psychology point of view. Therefore, the use of the application was not controlled or observed during the intervention period and no extra promotion regarding physical activity was performed by the researchers or the teachers. Whereas the control group continued their physical activity habits as before, all the students in the intervention group reported to have been using the activity tracker during the intervention period in the most suitable way for them. In both the control and intervention groups, the level of participants' physical activity varied from almost sedentary to an athletic level. In the beginning of the study, most of the participants in both groups reported being somewhat familiar with sport and wellness technology, though for most of them, prior experience was restricted only to occasional usage.

After the intervention period, the intervention group participants were asked about their application usage. The average self-reported usage of the application was 2–3 times per week. The usage levels varied from as few as a couple of times per month to as frequently as daily usage. Most participants reported using the workout tracking and training log features, whereas the social media sharing was not used by most participants.

The Application Used in This Study

The sport and wellness technology application used in this study was called Sports Tracker, of which the study used the premium version as it is ad-free and has more features (Sports Tracker, 2018). Sports Tracker is a fitness app for smart phones. The app functions as a workout tracking app, training log, and social media platform for the app's users. The app serves three main functions. First, it is an exercise tracking app, utilizing a smart phone's GPS signal to track the user's route and provide speed and distance data in real-time. At the end of the workout, the app provides information on the distance the user covered, their speed, elevation gain, steps taken, and several other measurements. The app also presents a map of the user's route and a calculation of the burned calories.

The second function is that the app serves as a training log. All of the workouts a user performs with the app are stored in the cloud and can be reviewed at any time. Further, the app can present cumulative workout data, such as measuring how much training has been done in the past week or how many calories have been burned in the past month. A user may optionally use a previous workout to set a route for an upcoming workout, and the app will provide directions to follow this route. A target speed for the route is given. A user may additionally create a "ghost" workout, enabling them to race themselves from a previous workout, and be given feedback in real-time on how their performance compares to their "ghost", i.e., past performance.

Third, the app enables users to share their routes with other users of the app. Users may optionally make their route available to others, either specific people or publicly. Others can then give a "thumbs up" or give comments. A user can also post photos or videos of their route. Conversely, users can also explore posted workouts from other users, create a ghost workout similar to that described above, or explore a map showing routes other users have posted. Users may also follow specific people and receive updates in the app when those people have posted new workouts.

The application was suitable for the study since it consisted of basic tracking functions as well the ability to be used in Finnish language. The application can be used with various sports and activities, which were suitable for the target group.

Data Analysis

The collected data was analyzed by using structural equation modelling. The data was collected from two points in time instead of one. Because of this, the approach suggested by Roemer (2016) was used, in which the model constructs were operationalized as change constructs that capture the potential change in their values between the two surveys. The indicators of these constructs were formed by subtracting the value of the specific indicator in the first survey from the value of that same indicator in the second survey.

Because of the small sample size, variance-based partial least squares (PLS), instead of the covariance-based approach, was used as the structural equation modelling approach for estimating the models. However, by following the rough "ten times rule of thumb" (Chin, 1998; Hair et al., 2016), which suggests a minimum sample size of ten times the largest number of indicators used to measure a construct with a formative measurement model or ten times the largest number of structural paths directed at a specific construct in the structural model, the sample size can still be considered as large enough in order to estimate separate models for the intervention group and the control group.

The model estimation was done with the SmartPLS 3.2.7 software (Ringle et al., 2015) and by following the guidelines given by (Hair et al., 2017) for running the analyses and reporting the results in the IS context. For example, in the model estimation, path weighting was used as the weighting scheme and +1 as the initial weights, while the statistical significance of the model estimates was tested by using bootstrapping with 2,500 subsamples and individual sign changes. As the limit for statistical significance, the study used $p < 0.05$. When estimating the models, all the constructs were specified as mode A (Roemer, 2016) constructs measured by a reflective measurement model. Also, subjective norm was specified as a latent construct but measured by only single indicator whose loading and weight were fixed to one. Because the proportions of missing values were very low (about 2.1% of the values in the intervention group and about 2.4% of the values in the control group), they were handled by using simple mean replacement.

The comparisons between the intervention group and the control group were based on first establishing an adequate level of measurement invariance by using the three-step MICOM (measurement invariance of composite models) procedure by Henseler et al. (2016). More specifically, the MICOM procedure posits that both configural and compositional invariance have to hold across the groups before any tests concerning the equality of their construct means, construct variances, and path coefficients can be meaningfully conducted.

The qualitative data received from the questionnaires were analyzed using thematic analysis, which is a method for "identifying, analyzing, and reporting patterns (themes) within data" (Braun & Clarke, 2006, p. 79). Thematic analysis is the most widely used analysis method in qualitative research (Braun & Clarke, 2006). Thematic analysis enables organizing and describing the data in rich detail and to interpret various aspects of the research topic (Braun & Clarke, 2006). To assist in conducting the analysis, guidelines by Braun and Clarke (2006) were applied, and as suggested, these guidelines were applied flexibly to fit the research questions and the collected data.

Background of the Participants

The participants' physical activity background varied. 19% of the participants reported being physically active less than seven hours per week, 48% of the participants reported to be active 7–10 hours per week, and the remaining 33% reported to be physically active more than ten hours on a weekly basis. The reported physical activity time included active time in commuting to school, physical education classes as well as physical activity done in leisure time. In Finland the physical activity recommendation for teenagers (ages 12-18) is 1–1,5 hours per day, which equals 7–10 hours per week (Husu et al., 2001). Despite the fact that around 80% of the participants reported being physically active enough to meet this recommendation, 39% of the participants felt they needed to increase their general physical activity levels.

The main motivation for participants to be physically active was the good feeling associated with physical activity, as illustrated by the following quote: "exercising makes me feel good and it is fun". This intrinsic type of motivation was reported to be the main reason for exercising for 53% of the participants. The next most important motivation for exercising was gaining and maintaining better physical condition, followed by having spending time with friends or even getting new friends via physical activities. Other, less frequently mentioned sources of exercise motivation were related to personal appearance and weight loss, being able to challenge and develop oneself, a love for a particular sport, and the possibility to relax and reduce stress with exercising. Only three participants reported being physically active because they wanted to ensure they would stay healthy in the future.

RESULTS

For the quantitative results, the study will first report the results of model estimation as well as the evaluations of model reliability and validity separately for both the intervention group and the control group. After this, the study will report the results of the group comparisons in terms of construct means, construct variances, and path coefficients. After these, the qualitative results will be presented in the last sub-section.

Model Estimation

Figure 2 reports the results of model estimation in terms of standardized path coefficients, their statistical significance, and the proportion of explained variance (R2) for both the intervention group (left side) and the control group (right side). In both groups, the effects of attitude, subjective norm, and self-efficacy on intention were found as positive, but there were considerable differences in the effect sizes and statistical significance of the effects between the two groups. In the intervention group, both self-efficacy and attitude had a statistically significant effect on intention, and the model explained about 65.0% of the variance in intention. In contrast, in the control group, all the effects were statistically not significant, and the model explained about 19.5% of the variance in intention.

Figure 2. Results of model estimation (left = intervention group, right = control group, *** = p < 0.001, ** = p < 0.01, * = p < 0.05)

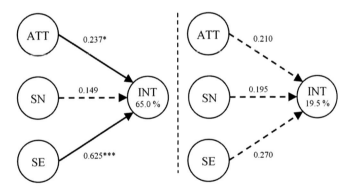

Reliability, Validity, and Goodness-of-Fit

The reliability and validity of the estimated models for both the groups were evaluated at the indicator and construct levels. Indicator reliabilities and validities were evaluated by using the standardized loadings of the indicators. In a typical case in which each indicator loads only on one construct, it is commonly expected that the standardized loading of each indicator should be statistically significant and greater than or equal to 0.707 (Fornell & Larcker, 1981). However, in some prior IS studies, even standardized loadings of as low as 0.4 have been seen as acceptable (Gefen et al., 2000). In this study, as a compromise, the standardized loading of 0.6 was used as the criterion for acceptance. The standardized loadings of

Table 2. Indicator means, standard deviations (SD), and loadings (*** = p < 0.001, ** = p < 0.01, * = p < 0.05, a = fixed to one)

	Intervention Group			Control Group		
	Mean	**SD**	**Loading**	**Mean**	**SD**	**Loading**
INT1	-0.029	1.749	0.863***	0.267	1.081	0.886***
INT2	-0.206	1.789	0.881***	0.233	1.073	0.853***
INT3	-0.029	1.732	0.893***	0.533	1.252	0.829***
ATT1	0.118	0.769	0.776**	-0.241	0.857	0.678**
ATT2	-0.091	0.668	0.651**	0.379	1.064	0.821**
ATT3	0.091	0.668	0.878***	-0.036	0.928	0.810***
SN1	0.419	1.343	1.000[a]	0.233	1.194	1.000[a]
SE1	-0.636	2.772	0.891***	-0.500	1.776	0.818***
SE2	-0.212	2.280	0.845***	-0.367	3.168	0.784***
SE3	0.545	2.536	0.766***	-0.241	2.873	0.872***

the indicators for both the groups are reported in Table 2, along with their mean and standard deviation (SD). As can be seen, the criterion was met by all the indicators.

Construct reliabilities were evaluated by checking that the composite reliability (CR) of each construct was greater than or equal to 0.7 (Fornell & Larcker, 1981; Nunnally & Bernstein, 1994). The CR of the constructs is reported in the first column of Table 3 for the intervention group and Table 4 for the control group. As shown, all the constructs met this criterion. Construct validities were evaluated by examining the convergent and discriminant validity of each construct by using the two criteria based on the average variance extracted (AVE) of the constructs, which refers to the average proportion of variance a construct explains in its indicators (Hair et al., 2017). To have acceptable convergent validity, the first criterion requires that each construct have an AVE greater than or equal to 0.5, meaning that, on average, each construct should explain at least half of the variance of its indicators. The AVE of the constructs is reported in the second column of Table 3 for the intervention group and Table 4 for the control group. As shown, all the constructs met this criterion.

Table 3. Construct reliabilities (CR), average variances extracted (AVE), and construct correlations for the intervention group

	CR	**AVE**	**INT**	**ATT**	**SN**	**SE**
INT	0.911	0.773	0.879			
ATT	0.815	0.599	0.549	0.774		
SN	1.000	1.000	0.304	0.178	1.000	
SE	0.874	0.698	0.760	0.457	0.181	0.835

Table 4. Construct reliabilities (CR), average variances extracted (AVE), and construct correlations for the control group

	CR	AVE	INT	ATT	SN	SE
INT	0.892	0.733	0.856			
ATT	0.815	0.597	0.245	0.773		
SN	1.000	1.000	0.337	0.375	1.000	
SE	0.865	0.682	0.287	-0.140	0.235	0.826

In order to have acceptable discriminant validity, the second criterion requires that each construct should have a square root of AVE greater than or equal to its absolute correlation with the other constructs. This means that, on average, each construct should share at least an equal proportion of variance with its indicators than it shares with the other constructs. The square root of AVE of the constructs (on-diagonal cells) and the correlations between the constructs (off-diagonal cells) are reported in the remaining columns of Table 3 for the intervention group and Table 4 for the control group. As shown, all constructs also met this criterion.

In addition, the discriminant validity was evaluated by examining the cross loadings of the indicators. Here, in both the groups, all the indicators were found to have the highest loadings on the constructs that they were intended to measure, thus offering further support for acceptable discriminant validity.

Finally, although not in the guidelines by Hair et al., (2017) and perhaps more common in the case of models estimated with consistent partial least squares (PLSc) (Dijkstra & Henseler, 2015a; Dijkstra & Henseler, 2015b) rather than with the traditional PLS, the goodness-of-fit of the estimated models were also evaluated for both the groups in line with Henseler et al. (2016). This was done by checking whether the standardized root mean square residual (SRMR), the geodesic discrepancy dG and the unweighted least squares discrepancy dULS (Dijkstra & Henseler, 2015a) of the estimated models as well as the saturated models with freely estimated correlations between the constructs were all within their 95% confidence intervals obtained from the Bollen-Stine (Bollen & Stine, 1992) bootstrapping. As this was found to be the case, it can be concluded that the discrepancy indicated by the aforementioned fit indices between the empirical covariance matrices and the covariance matrices implied by the estimated models is quite likely to result from sampling error rather than from a bad fit with the estimated models and the data. Therefore, the estimated models should not be rejected. However, this conclusion should be taken with caution as the value of evaluating the goodness-of-fit in the case of PLS still remains an open question (Hair et al., 2016).

Group Comparisons

As already discussed above, the group comparisons and the investigation of measurement invariance were based on the three-step MICOM procedure (Henseler et al., 2016). First, configural invariance between the groups was found to hold because both groups employed an identical set of indicators to measure the constructs. In addition, the data treatment and the algorithm settings in both groups were identical.

Second, compositional invariance was assessed by examining whether the indicator weights estimated for the two groups are equal. One way to do this is through testing whether the correlation of the composite scores calculated for each study participant by using the indicator weights estimated for

Table 5. Testing compositional invariance

	c	95% CI of c	p (c = 1)
INT	0.987	[0.986, 1.000]	0.051
ATT	0.917	[0.521, 1.000]	0.533
SN	1.000	[1.000, 1.000]	1.000
SE	0.996	[0.917, 1.000]	0.766

the intervention group with the composite scores calculated for the each study participant by using the indicator weights estimated for the control group (c = cor(ξIntervention, ξControl)) is equal to one. As a statistical test for this, a permutation test with 5,000 permutations was used (Henseler et al., 2016). The results of these tests in terms of the test statistic c, the 95% confidence interval (CI) of the test statistic c, as well as the p value of the null hypothesis c = 1 are reported in Table 5. As can be seen, compositional invariance between the two groups was found to hold for all the constructs. Thus, the construct scores of the study participants can also be calculated by using the indicator weights estimated for the pooled sample instead of using the indicator weights estimated separately for each group.

Third, the equivalence of the means and variances of the constructs was assessed by first calculating the construct scores of each study participant by using the indicator weights estimated for the pooled sample and then testing whether the difference in mean of the construct scores calculated for the intervention group and the mean of the construct scores calculated for the control group (m = mean ξIntervention – mean ξControl) as well as the logarithm of the ratio of the variance of the construct scores calculated for the intervention group to the variance of the constructs scores calculated for the control group (v = log(var ξIntervention / var ξControl)) is zero. As a statistical test for this, a permutation test with 5,000 permutations was used (Henseler et al., 2016). The results of these tests in terms of the test statistics m and v, their 95% confidence interval of the test statistics m and v, as well as the p value of the null hypotheses m = 0 and v = 0 are reported in Table 6 in the case of the equivalence of means and in Table 7 in the case of the equivalence of variances. As shown, in the case of all constructs, the 95% confidence interval of both test statistics included zero, supporting the null hypothesis that there were no differences in the means or variances of any of the constructs between the groups.

Table 6. Testing the equality of construct variances

	m	95% CI of m	p (m = 0)
INT	-0.326	[-0.509, 0.478]	0.194
ATT	0.050	[-0.518, 0.482]	0.843
SN	0.148	[-0.471, 0.476]	0.565
SE	0.067	[-0.481, 0.490]	0.788

Finally, the equivalence of the path coefficients was tested. The study used the bias-corrected 95% confidence intervals according to Shi (1992) in line with the procedure proposed by Sarstedt et al., (2011), in which it is checked whether the effect sizes estimated for the intervention group are within the

Table 7. Testing the equality of construct means

	v	95% CI of v	p (v = 0)
INT	0.901	[-0.983, 1.010]	0.079
ATT	-0.625	[-0.954, 1.044]	0.221
SN	0.239	[-0.859, 0.893]	0.601
SE	0.289	[-0.957, 0.990]	0.556

corresponding 95% bias-corrected confidence intervals of the control group and vice versa. If there is no overlap, this means that there is a statistically significant difference in the path coefficients between the two groups. The effect sizes and their 95% bias-corrected confidence intervals (CI) for both groups are reported in Table 8. As shown, a statistically significant difference in the path coefficients was found only in the effect of self-efficacy on intention, which was found to be much stronger in the intervention group. The study also replicated the analysis while using no sign changes in bootstrapping, but this did not change the results.

Table 8. Testing the equality of path coefficients

Effect	Group	Effect Size	95% CI
ATT ® INT	Intervention	0.237	[0.013, 0.394]
ATT ® INT	Control	0.210	[0.000, 0.377]
SN ® INT	Intervention	0.149	[0.009, 0.334]
SN ® INT	Control	0.195	[0.003, 0.512]
SE ® INT	Intervention	0.625	[0.397, 0.801]
SE ® INT	Control	0.270	[0.005, 0.553]

Teenagers and Sport and Wellness Technology – Qualitative Findings

Before the study, 70% of the participants had some previous experience with sport and wellness technology. However, in most cases the experience did not include longer-term usage but was limited to a shorter period of time or was used less consistently. The participants who reported using sport and wellness technology on almost a daily basis were usually using a mobile phone application to keep track of their daily steps.

Most of the participants had used either step counters or other exercise and health applications that were included on their mobile phones. Only a few of the participants were using or had used wearable fitness trackers, sport watches, or heart rate monitors to measure their physical activity.

The main reasons reported for using sport and wellness technology was the desire to see actual data regarding their own exercising and to keep track of how much they have exercised. For some participants this meant paying attention to their step count or the number of kilometers walked, keeping an exercise diary, or comparing their fitness results to previous results. Some of the participants said the main reason to use sport and wellness technology is because it is entertaining and makes exercising more fun, whereas other participants said including technology into training makes exercising easier and more comfortable. There were also a few participants who used sport and wellness technology to track their sleep or to increase their training efficiency by staying in the right heart rate zone.

Participants were also asked whether they thought using sport and wellness technology has potential in increasing people's exercise motivation. Almost all thought technology can increase motivation towards physical activity. The reasons behind this perception varied between participants, including for example, being able to follow one's performance and progress with the help of technology, being able to set specific goals, being able to compete against oneself by trying to increase the level of personal performance, having an encouraging reminder to exercise, having a tool to bring more variety to exercise and having something that can provide instructions on what to do. Some participants also stated that technology is part of everyday life and therefore it is natural to use it as a part of physical activity and exercising. However, it was also stated that in order to make sport and wellness technology more attractive, they should have enough variety to keep the user interested. At the same time, the technology should also be easy to use. Some participants also believed that having an interest towards a sport technology device or application might be the needed first motivation for a sedentary teenager to start doing physical activity.

In the end of the study, the intervention group participants were asked whether using the Sports Tracker application had had any influence on their exercise motivation. 53% of the participants stated that the use of the application had increased their motivation towards physical activity and exercise, whereas 38% of the participants stated the technology had not increased their motivation. The remaining 9% were not sure. The most common features related to increased motivation were goal setting, gamification features, and the ability to track one's results and performance. Despite the positive perceptions, teenagers felt that sport and wellness technology might have a negative effect for exercising. The main negative issue was focusing too much on the data and results instead of the actual activity. This might make exercising too performance oriented and competitive, and could also be distracting during the exercise. Other presented negative issues were the need to carry the phone during the exercise, and that sharing exercise data can lead to social comparison, which may lead to feelings of inferiority and subsequently decrease the motivation to be physically active or to exercise.

The participants seemed to have relatively high trust towards the information provided by sport and wellness technology in general. They also had high confidence in themselves when it came to learning to use new sport and wellness technology devices and applications. While the high level of trust towards technology was almost equal between boys and girls, the level of self-efficacy regarding using new sport and wellness technology devices and applications was slightly higher among boys.

DISCUSSION AND RECOMMENDATIONS

This study used a mixed methods approach to study the impact of using sport and wellness technology on teenagers and their physical activity. The study was conducted as a five-week-long intervention study including 64 teenage participants divided into an intervention group and a control group. The theoretical model used in the study was based on the TPB combined with the concept of self-efficacy. The aim was to quantitatively find out whether a sport and wellness technology application can affect the constructs and their interrelationships in the theoretical model and subsequently influence the physical activity behavior of teenagers. In addition, qualitative data was collected to investigate teenagers' perception towards sport and wellness technologies.

Regarding the quantitative investigation, there were two main findings. First, no statistically significant differences between the two groups in terms of the means and variances of the four change constructs (attitude, subjective norm, self-efficacy, and intention) were found. This means that the average attitude, subjective norm, self-efficacy, and intention of the study participants towards physical activity and exercising did not increase or decrease due to the intervention, and the intervention also did not increase or decrease the variance between the study participants in these respects. Second, no statistically significant differences between the groups in the effects of attitude and subjective norm on intention were found, but a statistically significant difference was found in the effect of self-efficacy on intention. This effect was found to be considerably stronger in the intervention group than in the control group. This suggests that the intervention strengthened the causal relationship between self-efficacy and intention so that positive changes in self-efficacy were likely to result in positive changes in intention, whereas negative changes in self-efficacy were likely to result in negative changes in intention. In other words, although the intervention did not affect self-efficacy or intention itself, it seemed to moderate their interrelationship.

Regarding the qualitative investigation, the main findings were that the use purposes varied a lot between the participants. However, the most important reason for using sport and wellness technology seemed to be the desire to see actual data regarding one's own exercising and keeping track of one's own physical activities and performances. Further, most participants perceived sport and wellness technology, in general, as having potential in increasing motivation towards physical activity and exercise. Indeed, over half of the intervention group participants stated that the use of the application had increased their motivation towards physical activity and exercise during the intervention. However, despite all the positive perceptions, the participants also saw potential negative issues in using these technologies, most notably focusing too much on the data instead of the actual physical activity, and the possible negative feelings resulting from social comparison.

From a theoretical point of view, the findings suggest that the use of sport and wellness technology, with self-monitoring of behavior as an intervention tool, can promote the relationship between exercise self-efficacy and exercise intention. The results contribute to previous research (Hagger et al., 2001) highlighting the role of sport and wellness technology as a mediator between self-efficacy and intention. The sport and wellness technology application was able to activate cognitive mechanisms for the behavior. However, it seems that other significant determinants such as planning or environmental influences were not activated, which suggests that a basic physical activity tracker needs other supporting additional intervention techniques to be effective for teenagers.

When comparing the results from the qualitative and quantitative data, it can be seen that even though teenagers perceive sport and wellness technology in general having potential to increase exercise motivation, the quantitative results showed no statistically significant change in exercise intention. This could mean that even though the particular sport and wellness technology application used in this study was not perceived to affect motivation, other types of sport and wellness technology still might. It can also be that the particular sport and wellness technology device used in this study was able to temporarily increase participant's exercise motivation but did not lead to significant changes in longer term motivation.

Although the reason for the intervention promoting the relationship between self-efficacy and intention cannot be explained by the research data, from a practical point of view, by having a sport and wellness technology application, the teenagers had a chance to see their exercise performance through numeric data and follow their exercise routines. This could have increased their awareness regarding their own physical activity. As highlighted by Hagger et al., (2001), exercise data can help teenagers get personal control over their exercising. Further, the information from the activity tracker, received via self-monitoring, may have affected the user's self-efficacy, which relates to having increased or decreased intentions for physical activity. An association between exercise self-efficacy and self-regulation techniques, such as self-monitoring, has been found in previous research (Belmon et al., 2015; Zimmermann, 2000). The feeling of psychological capability (self-efficacy) is an important element in behavioral change processes (Michie et al., 2014). However, it is important to note that there are other elements, such as physical capability, motivation, and social and physical opportunity that affect the intention and behavior.

Sport and wellness technology has been found to affect the levels of physical intention among adults (Hurling et al., 2007). However, according to an intervention study among teenagers by Gaudet et al., (2017), activity trackers are not able to affect the physical activity levels in general but can affect participants who have a more positive attitude towards physical activity. Other previous studies done among Finnish teenagers have also found potential in using sport and wellness technology, although they have not focused on testing psychological determinants (Schaefer et al., 2016; Ridgers et al., 2016: Ng et al., 2017; Kettunen & Kari, 2018). The results of this study are in line with previous research showing that the use of sport and wellness technology in teenage-targeted interventions can have the potential to influence physical activity intentions, but the technology should be accompanied with other intervention tools for better effectiveness. Since teenagers are an important target group, it is important to study the preferences of teenagers to make the physical activity interventions more successful.

Limitations

This study has a few notable limitations. First, the size of the study sample was relatively small with 64 participants. Regardless, a strong and statistically significant moderation effect was found in the interrelationship between self-efficacy and exercise intention. In the future, it would be valuable to do similar studies with a larger data set as well as combining and comparing the psychological data with actual physical activity data. Second, the intervention period was approximately five weeks long – a relatively short period. This limits the findings to short-term effects. Future similar studies should be conducted with longer durations. Third, the participants in this study self-reported to be more physically active (80% meeting PA recommendations) than the general teenage population (40% meeting PA recommendations) in Finland. However, in reality, this difference might not be so big considering the known challenges of research participants intentionally reporting their behavior more positively than reality (Sirard & Pate, 2001). Still, this can affect the generalizability of the results. Similarly, because the usage levels of the application were not tracked using the application itself, the self-reported usage data cannot be compared to any other physical activity data.

FUTURE RESEARCH DIRECTIONS

The sport and wellness technology device used in this study was relatively simple, consisting only of elements related to basic physical activity and exercise tracking. In the future, similar studies could be done using more advanced devices or applications, for example, ones that include gamification (Kettunen & Kari, 2018; Kari et al., 2016) or exergaming (Kari & Makkonen, 2014) elements. Focus could also be in personalized instructions and feedback (e.g., digital coaching) elements as suggested by previous research done among teenagers in Finland (Ng et al., 2017; Kettunen & Kari, 2018). These elements could make the sport and wellness technology more interesting for teenagers so that they would want to continue using them for longer, which could subsequently promote physical activity and a healthier lifestyle. Future research could also focus on determining which application-based interventions are most effective in increasing positive feelings towards physical activity.

CONCLUSION

To summarize, based on the findings, adding a sport and wellness technology device or application to a physical activity intervention can increase the connection between self-efficacy and physical activity intentions. However, using activity-tracking sport and wellness technology applications is not necessarily enough to induce actual changes in the physical activity intentions or behaviors. Therefore, based on the findings, adding some additional motivational elements into the interventions to affect the exercise intention and behavior could prove worthwhile. Adding additional motivational elements to basic activity trackers or using sport technology along with other kinds of intervention tools such as a human or digital coach is recommended.

ACKNOWLEDGMENT

This research received no specific grant from any funding agency in the public, commercial, or not-for-profit sectors.

REFERENCES

Ajzen, H., & Fishbein, M. (1980). *Understanding attitudes and predicting social behavior*. Academic Press.

Ajzen, I. (1985). From intentions to actions: A theory of planned behavior. In *Action control* (pp. 11–39). Springer. doi:10.1007/978-3-642-69746-3_2

Ajzen, I. (1991). The theory of planned behavior. *Organizational Behavior and Human Decision Processes*, *50*(2), 179–211. doi:10.1016/0749-5978(91)90020-T

Bandura, A. (1986). Social foundations of thought and action. Academic Press.

Bandura, A. (1991). Self-efficacy mechanism in physiological activation and health-promoting behavior. *Neurobiology of learning, emotion and affect*, 229-269.

Bandura, A. (1998). Health promotion from the perspective of social cognitive theory. *Psychology & Health*, *13*(4), 623–649. doi:10.1080/08870449808407422

Belmon, L. S., Middelweerd, A., te Velde, S. J., & Brug, J. (2015). Dutch young adults ratings of behavior change techniques applied in mobile phone apps to promote physical activity: A cross-sectional survey. *JMIR mHealth and uHealth*, *3*(4), e103. doi:10.2196/mhealth.4383 PMID:26563744

Bollen, K. A., & Stine, R. A. (1992). Bootstrapping goodness-of-fit measures in structural equation models. *Sociological Methods & Research, 21*(2), 205–229. doi:10.1177/0049124192021002004

Braun, V., & Clarke, V. (2006). Using thematic analysis in psychology. *Qualitative Research in Psychology, 3*(2), 77–101. doi:10.1191/1478088706qp063oa

Brodersen, N. H., Steptoe, A., Boniface, D. R., Wardle, J., & Hillsdon, M. (2007). Trends in physical activity and sedentary behaviour in adolescence: Ethnic and socioeconomic differences. *British Journal of Sports Medicine, 41*(3), 140–144. doi:10.1136/bjsm.2006.031138 PMID:17178773

Carrino, S., Caon, M., Khaled, O. A., Andreoni, G., & Mugellini, E. (2014, June). Pegaso: Towards a life companion. In *International Conference on Digital Human Modeling and Applications in Health, Safety, Ergonomics and Risk Management* (pp. 325-331). Springer.

Carrion, C., Caon, M., Carrino, S., Moliner, L. A., Lang, A., Atkinson, S., . . . Espallargues, M. (2015, September). Wearable lifestyle tracking devices: are they useful for teenagers? In *Adjunct Proceedings of the 2015 ACM International Joint Conference on Pervasive and Ubiquitous Computing and Proceedings of the 2015 ACM International Symposium on Wearable Computers* (pp. 669-674). Academic Press.

Chin, W. W. (1998). The partial least squares approach to structural equation modeling. *Modern methods for business research, 295*(2), 295-336.

Courneya, K. S., & Friedenreich, C. M. (1999). Utility of the theory of planned behavior for understanding exercise during breast cancer treatment. Psycho-Oncology: Journal of the Psychological. *Social and Behavioral Dimensions of Cancer, 8*(2), 112–122. PMID:10335555

Craig, S., Goldberg, J., & Dietz, W. H. (1996). Psychosocial correlates of physical activity among fifth and eighth graders. *Preventive Medicine, 25*(5), 506–513. doi:10.1006/pmed.1996.0083 PMID:8888317

Dijkstra, T. K., & Henseler, J. (2015). Consistent and asymptotically normal PLS estimators for linear structural equations. *Computational Statistics & Data Analysis, 81*, 10–23. doi:10.1016/j.csda.2014.07.008

Dijkstra, T. K., & Henseler, J. (2015). Consistent partial least squares path modeling. *Management Information Systems Quarterly, 39*(2), 297–316. doi:10.25300/MISQ/2015/39.2.02

Direito, A., Jiang, Y., Whittaker, R., & Maddison, R. (2015). Smartphone apps to improve fitness and increase physical activity among young people: Protocol of the Apps for IMproving FITness (AIM-FIT) randomized controlled trial. *BMC Public Health, 15*(1), 635. doi:10.118612889-015-1968-y PMID:26159834

Dos Santos, H., Bredehoft, M. D., Gonzalez, F. M., & Montgomery, S. (2016). Exercise video games and exercise self-efficacy in children. *Global pediatric health, 3*, 2333794X16644139.

Feltz, D. L., & Lirgg, C. D. (2001). Self-efficacy beliefs of athletes, teams, and coaches. Handbook of sport psychology, 2(2001), 340-361.

Fishbein, M., & Ajzen, I. (1975). *Belief, attitude, intention, and behavior: An introduction to theory and research*. Addison-Wesley.

Fishbein, M., & Ajzen, I. (2010). *Predicting and Changing Behavior: The Reasoned Action Approach.* Taylor & Francis.

Fishbein, M., & Cappella, J. N. (2006). The role of theory in developing effective health communications. *Journal of Communication, 56*(suppl_1), 1–17. doi:10.1111/j.1460-2466.2006.00280.x

Foley, L., Prapavessis, H., Maddison, R., Burke, S., McGowan, E., & Gillanders, L. (2008). Predicting physical activity intention and behavior in school-age children. *Pediatric Exercise Science, 20*(3), 342–356. doi:10.1123/pes.20.3.342 PMID:18714123

Fornell, C., & Larcker, D. F. (1981). Evaluating structural equation models with unobservable variables and measurement error. *JMR, Journal of Marketing Research, 18*(1), 39–50. doi:10.1177/002224378101800104

Gaudet, J., Gallant, F., & Bélanger, M. (2017). A bit of fit: Minimalist intervention in adolescents based on a physical activity tracker. *JMIR mHealth and uHealth, 5*(7), e92. doi:10.2196/mhealth.7647 PMID:28684384

Gefen, D., Straub, D., & Boudreau, M. C. (2000). Structural equation modeling and regression: Guidelines for research practice. *Communications of the Association for Information Systems, 4*(1), 7.

Godin, G. (1994). Theories of reasoned action and planned behavior: Usefulness for exercise promotion. *Medicine and Science in Sports and Exercise, 26*(11), 1391–1394. doi:10.1249/00005768-199411000-00014 PMID:7837960

Guest, G., MacQueen, K. M., & Namey, E. E. (2012). *Applied Thematic Analysis.* SAGE. doi:10.4135/9781483384436

Hagger, M. S., Chatzisarantis, N., & Biddle, S. J. (2001). The influence of self-efficacy and past behaviour on the physical activity intentions of young people. *Journal of Sports Sciences, 19*(9), 711–725. doi:10.1080/02640410152475847 PMID:11522147

Hair, J., Hollingsworth, C. L., Randolph, A. B., & Chong, A. Y. L. (2017). An updated and expanded assessment of PLS-SEM in information systems research. *Industrial Management & Data Systems, 117*(3), 442–458. doi:10.1108/IMDS-04-2016-0130

Hair, J. F. Jr, Hult, G. T. M., Ringle, C., & Sarstedt, M. (2016). *A primer on partial least squares structural equation modeling (PLS-SEM).* Sage publications.

Hausenblas, H. A., Carron, A. V., & Mack, D. E. (1997). Application of the theories of reasoned action and planned behavior to exercise behavior: A meta-analysis. *Journal of Sport & Exercise Psychology, 19*(1), 36–51. doi:10.1123/jsep.19.1.36

Henseler, J., Hubona, G., & Ray, P. A. (2016). Using PLS path modeling in new technology research: Updated guidelines. *Industrial Management & Data Systems, 116*(1), 2–20. doi:10.1108/IMDS-09-2015-0382

Henseler, J., Ringle, C. M., & Sarstedt, M. (2016). Testing measurement invariance of composites using partial least squares. *International Marketing Review, 33*(3), 405–431. doi:10.1108/IMR-09-2014-0304

Hurling, R., Catt, M., De Boni, M., Fairley, B., Hurst, T., Murray, P., Richardson, A., & Sodhi, J. (2007). Using internet and mobile phone technology to deliver an automated physical activity program: Randomized controlled trial. *Journal of Medical Internet Research*, 9(2), e7. doi:10.2196/jmir.9.2.e7 PMID:17478409

Husu, P., Paronen, O., Suni, J., & Vasankari, T. (2011). *Suomalaisten fyysinen aktiivisuus ja kunto 2010: terveyttä edistävän liikunnan nykytila ja muutokset* [The Physical Activity Levels of Finns, 2010]. Opetus ja Kulttuuriministeriön Julkaisuja.

Kari, J. T., Pehkonen, J., Hutri-Kähönen, N., Raitakari, O. T., & Tammelin, T. H. (2017). Longitudinal associations between physical activity and educational outcomes. *Medicine and Science in Sports and Exercise*, 49(11), 2158–2166. doi:10.1249/MSS.0000000000001351 PMID:29045322

Kari, J. T., Tammelin, T. H., Viinikainen, J., Hutri-Kähönen, N., Raitakari, O. T., & Pehkonen, J. (2016). Childhood physical activity and adulthood earnings. *Medicine and Science in Sports and Exercise*, 48(7), 1340–1346. doi:10.1249/MSS.0000000000000895 PMID:26871991

Kari, T., & Makkonen, M. (2014). Explaining the usage intentions of exergames. *35th International Conference on Information Systems, Auckland 2014. Association for Information Systems (AIS)*.

Kari, T., Piippo, J., Frank, L., Makkonen, M., & Moilanen, P. (2016). To gamify or not to gamify? Gamification in exercise applications and its role in impacting exercise motivation. *BLED 2016: Proceedings of the 29th Bled eConference Digital Economy*.

Kettunen, E., & Kari, T. (2018). Can Sport and Wellness Technology be My Personal Trainer?: Teenagers and Digital Coaching. In *Bled eConference*. University of Maribor Press. doi:10.18690/978-961-286-170-4.32

Knell, G., Durand, C. P., Kohl, H. W., Wu, I. H., & Gabriel, K. P. (2019). Prevalence and likelihood of meeting sleep, physical activity, and screen-time guidelines among US youth. *JAMA Pediatrics*, 173(4), 387–389. doi:10.1001/jamapediatrics.2018.4847 PMID:30715096

Kroll, T., Kehn, M., Ho, P. S., & Groah, S. (2007). The SCI exercise self-efficacy scale (ESES): Development and psychometric properties. *The International Journal of Behavioral Nutrition and Physical Activity*, 4(1), 34. doi:10.1186/1479-5868-4-34 PMID:17760999

Kumar, B., Robinson, R., & Till, S. (2015). Physical activity and health in adolescence. *Clinical Medicine*, 15(3), 267–272. doi:10.7861/clinmedicine.15-3-267 PMID:26031978

Masteller, B., Sirard, J., & Freedson, P. (2017). The Physical Activity Tracker Testing in Youth (PATTY) Study: Content Analysis and Children's Perceptions. *JMIR mHealth and uHealth*, 5(4), e55. doi:10.2196/mhealth.6347 PMID:28455278

McAuley, E., & Blissmer, B. (2000). Self-efficacy determinants and consequences of physical activity. *Exercise and Sport Sciences Reviews*, 28(2), 85–88. PMID:10902091

McAuley, E., Szabo, A., Gothe, N., & Olson, E. A. (2011). Self-efficacy: Implications for physical activity, function, and functional limitations in older adults. *American Journal of Lifestyle Medicine*, 5(4), 361–369. doi:10.1177/1559827610392704 PMID:24353482

Michie, S., Atkins, L., & West, R. (2014). *The behaviour change wheel: a guide to designing interventions.* Silverback Publishing.

Ng, K., Tynjälä, J., & Kokko, S. (2017). Ownership and use of commercial physical activity trackers among Finnish adolescents: Cross-sectional study. *JMIR mHealth and uHealth, 5*(5), e61. doi:10.2196/mhealth.6940 PMID:28473304

Nunnally, J. C. (1994). *Psychometric theory 3E.* Tata McGraw-Hill Education.

Plotnikoff, R. C., Lubans, D. R., Costigan, S. A., Trinh, L., Spence, J. C., Downs, S., & McCargar, L. (2011). A test of the theory of planned behavior to explain physical activity in a large population sample of adolescents from Alberta, Canada. *The Journal of Adolescent Health, 49*(5), 547–549. doi:10.1016/j.jadohealth.2011.03.006 PMID:22018572

Ridgers, N. D., McNarry, M. A., & Mackintosh, K. A. (2016). Feasibility and effectiveness of using wearable activity trackers in youth: A systematic review. *JMIR mHealth and uHealth, 4*(4), e129. doi:10.2196/mhealth.6540 PMID:27881359

Ringle, C. M., Wende, S., & Becker, J. M. (2015). *SmartPLS 3.* Boenningstedt: SmartPLS GmbH. Retrieved from http://www.smartpls.com

Roemer, E. (2016). A tutorial on the use of PLS path modeling in longitudinal studies. *Industrial Management & Data Systems, 116*(9), 1901–1921. doi:10.1108/IMDS-07-2015-0317

Sarstedt, M., Henseler, J., & Ringle, C. M. (2011). Multigroup analysis in partial least squares (PLS) path modeling: Alternative methods and empirical results. *Adv Int Mark, 22,* 195–218. doi:10.1108/S1474-7979(2011)0000022012

Schaefer, S. E., Ching, C. C., Breen, H., & German, J. B. (2016). Wearing, thinking, and moving: Testing the feasibility of fitness tracking with urban youth. *American Journal of Health Education, 47*(1), 8–16. doi:10.1080/19325037.2015.1111174

Shi, S. G. (1992). Accurate and efficient double-bootstrap confidence limit method. *Computational Statistics & Data Analysis, 13*(1), 21–32. doi:10.1016/0167-9473(92)90151-5

Sirard, J. R., & Pate, R. R. (2001). Physical activity assessment in children and adolescents. *Sports Medicine (Auckland, N.Z.), 31*(6), 439–454. doi:10.2165/00007256-200131060-00004 PMID:11394563

Terry, D. J., & O'Leary, J. E. (1995). The theory of planned behaviour: The effects of perceived behavioural control and self-efficacy. *British Journal of Social Psychology, 34*(2), 199–220. doi:10.1111/j.2044-8309.1995.tb01058.x PMID:7620846

TrackerS. (n.d.). Retrieved from: https://www.sports-tracker.com

Wartella, E., Rideout, V., Montague, H., Beaudoin-Ryan, L., & Lauricella, A. (2016). Teens, health and technology: A national survey. *Media and communication, 4*(3), 13-23.

World Health Organization. (2018). *Physical Activity Fact Sheet.* Retrieved from http://www.who.int/mediacentre/factsheet

Zimmerman, B. J. (2000). Self-efficacy: An essential motive to learn. *Contemporary Educational Psychology*, *25*(1), 82–91. doi:10.1006/ceps.1999.1016 PMID:10620383

ADDITIONAL READING

Ajzen, I. (1991). The theory of planned behavior. *Organizational Behavior and Human Decision Processes*, *50*(2), 179–211. doi:10.1016/0749-5978(91)90020-T

Bandura, A. (1986). *Social foundations of thought and action.*

Hagger, M. S., Chatzisarantis, N., & Biddle, S. J. (2001). The influence of self-efficacy and past behaviour on the physical activity intentions of young people. *Journal of Sports Sciences*, *19*(9), 711–725. doi:10.1080/02640410152475847 PMID:11522147

Kettunen, E., & Kari, T. (2018). Can Sport and Wellness Technology be My Personal Trainer?: Teenagers and Digital Coaching. In *Bled eConference*. University of Maribor Press. doi:10.18690/978-961-286-170-4.32

KEY TERMS AND DEFINITIONS

Exercise Psychology: Exercise psychology involve the scientific study of the psychological factors associated in sport, exercise, and physical activity.

Self-Efficacy: A person's beliefs in his/her capabilities of performing a specific task.

Sport and Wellness Technology: Technological device or application used in the support of a person's pursuit of their health, fitness, physical activity goals.

Teenager/Adolescent: In this study, the definition includes people between ages 13-17 years.

Theory of Planned Behavior (TPB): The theory states that intention toward attitude, subject norms, and perceived behavioral control, together shape an individual's behavioral intentions and behaviors.

Chapter 16
Using Health 4.0 to Enable Post-Operative Wellness Monitoring:
The Case of Colorectal Surgery

Nilmini Wickramasinghe
(iD) https://orcid.org/0000-0002-1314-8843
Swinburne University, Australia & Epworth HealthCare, Australia

Vijay Geholt
Vilanova University, USA

Elliot Sloane
Vilanova University, USA

Philip James Smart
Austin Health, Australia

Jonathan L. Schaffer
Cleveland Clinic, USA

ABSTRACT

Healthcare delivery is facing multiple orthogonal challenges around escalating costs and providing quality care, especially in OECD countries. This research examines the opportunity to leverage Health 4.0 technology and techniques to address the post-operative discharge phase of the patient journey. In so doing it serves to proffer a technology enabled model that supports not only a quality care experience post discharge but also prudent management to minimize costly unplanned readmissions and thereby subscribe to a value-based care paradigm. The chosen context is stoma patients but the solution can be easily generalized to other contexts. Next steps include the conducting of clinical trials to establish proof of concept, validity, and usability.

DOI: 10.4018/978-1-5225-6067-8.ch016

1. INTRODUCTION

Given the challenges facing private healthcare today and moving forward there is increasing pressure on private healthcare organizations to provide high value, high quality patient-centered care across the acute-care continuum (ACSQH 2010). While the recognition for the need of care delivery to be patient-centric is growing, the appropriateness of the approaches adopted to achieving this endeavor remain questionable (Kitson et al. 2013).

An integral enabler is without question Information Technology (IT) solutions (see for example Hibbard and Greene 2013, Wildevuur and Simonse 2015, Middleton et al. 2013). The limitation with many current systems is their limited coverage across the acute-care continuum (Collin 2015, Audet et al. 2014), where both pre-admission and post-discharge phases are not seamlessly connected to the hospitalization phase in the patient journey.

In Australia, as in other OECD countries like the US, unplanned readmissions are now being more carefully scrutinized. In most instances in Australia, unplanned readmissions are not reimbursed. i.e., readmissions within 28 days of discharge are considered to be related to the primary diagnosis/treatment, so the added cost must be borne by the provider (AIHW 2017). We believe it is possible to reduce the number of unplanned readmission by developing precision post discharge wellness monitoring solutions, and the following serves to outline this solution and answer the research question: "How can we design a suitable technology solution to support post discharge monitoring?"

We select stoma patients as a pilot study for this solution because we note that based on hospital data gathered from a large not-for-profit tertiary institute in Melbourne, Australia a common and avoidable unplanned readmission relating to stoma patients is due to inadequate hydration. This is particularly problematic during the hot dry Australian summer months.

This paper proposes a generic, open-source-based starting point for a customizable modeling, simulation and testing framework for mobile Patient Care Devices (PCDs) that can support relatively complex coordination of care for post-surgical patients. This system uses an architecture that can be modified to suit each patient's precise needs or widely differing clinical protocols. These tools allow simulation of expected ranges of safe and reliable performance and can also be used to explore or simulate likely failure modes and potential safety or health risks due to communication system or staffing overload, errors, or other complications.

2. BACKGROUND

In a recent study by the International Surgical Group on the dynamics of surgery across the globe, the findings indicated that over 320 million people globally have undergone surgical procedures; approximately 17% of these patients develop several complications and among them nearly 2.8% pass away due to these complications. It can, therefore, be estimated that approximately 1.5 million patients annually or three patients per day die due to post-operative complications. For instance, Bartels et al (2013) argue that in America, if the postoperative mortality was to be included in the official statistics as per the data from the Centers for Disease Control and Prevention, it would depict the third leading cause of death after heart illness and cancer (Bartels et al. 2015). Succinctly, many patients die in the ward or post discharge, where the doctor to patient ratio is low and where the individuals are not continuously monitored. Monitoring patients beyond the operating room and ICU may enable early detection of medical deterioration and timely interventions (Michard et al., 2015). Michard et al. (2015) notes that postoperative complications are not only a human burden but also a dramatic increase in the hospital expenses. As a result of this clinical and economic burden, a number of initiatives have been developed to offer an advanced quality of surgical care, including clear surgical safety specifications, minimally-invasive surgical procedures, protecting mechanical ventilation, and improved post-surgical recovery initiatives (Bartels et al., 2013). Due to recent technological advancements and innovations in healthcare systems it is becoming easier to monitor patients in the ward and post discharge and this in turn serves to improve patient satisfaction and overall outcomes.

"Prehabilitation" is one of the elements that are thought to have a great influence on the postoperative outcome. Ideally, preoperative improvements in the physical status in addition to better control of risk factors can be enhanced by digital tools and smart applications which are downloaded on smartphones and in tablets (Michard et al., 2017). According to Michard et al. (2017), the connected devices including brachial cuffs as well as electronic scales are often used for self-monitoring of blood pressure and weight, better control of hypertension and weight gain, and the visualization of the surgical trends over time.

However, a growing area of focus is now on post discharge and rehabilitation monitoring. Numerous sensors and monitoring systems are being designed and developed for proactive post operated patients as well as ambulatory patients. According to Michard et al. (2017), smart software has been developed to prevent alarm fatigue, to filter artifacts, and to fuse vital signs into the postoperative wellness indexes or the warning scores that are used for easy and visual identification of health deterioration, or even the prediction of hostile events beforehand (Pinsky et al., 2016).

Intraoperative fluid monitoring is one of the major determinants of postoperative outcome (Pinsky et al. 2016). Over the years, fluid overload has been known to be a major factor responsible for complications that are related to tissue oeadema such as prolonged mechanical ventilation along with anastomotic leak (ibid). Thus, fluid restrictions have been encouraged to some extent. Nevertheless, recent researches such as the one by Thacker et al (2016) have clearly illustrated that insufficient fluid management is linked to a considerable increase in postoperative complications (Thacker et al (2016). According to Michard et al. (2017), titrating and modifying fluid management to patient's needs is highly desirable to make certain that patients receive the correct amount of fluid at the appropriate time. Multiple noninvasive hemodynamic monitoring interventions are currently available, including bio-impedance tracheal tubes, volume clamp approaches, application tonometry and bio-reactance surface electrodes (Michard et al. 2017). These offer physicians an opportunity to measure and track any change in the blood flow during the therapeutic programs and to rationalize fluid management. Benes et al. (2014) state that precluding unjustified fluid management by detecting fluid unresponsiveness has been considered to be important to minimize postoperative morbidity, hospitalization time, and cost (Benes et al. 2014). Some of the noninvasive parameters, including pulse pressure variation from volume clamp approaches and SpO2 variability index from the pulse oximeters, are helpful in detecting fluid unresponsiveness (Benes et al. 2014).

Pulse oximeters were used to continuously monitor the SpO2 as well as heart rate among 2,841 orthopedic patients. According to Taenzer et al. (2010), this use was linked to a significant decline in the number of rescue events and ICU transfers. Piezoelectric contact-free sensors placed under the mattress aids in the continuous monitoring of heart rate and respiratory rate among 2,314 medico-surgical patients (Taenzer et al. 2010). This patients' population has been linked to a significant decrease in the number of calls for hospitalization and cardiac arrest (Brown et al., 2014).

Subbe et al. (2017) contend that wireless sensors have been invented recently to help in monitoring vital signs such as the heart rate, respiratory rate, SpO2, and blood pressure. Such solutions automatically calculate an early warning score, and then alert nurses if deterioration has been detected (Subbe et al. 2017). This can be associated with a considerable decrease in the number of cardiac arrests and mortality rates.

There has been a strong correlation between intraoperative hypotension and postoperative difficulties such as acute kidney injury, stroke, and myocardial injury. It has been established that intermittent blood pressure measurements fail capture every patient's hypotension events in a timely manner (Chen et al., 2012). According to Chen et al (2012) clinicians may miss nearly seven minutes of hypertension per hour during a three hour orthopedic or abdominal procedures, especially when using the intermittent blood pressure measurement. Recently, it has been suggested that only a minimal number of minutes of hypertension can significantly affect the postoperative outcome. Thus, though fatality from intraoperative hypotension and postoperative difficulties has not yet been identified, it appears desirable hypotension events as much possible (Salmasi et al. 2017). This may need a more rational as well as controlled use of the anesthetic agents, especially during induction. It may also require continuous monitoring of blood pressure with the non-invasive methods for the immediate detection and correction of any considerable blood pressure drop.

Taken together, we can see there is a trend and potential to embrace technology solutions for post-operative monitoring; however, what is key is to have focused solutions. This paper tries to address this and identify critical issues for the design and development of post discharge monitoring of stoma patients.

3. CLINICAL USE CASE

In order to provide proactive patient care post-discharge following stoma surgery, several remote medical devices can be employed. For example, elevated patient temperature or pulse can indicate an emerging infection at home which might easily and inexpensively be treated by early intervention with an appropriate antibiotic. High blood pressure and pulse might be an indicator of patient pain or discomfort, which might be initially treated with basic over-the-counter anti-inflammatory medications. Low blood pressure and elevated pulse might be predictors of dehydration, which might readily be treated by drinking more fluids and electrolytes. The stoma bag may also be monitored with simple sensors that keep track of filling and emptying rates, providing an indication of inadequate food and liquid intake.

In all cases, the monitored patient wellness parameters can be routed to a central patient homecare coordination team. The care coordination team can invoke appropriate rules and treatment actions. For example, a care coordinator could call the patient/ family, provide remediation guidance, education, and/ or prescriptions. If needed, a visiting nurse or physician could be dispatched to provide in-home care.

In addition, the monitors and the data monitoring systems can have alarm and/or alert level triggers pre-set or remotely adjusted. Thus, if a low-grade fever appears to be emerging, the patient, family, or care coordination team could increase the temperature alarm by one degree, to notify them if/when the fever becomes more severe. Similarly, a high and low blood pressure alarm could be pre-established based on the patient's discharge condition, in order to alert caregivers of unusual emerging risks.

Once a patient's physiological data is available to the care coordination system and team, clinical decision support algorithms and systems can be used to enhance, accelerate, and escalate emerging patient risks to staff who are appropriately trained to support high-quality, safe home care for discharged patients.

Intervention at the home will usually be far, far less expensive than re-admission to the hospital, and care plan changes can often occur quickly. The care coordination team will be able to arrange emergency care or transport if home-care turns out to be inadequate for a specific patient situation.

Because many physiologic monitoring devices are now becoming rather inexpensive and ubiquitous, and they rely on consumer-grade internet or cellular communication channels, the incremental cost of deploying such systems is falling rapidly. In addition, many of these devices can be cleaned and re-used for subsequent patients.

In the following sections, we illustrate the system design and simulation of a flexible home-care monitoring and care coordination system. We identify representative monitoring devices, but the model is extensible. Additional monitoring devices and data can easily be added. e.g., in some cases patient weight may be a valuable indicator of dehydration, or of congestive heart failure complications. Adding a patient scale and decision support rules is very easy with this system.

In addition, this system could easily be extended to include patient co-morbidities. For example, a severe industrial or automobile trauma patient could conceivably be sent home with both a stoma bag and a hip replacement. If that were the situation, additional physiologic channels may be added, such as gait and PT/exercise/mobility tracking and analysis.

4. MODELING APPROACH AND METHOD

Our focus is to create a simulation model based flexible framework to assess and validate various protocols and workflows for post-operative and post-discharge care. Towards this end, we are using the Colored Petri Nets (CPN) modeling and simulation approach (Jensen and Kristensen 2009, Gehlot and Nigro 2010, Sloane and Gehlot 2007).

CPNs are extensions of the widely studied Petri Net formalism, which is a graphical notation for modeling systems (Reisig 2013). CPNs combine the graphical components of Petri Nets with the strengths of a high level programming language, making them suitable for modeling complex systems. Petri Nets provide the foundation for modeling concurrency, communication, synchronization and resource sharing constraints, while a high-level programming language provides the foundation for the definition of data types and the manipulations of data values. As we show later on, support for compound data types is crucial for representing and processing different data details of a variety of monitoring devices. The CPN language allows the model to be represented as a set of modules, allowing complex nets (and systems) to be represented in a hierarchical manner.

CPNs allow for the creation of both timed and untimed models. Simulations of untimed models are usually used to validate the logical correctness of a system, while simulations of timed models are used to evaluate the performance of a system. Timed activities play an important role in home-care monitoring and care coordination systems.

5. SIMULATION MODEL

As mentioned above, we use CPNs to create a flexible framework for postoperative wellness monitoring. In particular, we use the hierarchical approach of the CPNs. Figure 1 depicts the top-level system view of this model.

In Figure 1 we have also explicitly identified care coordination and vigilance as separate layers: "Community Care Coordination Hub" and "Home Data and Alerting Aggregation System". These layers abstract away clinical vigilance alerting rules that are needed for various clinical care coordination categories, allowing customization to suit the situation. For example, systolic and diastolic high blood pressure alert limits might trigger when any patient's BP exceeds either 180 mmHg systolic or 140 mmHg diastolic, but individual patient overrides are likely needed. There should be care coordination rules to set personal limits higher or lower based on medication and clinical situation. Automatic implementation rules may also require the ability to fetch relevant data from an EHR.

Each of the six rectangles with double border in Figure 1 are called Substitution Transitions. Each of these Substitution Transitions represents a distinct page/layer/module/subsystem that becomes integrated into the entire model. For the purposes of this paper, we will use the term Submodule net to refer to these Substitution Transitions. In essence, each Submodule net can be evolved into a complex CPN subsystem if/as needed, facilitating modular design and testing. In each referenced Submodule net, we can assemble all needed details to support the underlying activity or sub-system.

In defining this framework, we have chosen a general scenario where patients condition is monitored by a variety of devices. This is consistent with the basic architecture used in IHE International's Patient Care Device Domain (IHE-PCD) standards (www.IHE.net, and the HITSP IS-77 and TN-905 at www. HITSP.org). Each PCD (device) functions like a stand-alone IoT device. In the HITSP documents above, two architectures are offered: the discrete device model and the local patient data aggregation hub model that is embodied in the Continua and the ICE/OpenICE (Integrated Health Environment) standard. In this second architecture, a home data aggregation hub stores data until it is polled (store-and-forward). We model the second approach. Thus, as shown in Figure 1, the data from these devices is sent to a *Home Data and Alerting Aggregation System* via the underlying *Home Network*.

The component *Monitored Patients* consists of three categories of PCD monitors, sensors, and/or apps: Wearable Sensors, Homecare Sensors/Apps, and Mobile Self-Reporting Apps. Figure 2 shows the subcomponent associated with Wearable Sensors.

Each category allows any number of patients and devices. This is achieved by modeling each device behavior as a generic net and then populating that net with unique patient IDs and unique device IDs. For example, Figure 3, below, shows the net associated with a blood pressure monitoring device.

As mentioned before, the single CPN submodule net that is shown in Figure 3 can keep track of any number of patient-device pairs. We achieve this by defining a color set (i.e., a data type) consisting of a PatientID and a DeviceID. Assuming we have an stoma patient [PatientID_1] wearing a blood pressure monitoring device [DeviceID_1], and an ortho patient [PatientID_2] wearing a different blood pressure monitoring device [DeviceID_2], the initial marking *1`(1,2)@5+++1`(2,1)@10* depicted on place *Patient Data Trigger* will initialize the net with two timed tokens. The first one will trigger a reading at simulation time 5 and the second one will trigger a reading at time 10. The depicted function *bpTrigger(pd)* is a customizable function that sets the trigger for the next reading. The current blood pressure reading is sent by the firing of the transition *Send BP Data* and the associated data is generated by *bpData(pd)*. For example, the current token depicted in green residing in place *From Devices* shows that a reading for PatientID_1 of 195/62 was generated at time 143 by DeviceID_1. This data packet will be sent over the home network to *Home Data and Alerting Aggregation System*. As mentioned before, this system is responsible for collecting and storing data locally as part of a patient's Personal Health/Medical Record (PHR/PMR). The stored data may be polled remotely by a *Community Care Coordination Hub* or even by *Family and Caregivers* over a broadband network as shown in Figure 1. The aggregator/hub can itself

Figure 1. CPN model of our framework for post discharge care

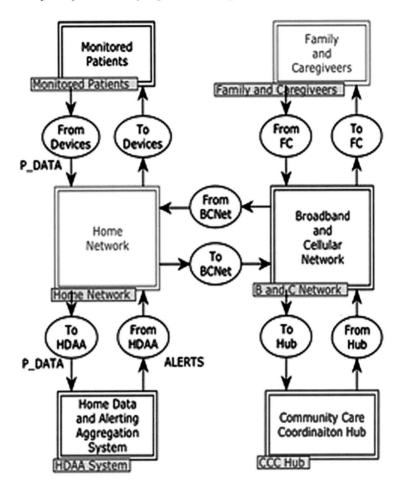

add vigilance, alerts, and other functionality depending on the underlying protocol for patient monitoring and care. Figure 4 shows the subnet associated with the *Home Data and Alerting Aggregation System* in our CPN model.

In this net, the place PMR collects and aggregates patient data. The current token shown in green, depicts the various device data that has been collected for each of the two patients. For example, the entry *(4,25,TEMP(97))* means at time 25, a temperature reading of 97 was recorded for PatientID_1 and the reading was generated by DeviceID_4. Similarly, the entry *(11,120,P(5))* means at time 120 PatientID_2 reported a pain level of 5 via a Self-reporting_appID_11.

Figure 5 below shows the subnet associated with an ostomy bag that has a "bag full" alarm built into it. Since only patient 1 is a stoma patient, the net is initialized only with patient ID 1. Thus, our framework and model allow flexibility both in terms of number of devices as well as type of devices associated with a patient to be monitored.

The net monitors the current level and generates an "ostomy bag full" alarm if the level reaches a defined alert level via the firing of the transition *Send OBag Alert*. The level is checked and alert is

Figure 2. Wearable Sensors model component depicting various sensors that may be worn by a patient

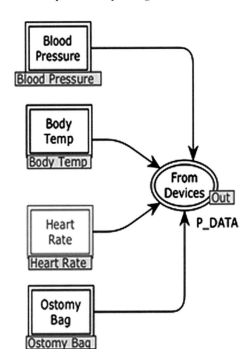

generated by function *bagAlarm(pd,l)*. The current green token in place *OBag Level* shows the current level to be 3.

The CPN Tool models provide an important additional opportunity: when ready for clinical testing, each Sublayer net may be replaced with functional programs and/or real devices and sensors can be interfaced to feed actual patient data directly into the model. That allows incremental conversion of the CPN model from a simulation to a functional clinical tool. This facilitates straight-forward pilot testing, functional validation, and full system scalability verification prior to widespread clinical deployment.

Figure 3. The net describing the behavior of a blood pressure monitoring device

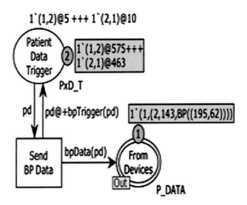

Figure 4. Patient device data aggregator and alerting system

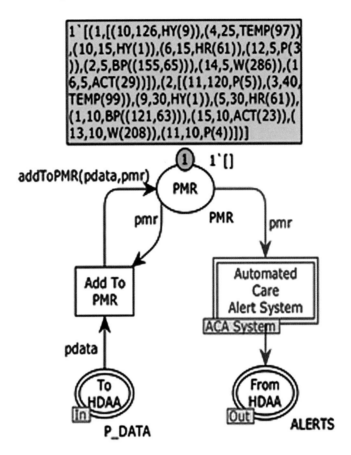

In addition, different clinical decision support systems and rules can be substituted without disturbing the rest of the system, enabling customization and research to match evolving needs.

6. RESULTS AND DISCUSSIONS

The previous section proffers a solution that leverages the capabilities of various technologies. The aim is to monitor patients as unobtrusively as possible so that alerts can be triggered to inform the designated healthcare professional if a trigger incident has occurred that should be addressed. In this way, the patient is able to navigate the post-discharge phase of their treatment effectively and efficiently, with the highest level of positive patient and caregiver experience. In addition, by having alerts promptly triggered if a problem arises it is also possible to act as quickly as possible, thereby averting a more complicated, dangerous, and/or expensive problem further down the track. In this way, we believe we are addressing two critical objectives of healthcare delivery simultaneously; namely providing a high-quality patient experience as well as providing a high value solution as we are trying to mitigate the need for unplanned readmissions by catching trigger situations as early as possible and then addressing them.

Figure 5. Net associated with ostomy bag

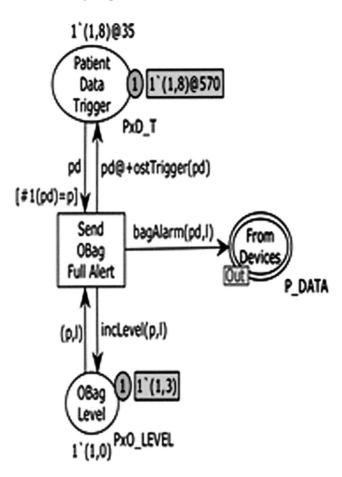

The next step is to run a two arm non-blinded clinical trial to test the full benefits of the proposed solution. The control arm will continue to have patients exposed to standard practices around discharge and post discharge follow up and monitoring while the intervention arm will focus on using the developed technology solution in addition to standard care practices around discharge and post-discharge management. In particular, we plan to monitor levels of hydration, using triggers of blood pressure, pulse and weight to trigger levels going below an appropriate threshold. In addition, patients will receive via their mobile phones education, reminders and other important information about maintaining appropriate levels of hydration. We focus on hydration as this has been identified as the singular most frequent reason for unplanned readmission with stoma patients at the chosen healthcare facility. We have secured ethics committee approval, and plan to run this trial as soon as final clinical post-discharge protocols are complete, validated, and approved and patient recruitment is complete.

For model validation, we adopt the approach described in (Sargent 2011). Figure 6 illustrates the overall approach to model verification and validation. In this figure, *Conceptual Model* refers to a non-executable model notation whereas *Computerized Model* refers to a software implementation of such a model. However, in our case, a CPN model is both a conceptual model as well as a computerized model since CPN models themselves are executable. According to (Sargent 2011), model verification is the

Figure 6. Model validation approach
(Sargent 2011)

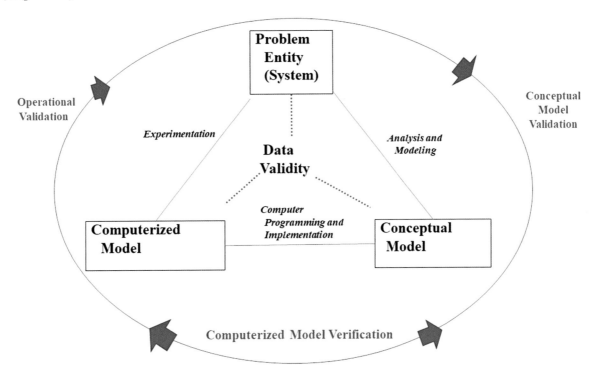

process of determining that a model implementation accurately represents the conceptual description and specifications whereas model validation is the process of determining the degree to which a model is an accurate representation of the real world. In particular, "…operational validation is carried out to determine the simulation model's output behavior has the accuracy required for the model's intended purpose over the domain of the model's intended applicability."

For data generation and validation purposes, CPN software provides an extensive monitoring and simulation report generation facility (Lindstrøm and Wells 2002). Simulation report provides a complete execution trace of the model whereas a monitor is a mechanism in the CPN software that is used to observe, inspect, control, or even modify a simulation of a CPN. A variety of monitors can be defined for a given net. Monitors can inspect both the markings of places and enabling of transitions during a simulation, and they can take appropriate actions based on the observations as well as extract relevant data. Table 1 depicts a sample simulation report generated by the model under consideration for a sample run. Even in absence of any device data in the shown simulation report, the sequence of activities alone provides a good insight into the system behavior. Typically, such runs are useful in identifying any unsafe or undesirable behaviors. For situations where device and other data is crucial, the aforementioned monitoring facilities can be used to log necessary data during simulation.

Table 1. Sample simulation report generated by CPN software

Step	Time	Transition Occurrence
1	5	Send_Activity_Data @ (1:Activity)
2	5	Send_Weight_Data @ (1:Weight)
3	5	Send_Pain_Data @ (1:Pain)
4	5	Forward_To_HDAA @ (1:Home_Network)
5	5	Add_To_PMR @ (1:HDAA_System)
6	5	Forward_To_HDAA @ (1:Home_Network)
7	5	Add_To_PMR @ (1:HDAA_System)
8	5	Forward_To_HDAA @ (1:Home_Network)
9	5	Add_To_PMR @ (1:HDAA_System)
10	5	Send_BP_Data @ (1:Blood_Pressure)
11	5	Forward_To_HDAA @ (1:Home_Network)
12	5	Add_To_PMR @ (1:HDAA_System)
13	10	Send_Pain_Data @ (1:Pain)
14	10	Send_Activity_Data @ (1:Activity)
15	10	Send_BP_Data @ (1:Blood_Pressure)
16	10	Forward_To_HDAA @ (1:Home_Network)
17	10	Add_To_PMR @ (1:HDAA_System)
18	10	Forward_To_HDAA @ (1:Home_Network)
19	10	Send_Weight_Data @ (1:Weight)
20	10	Forward_To_HDAA @ (1:Home_Network)
21	10	Add_To_PMR @ (1:HDAA_System)
22	10	Forward_To_HDAA @ (1:Home_Network)
23	10	Add_To_PMR @ (1:HDAA_System)
24	10	Add_To_PMR @ (1:HDAA_System)
25	15	Send_Hyd_Data @ (1:Hydration)
26	15	Forward_To_HDAA @ (1:Home_Network)
…	…	…
44	160	Send_Pain_Data @ (1:Pain)
45	160	Forward_To_HDAA @ (1:Home_Network)
46	160	Add_To_PMR @ (1:HDAA_System)
47	162	Send_Temp_Data @ (1:Body_Temp)
48	162	Forward_To_HDAA @ (1:Home_Network)
49	162	Add_To_PMR @ (1:HDAA_System)
50	182	Send_Weight_Data @ (1:Weight)
51	182	Forward_To_HDAA @ (1:Home_Network)

7. CONCLUSION

This research in progress paper has served to proffer a solution to address the post discharge phase of stoma patients and thus begin to answer the posed research question. The proffered technology enabled solution supports both a high-quality patient experience as well as a value-based care paradigm. We contend that such solutions are not just useful in the context as we have presented; i.e., stoma patients, but can be applied more generally so that the post dis-charge phase of the patient journey is also monitored and managed, enabling both a high-quality patient experience as well as prudent management of likely trigger situations that may if not addressed lead to unplanned readmissions. Given the challenges faced by all OECD countries with respect to the exponential costs to provide quality care and the increasing pressures on healthcare organizations to deliver high quality and high value care we believe such technology solutions are strategic necessities and must be carefully considered. Hence, our study has significant and far reaching contributions to both theory and practice around enabling high value, high quality care to continue in the post discharge phase of the patient journey. Our future work will focus on conducting clinical trials to establish the validity, usability and proof of concept of the proffered solution.

REFERENCES

Audet, A. M., Squires, D., & Doty, M. M. (2014). Where are we on the diffusion curve? Trends and drivers of primary care physicians' use of health information technology. *Health Services Research*, *49*(1 Pt 2), 347–360. doi:10.1111/1475-6773.12139 PMID:24358958

Australian Commission on Safety and Quality in Healthcare (ACSQH). (2010). *Patient-Centered Care: Improving Quality and Safety by Focusing Care on Patients and Consumers Discussion Paper*. Department of Health and Ageing, Sydney.

Australian Institute of Health and Welfare (AIHW). (2017). *Variation in hospital admission policies and practices: Australian hospital statistics*. Available at https://www.aihw.gov.au/reports/hospitals/variation-hospital-admission-policies-practices/contents/table-of-contents

Bartels, S. J., Pratt, S. I., Aschbrenner, K. A., Barre, L. K., Jue, K., Wolfe, R. S., Xie, H., McHugo, G., Santos, M., Williams, G. E., Naslund, J. A., & Mueser, K. T. (2013). Clinically significant improved fitness and weight loss among overweight persons with serious mental illness. *Psychiatric Services (Washington, D.C.)*, *64*(8), 729–736. doi:10.1176/appi.ps.003622012 PMID:23677386

Benes, J., Giglio, M., Brienza, N., & Michard, F. (2014). The effects of goal-directed fluid therapy based on dynamic parameters on post-surgical outcome: A meta-analysis of randomized controlled trials. *Critical Care (London, England)*, *18*(5), 584–594. doi:10.118613054-014-0584-z PMID:25348900

Brown, H., Terrence, J., Vasquez, P., Bates, D. W., & Zimlichman, E. (2014). Continuous Monitoring in an Inpatient Medical-Surgical Unit: A Controlled Clinical Trial. *The American Journal of Medicine*, *127*(3), 226–232. doi:10.1016/j.amjmed.2013.12.004 PMID:24342543

Chen, G., Chung, E., Meng, L., Alexander, B., Vu, T., Rinehart, J., & Cannesson, M. (2012, April). (212). Impact of non invasive and beat-to-beat arterial pressure monitoring on intraoperative hemodynamic management. *Journal of Clinical Monitoring and Computing, 26*(2), 133–140. doi:10.100710877-012-9344-2 PMID:22382920

Collen, M. F. (2015). *A history of medical informatics in the United States* (M. J. Ball, Ed.). Springer. doi:10.1007/978-1-4471-6732-7

Gehlot, V., & Nigro, C. (2010). An Introduction to Systems Modeling and Simulation with Colored Petri Nets. *Proceedings of the 2010 Winter Simulation Conference,* 104-118. 10.1109/WSC.2010.5679170

Hibbard, J. H., & Greene, J. (2013). What the evidence shows about patient activation: Better health outcomes and care experiences; fewer data on costs. *Health Affairs, 32*(2), 207–214. doi:10.1377/hlthaff.2012.1061 PMID:23381511

Jensen, K., & Kristensen, L. M. (2009). *Coloured Petri Nets: Modelling and Validation of Concurrent Systems.* Springer-Verlag. doi:10.1007/b95112

Kitson, A., Marshall, A., Bassett, K., & Zeitz, K. (2013). What are the core elements of patient-centred care? A narrative review and synthesis of the literature from health policy, medicine and nursing. *Journal of Advanced Nursing, 69*(1), 4–15. doi:10.1111/j.1365-2648.2012.06064.x PMID:22709336

Lindstrøm, B., & Wells, L. (2002). Towards a Monitoring Framework for Discrete-Event System Simulations. In *Proceedings of the Sixth International Workshop on Discrete Event Systems (WODES'02),* (pp. 127–134). IEEE Computer Society. 10.1109/WODES.2002.1167679

Michard, F., Giglio, M. T., & Brienza, N. (2017). Perioperative goal-directed therapy with uncalibrated pulse contour methods: Impact on fluid management and postoperative outcome. *British Journal of Anaesthesia, 119*(1), 22–30. doi:10.1093/bja/aex138 PMID:28605442

Michard, F., Mountford, W. K., Krukas, M. R., Ernst, F. R., & Fogel, S. L. (2015). Potential return on investment for implementation of perioperative goal-directed fluid therapy in major surgery: A nationwide database study. *Perioperative Medicine (London, England), 4*(1), 11. doi:10.118613741-015-0021-0 PMID:26500766

Middleton, B., Bloomrosen, M., Dente, M. A., Hashmat, B., Koppel, R., Overhage, J. M., & Zhang, J. (2013). Enhancing patient safety and quality of care by improving the usability of electronic health record systems: Recommendations from AMIA. *Journal of the American Medical Informatics Association: JAMIA, 20*(e1), e2–e8. doi:10.1136/amiajnl-2012-001458 PMID:23355463

Pinsky, M. R., Clermont, G., & Hravnak, M. (2016). Predicting cardiorespiratory instability. *Critical Care (London, England), 20*(1), 70–77. doi:10.118613054-016-1223-7 PMID:26984263

Reisig, W. (2013). *Understanding Petri Nets.* Springer-Verlag. doi:10.1007/978-3-642-33278-4

Salmasi, V., Maheshwari, K., Yang, D., Mascha, E. J., Singh, A., Sessler, D. I., & Kurz, A. (2017). Relationship between Intraoperative Hypotension, Defined by Either Reduction from Baseline or Absolute Thresholds, and Acute Kidney and Myocardial Injury after Noncardiac Surgery: A Retrospective Cohort Analysis. *Anesthesiology: The Journal of the American Society of Anesthesiologists, 126*(1), 47–65. doi:10.1097/ALN.0000000000001432 PMID:27792044

Sargent, R. D. (2011). Verification and validation of simulation models. *Proceedings of the 2011 Winter Simulation Conference*, 183–198. 10.1109/WSC.2011.6147750

Sloane, E. B., & Gehlot, V. (2007). Use of Coloured Petri Net models in planning, design, and simulation of intelligent wireless medical device networks for safe and flexible hospital capacity management. *International Journal of Networking and Virtual Organisations, 4*(2), 118–129. doi:10.1504/IJNVO.2007.013538

Subbe, C. P., Duller, B., & Bellomo, R. (2017). Effect of an automated notification system for deteriorating ward patients on clinical outcomes. *Critical Care (London, England), 21*(1), 52–60. doi:10.118613054-017-1635-z PMID:28288655

Taenzer, A. H., Pyke, J. B., McGrath, S. P., & Blike, G. T. (2010). Impact of Pulse Oximetry Surveillance on Rescue Events and Intensive Care Unit Transfers: A Before-and-After Concurrence Study. *Anesthesiology, 112*(2), 282–287. doi:10.1097/ALN.0b013e3181ca7a9b PMID:20098128

Thacker, J. K. M., Mountford, W. K., Ernst, F. R., Krukas, M. R., & Mythen, M. G. (2016). Perioperative Fluid Utilization Variability and Association with Outcomes: Considerations for Enhanced Recovery Efforts in Sample US Surgical Populations. *Annals of Surgery, 263*(3), 502–510. doi:10.1097/SLA.0000000000001402 PMID:26565138

Wildevuur, S. E., & Simonse, L. W. (2015). Information and communication technology–enabled person-centered care for the "big five" chronic conditions: Scoping review. *Journal of Medical Internet Research, 17*(3), e77. doi:10.2196/jmir.3687 PMID:25831199

Chapter 17
Protein Energy Malnutrition in Children:
Prevention System

Foluke Onaleye
Univesity of Illinois Chicago, USA

ABSTRACT

The current management to prevent Protein Energy Malnutrition (PEM) is examined and the use of technological tools such as Electronic Health Records (EHR) systems and mobile solutions are employed to prevent the development of PEM and its complications. Implementation of technological solutions in healthcare is a critical factor in achieving better health outcomes as documented in some parts of the world. Sub-Saharan Africa is behind on the adoption of electronic health records and other health information technology solutions due to several challenges such as lack of funding and infrastructure required to implement its use. Recent studies show that Sub-Saharan Africa is slowly gravitating towards adoption of health information technology particularly EHR systems and mobile solutions because of the need to find solutions to its healthcare crisis. Development of a PEM prevention system using these tools to enhance the current management will improve patient health outcomes and decrease the mortality rate of PEM.

INTRODUCTION

According to World Health Organization (2020) Malnutrition refers to "deficiencies, excesses or imbalances in a person's intake of energy and/or nutrients. The term malnutrition covers two broad groups of conditions. One is 'undernutrition'—which includes stunting (low height for age), wasting (low weight for height), underweight (low weight for age) and micronutrient deficiencies or insufficiencies (a lack of important vitamins and minerals). The other is overweight, obesity and diet-related noncommunicable diseases." 52 million under-fives were suffering from wasting having a low weight for height, approximately 45% of deaths among children under five are due to under nutrition-WHO (2020). Several factors such as poverty, lack of education by the caregiver, culture and other socioeconomic reasons interplay

DOI: 10.4018/978-1-5225-6067-8.ch017

resulting in malnutrition, of these factors poverty was a major contributor. In 2015, the first goal of the United Nations Millenial Development Goal(MDG) was to eradicate extreme poverty and hunger. This is because of the burden of disease to public health, causing an increase in the number of undernourished people globally particularly in the developing countries of the world. United Nations set forth strategies to eradicate poverty since 1990, however in 2011, it was noted that all developing regions except sub-Saharan Africa had met the target of halving the proportion of people who live in extreme poverty. According to the 2015 MDG report, one third of undernourished children globally are from sub-Saharan Africa, this is not surprising because the world bank reported that in 2015, 27 countries out of the world's 28 poorest countries were located in Sub Saharan Africa. This indicates a possible correlation between poverty and malnutrition, as evidenced by the number of undernourished children in that region. Poverty alleviation and medical management has not significantly reduced the morbidity and mortality from malnutrition in children. Exploration of technological tools such as the implementation of an interoperable Electronic Medical System and the use of mobile solutions to increase the efficiency of the current management strategies in place is by creating a prevention system. It was shown that mobile health apps helped to improve the relationship between physicians and patients thereby resulting in better health outcomes and increased patient satisfaction (Lu et al, 2010). The implementation of such technological health monitoring tools will be achieved by creating a robust network that ensures that end users are actively involved by having access to the required systems. This will require a lot of effort from all the stakeholders to implement and sustain the systems. This chapter also provides a review of challenges and barriers to implementation, with the aim of developing an interoperable EHR and custom made mobile solutions based on the peculiarities of the community that will benefit from the Protein Energy Malnutrition prevention system that will be created.

BACKGROUND AND AIMS

Malnutrition in children is endemic in developing countries and nations like Sub-Saharan Africa. Protein Energy Malnutrition is a form of Malnutrition, an energy deficit caused by deficiency of macro and micronutrients. Protein Energy Malnutrition can be primary, which is caused by an inadequate nutrient intake or secondary resulting from disorders or drugs which affect the use of nutrients in the body. The type commonly seen in children is the primary Protein Energy Malnutrition. Protein Energy Malnutrition comprises 3 types namely, Kwashiokor, Marasmus and Marasmic Kwashiokor. Protein malnutrition is predominant in Kwashiokor, Marasmus is marked by a deficiency in calorie intake while Marasmic Kwashiokor is defined by a marked calorie insufficiency and marked protein deficiency. Marasmic Kwashiokor is the most severe form of malnutrition.

Marasmus is caused by a diet which is low in energy, protein and essential nutrients. In developing countries it is commonly seen in infants born to poor parents, due to a combination of undernutrition and poor hygiene. Some of the reasons are that the children are weaned too early or abruptly, inability to buy food and lack of access to potable water to cook leading to contamination by bacteria. This predisposes to illnesses and poor appetite which causes a depletion of the child's energy. Children with marasmus are thin, lack subcutaneous fat and muscles. Kwashiokor is mostly seen in the second year of life after the child is weaned from breast milk to a starchy diet low in protein. Usually symptoms are pronounced following an infection such as measles and severe malaria. The child is not thin as seen with marasmus and the abdomen protrudes. The skin is dry and wrinkled, hair color is altered, and falls out easily leaving the scalp hair thin. Generally, children with Protein Energy Malnutrtion are highly irritable and apathetic. Complications include diarrhea, hypothermia, hypoglycemia, encephalopathy, heart failure and infection.

The causes of Protein Energy Malnutrition have also been represented by the conceptual model for understanding the multifactorial causes of malnutrition, this model was illustrated by the United Nations International Children's Emergency Fund (UNICEF).

Figure 1. Conceptual model for understanding the causes of malnutrition.
UNICEF 2013

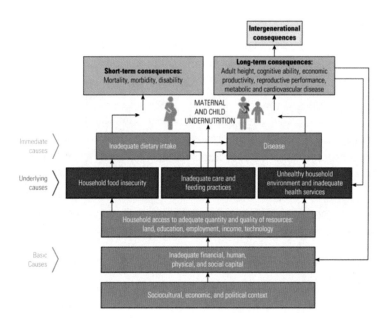

Immediate causes are mainly due to lack or insufficient food and disease, in this case the amount of nutrient required by the body is not absorbed due to having too little to eat or none, It could also be due to a disease state leading to lack of appetite or decreased absorption from the gut. These factors interplay and could run in a vicious cycle where malnutrition increases the risk of infections. This is referred to as the infection-malnutrition cycle. In Sub Saharan-Africa, Protein Energy Malnutrition could result as a complication of measles or severe malaria.

Underlying causes of malnutrition fall under three categories; i) inadequate household food security, this implies not having access to food, inability to utilize food or its unavailability. This is commonly seen during famines where food cannot be easily obtained. ii) inadequate care addresses caring practices by caregivers or parents in this context. Several factors such as religion, literacy, income, caregiver availability, and acceptance of perceived foreign culture(modern medicine) all play a part in determining the quality of care given to a loved one. Women are mostly the caregivers to children in Sub-Saharan Africa, majority of the women in the rural areas may not be educated or financially empowered to make informed decisions on child care. In cases where the woman may be financially empowered, cultural practices requires that the man makes important decisions on behalf of the family, instances such as this have resulted in lack of care when the father is away from the home for a prolonged period of time. iii) inadequate health services and unhealthy household environment; Access to health care is often a problem in Sub Saharan Africa, clinics and hospitals are sometimes located far away with no means of transportation to get the hospital. Inability to afford the means to travel to the healthcare center or pay for medical care is a challenge for some caregivers. Unhygienic environment and poor sanitary habits as commonly seen in overcrowded areas are breeding grounds for germs and other communicable diseases which may lead to malnutrition. Lack of potable water is still a problem in some parts of Africa, drinking unclean water causes conditions such as diarrhea which may also result in Protein Energy Malnutrition.

Basic causes include sociocultural, economic, and political factors that impact the nutritional status of individuals. This includes climate changes and how it may affect agriculture and availability of food, particularly in drought this becomes a serious issue leading to famine in some cases. In recent times there have been political unrest and civil wars in parts of Africa resulting to scarcity of essential commodities and food, this has resulted in malnutrition. Certain cultural practices causing food fads and fallacies impact the nutritional status of children, other cultural practices such as using traditional or no medication for a prolonged period of time when sick eventually leads to Protein Energy Malnutrition.

Determining the cause of Protein Energy Malnutrition requires a detailed history taking process keeping in mind the complexities of the causes and how they interplay. It is important to consider individual factors that may predispose a child to develop Protein Energy Malnutrition as well as a thorough physical examination to determine the type.

According to Haslett et al (1999), the following measures are in place to prevent Protein-Energy Undernutrition;

- "Growth monitoring- The parents keep a simple chart called the Road to Health card which is brought to clinic regularly for weighing and advice.
- Oral rehydration- This uses an electrolyte replacement therapy to save lives from gastroenteritis.
- Breastfeeding-Exclusive breast feeding is encouraged during the first six months of life in places where the sanitary conditions are poor and no facilities for hygiene.
- Immunization-This is to protect against common childhood infections such as Measles, Diphteria, Pertusis, Tetanus, Tuberculosis and Poliomyelitis."

Management includes prompt treatment of any underlying disease, it is also important to replace micronutrients such as vitamin A to prevent blindness which is one of the complications seen in measles. Replacement of macronutrients is part of the management, this involves a setting up a nutritional regimen and plan depending on the type of malnutrition.

Despite these measures, the incidence and mortality due to Protein Energy Malnutrition has not decreased in developing countries of the world. Some of the reasons include that there is not enough public awareness about Protein Energy Malnutrition and its complications, inadequate means of tracking and monitoring of children with common diseases that can predispose to the development of Protein Energy Malnutrition, such as malaria and measles. It is also difficult to track the immunization history of children to ensure that they have been immunized against common childhood infections amongst other reasons. Hence, an urgent need for more awareness campaigns by health care workers which can be provided through community education centers. This is where live classes can be held to educate the masses on how to get a balanced diet with locally made, inexpensive food items available. Education can also be through the use of pamphlets, posters and websites can be created to provide simplified details about

PEM and how to avoid it. The next area of focus is to identify at risk groups, this responsibility falls on the health care workers who come in direct contact with patients. It is important to point out that most of the hospitals in Northern Nigeria, Africa where I practiced do not use Electronic Medical Records, paper records are still the norm. Usually patients have a clinic card where doctors and other healthcare workers record patient encounters, sometimes patients go home with the cards and never return with the cards again, so there are no records of any previous encounter. In places where paper records are maintained in a file room, there have been instances where the patient's paper records are missing or lost. In view of these, there is an urgent need to implement the use of Electronic Medical Records hence the proposal for a Protein Energy Malnutrition prevention system.

METHODS

Review of relevant literatures on Protein Energy Malnutrition (PEM), Electronic Health Record(EHR) and Health Information Technology(HIT). Google Scholar searches were performed for relevant articles from PubMed, and PMC using the following keywords; Protein Energy Malnutrition, Malnutrition, Poverty, Electronic Medical Records, Telemedicine, Mobile solutions, Sub-Saharan Africa, Implementation, Prevention and Causes. About 28 literatures were reviewed, papers that did not reference sub-Saharan Africa were excluded with an exception to articles showing benefits of Electronic Medical Records, Mobile solutions and Clinical Monitoring Tools. Articles of interest were selected based on the clarity of the researcher(s) and the ability of the researcher to support their interpretation with enough information, references from identified publications were also reviewed. 17 articles were included in the final selection for review and analysis.

ASSESSMENT/EVALUATIONS

The goal is to develop a Protein Energy Malnutrition prevention system using a system where different Electronic Health Records in various facilities will be interoperable. An interoperable Electronic Health Record between facilities will be developed to store, use and retrieve data. Data will be stored using the relational database structure for ease of data retrieval. It is important to ensure that the system is easy to use with little or no formal training. The system will be well secured by generating user ID and passwords for each user. It is important to ensure protection of data by encryption of data, this eliminates unauthorized access to data. This system will possess an audit trail and must ensure that only the right users have access to the system.

In the past, developing countries like Nigeria have been slow to migrate to the use of Electronic Health Records due to challenges such as frequent power outage and internet services. The overwhelming positive health outcomes in places that have adopted the use of Electronic Health Records has proven it to be a necessity in the practice of medicine for better health outcomes and reduction in morbidity and mortality rates. It is important to ensure that this system is compliant to the health data protection laws of the country where it will be used. One of the strategies to make an efficient system is to embed a Clinical Decision Support System (CDSS) in the electronic health records system that will be used. "The CDSS alerts within the EHR inform the provider by a series of prompts on their computer screen that the patient they are currently seeing in their office is due for specific health maintenance screenings or chronic disease management based on the patient's age, gender, and comorbidities." (Amirfar et al, 2011). The system will ensure early identification of children with new cases of common childhood infections eliminating the risk of missed cases. An Electronic Health Records system will allow doctors and other healthcare workers to keep track of their patient's biodata, and previous encounters in order to identify children at risk of the disease rather than rely on the Health cards which is currently in use in parts of Sub Saharan Africa. The system will also serve as a means to store immunization records which are extremely vital in the prevention of Protein Energy Malnutrition. This will make it easy to track immunization history and reduce the issues of missed opportunities for immunization.

Wyatt and Sullivan(2005) stated that eHealth provides easier accessibility to healthcare and support services. It could serve as a platform for enhanced self expression for parents whose children have PEM. With the creation of the Protein Energy Malnutrition prevention system, information from different facilities pertaining to a patient can be accessed from one portal. The system will also address healthcare professional shortages in the region or communities by eliminating the need for referrals to the specialist or nutritionist by the General Practitioner (GP). In most third world countries, subjects are mostly seen by a General Practitioner, sometimes months could pass before they get a referral to see a specialist or nutritionist. This would save a lot of lives because the nutritionist who is regularly conducting surveillance, can quickly contact a patient considered at risk for developing Protein Energy Malnutrition and subsequently recommend the right meal plan for the patient.

Current management strategies for Protein Energy Malnutrition include the use of simple charts by parents and caregivers to capture relevant data such as weight. Caregivers are expected to measure the patient's weight daily and record it on the growth assessment chart. Failure to provide a consistent and accurate weight chart is a common finding. For most mothers who are usually the primary caregivers involved in care of their young ones when they are sick or have Protein Energy Malnutrition, this may be a cumbersome part of patient care during this stressful period. When caregivers are overwhelmed they fall short of certain expectations such as forgetting to capture relevant information, follow up in clinic as scheduled or may forget pertinent instructions provided by healthcare providers. These aspects in the management of a child with Protein Energy Malnutrition is very crucial in achieving positive outcomes and reducing the complications that may occur. This management process will improve significantly by the implementation of a mobile solution.

A mobile solution to the management of PEM will accelerate the recovery process through the involvement of caregivers in patient management. The use of mobile information applications developed using Node.js for cloud based healthcare applications will be a great asset for use by caregivers and patients. A user friendly mobile app will encourage patient independence by allowing the parents to take ownership of the management or treatment plan for their children since they are actively participating and may be held accountable for patient care in this situation. This will result in better healthcare and outcome since there is a sense of accountability by the caregivers at home. The concept is to keep the application simple, easy to operate without requiring professional assistance to operate it. Healthcare information regarding Protein Energy Malnutrition which is provided on the application must be legible, written clearly and easily comprehensible. Local languages, pictures and videos will be included to meet the demands of the target population. Mobile apps that are easy to use would enable patients to connect one on one with their healthcare provider. Patients can view appointments, referrals, test results and even medications using their mobile app. It is important to ensure that security and privacy issues are addressed during the development phase of the mobile applications, it must be encrypted and password secured. The app will include a growth assessment chart to record the daily weight by receiving prompts through a preset alarm within the app. After receiving such prompts the caregiver will weigh the patient, care givers can then upload the child's generated data such as the daily weight and height. The health care providers on the other hand will have access to this information in real time through which management strategies especially the dietary aspect, may be modified based on an increase or decrease in weight reported on the application. Nutritional regimens will be included on the mobile application, and with just a few information provided by the caregiver about the patient, a meal plan can be generated for the patient. This will reduce the care givers burden of trying to create new meals and at the same time ensure that the child is getting the right quantity and quality of nutrition that is needed for growth. The diet plan will consist of local recipes, portions required per meal and the time to administer the meal. Caregivers will receive frequent prompts or messages which will direct them to visit the app regularly as needed or when changes are implemented in the patient's dietary regimen. The app will include an Electronic diary or Electronic Medical Journal tracker which will help the caregiver to stay organized and also to capture relevant information that is required by the healthcare provider which will be needed for ongoing or future management of the patient.

Development of a Protein Energy Malnutrition prevention system is not without challenges in sub-Saharan Africa. Some of the barriers to Information and Communication Technology as noted by Wickramasinghe and Schaffer(2010) are also encountered in this scenario. Most of the developing countries have financial constraints and are generally poor. There is not enough funding available for healthcare, making it difficult to afford the cost of implementing and acquiring the technology needed for advancement in healthcare. Even when technology is adopted, implementation is stalled due to lack of funds. Human and Cultural barriers also play a big role in the adoption and implementation of technology. As previously noted in this project, paper health records have been used for decades in Africa, hence there have been resistance to EHR due to low computer literacy level of health care professionals and lack of prioritization of EHR. According to Odekunle et al(2017), a study conducted showed only about 26.7% of doctors in sub-Saharan Africa were familiar with computer tools to perform advanced tasks, this is relatively very low compared to the computer literacy level of doctors in the US which was reported as 91.4%. The relatively low literacy level of the public in developing countries plays a big role in the acceptance and usability of technological tools when implemented.

Lack of power supply and limited access to internet service makes it difficult to sustain technological tools in sub Saharan Africa. In some rural areas there is no power supply or internet service which makes the concept of technology completely foreign and almost unattainable. Corruption and poor coordination among the stakeholders has been cited by Pantuvo et al,2011.

These challenges can be overcome by implementing the web of Health Care Players Supplier, Health Care Organization, Regulator, Provider, Payor, Patient. These all interact to ensure a robust delivery of quality healthcare. According to Wickramasinghe and Schaffer(2010) healthcare organizations respond to these challenges by ensuring access to care for everyone at all times, providing effective and efficient delivery of healthcare and establishing integrated information repositories. A reliable, constant source of funding must be available from the government or non-governmental organization to implement technology. It was noted that most of the funding for EHR in sub-Saharan Africa was through foreign aid(Akanbi et al, 2012), there must be an understanding by the host institution of the need to understand the cost involved in the implementation and maintenance of technology, this will enable the management in planning and to assess if they can be financially ready for this change. It is important to note that implementation of Technology is a capital intensive project.

Figure 2. Web of Health Care Players

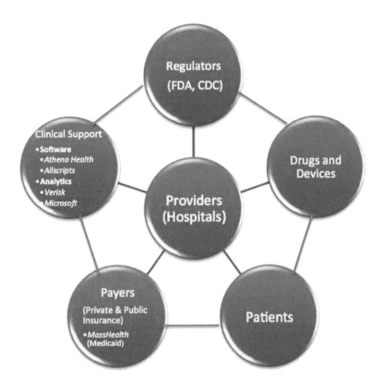

Training and education of health care personnel to use EHR or Clinical Decision Support System tools is required. In some cases there will be need to hire Information Technology experts to train healthcare workers in the institution, this will facilitate easier migration to technology such as EHR. It is recommended that training begins with the most interested healthcare workers who overtime will be responsible for assisting other personnel in the organization (Odekunle et al, 2012). For the mobile applications, informal training may occur by following prompts within the system, this maybe the only guidance needed to use the apps. Some of the challenges which will be encountered are resistance to use the app due to the difficulty of use, inability to understand terminologies used, the high cost and sustainability of use. Strategies to overcome the challenges include ensuring that only few steps are involved in the registration process, this will facilitate enrollment for use. It is also important to use terminologies that will be understood by the targeted population, familiarity with the local language and employment of colloquial forms of speech during the developmental stage of the application will be beneficial. Having a free trial period of use is necessary to encourage use of the app and if possible a subsidized mobile service fee should be offered to low income families after the trial period. Another limitation to use of a mobile app is poor service due to lack of coverage, network issues, or power outage. Having the government invest in the implementation and provide the necessary infrastructure to ensure these services are functional is a priority. Development of an offline app will serve users that have little or no access to service network due to their location.

Strategic planning by healthcare organisations is crucial to the implementation of this system. It is important to consider the financial and human resources available, current workflow and settings in which this change is anticipated(William and Boren, 2008). According to Pantuvo et al(2011), "a phased implementation is preferred for resource-constrained areas where the resources to tackle all issues that implementation will raise are not available, giving room to manage changes in small units and transfer lessons learned to other units."

CONCLUSION

The role of Information Technology in healthcare cannot be overemphasized, it has resulted in significant benefits leading to increased positive health outcomes. Studies have shown positive health outcomes in countries that have adopted the use of Electronic Medical Records and other technological tools such as mobile applications for healthcare. Protein Energy Malnutrition Prevention System will address some of the current issues that have led to an increase in morbidity and mortality due to Protein Energy Malnutrition. Despite the fact that such a system is capital intensive, adequate and sustainable funding from both government and non-governmental organizations for successful implementation will make it a reality. It is important to consider the peculiar situation of each pediatric patient in assessing what type of tools/apps that will be used in each case, this is to say that an online mobile app may not be used in certain communities due to their peculiarities such as extreme poverty, lack of power supply or internet service. In certain cases an offline version will be made available. It is also crucial to ensure that there is accountability among stakeholders, this will address the issue of corruption and lack of coordination. An interdisciplinary approach is used by involving various stakeholders such as doctors, nurses, nutritionist, dietitian, government officials, administrators and Information Technology specialists to form a platform to begin the work towards a Protein Energy Malnutrition prevention system.

REFERENCES

Akanbi, M. O., Ocheke, A. N., Agaba, P. A., Daniyam, C. A., Agaba, E. I., Okeke, E. N., & Ukoli, C. O. (2012). Use of Electronic Health Records in sub-Saharan Africa: Progress and challenges. *Journal of Medicine in the Tropics*, *14*(1), 1–6. PMID:25243111

Akombi, B. J., Agho, K. E., Merom, D., Renzaho, A. M., & Hall, J. J. (2017). Child malnutrition in sub-Saharan Africa: A meta-analysis of demographic and health surveys (2006-2016). *PLoS One*, *12*(5), e0177338. doi:10.1371/journal.pone.0177338 PMID:28494007

Amirfar, S., Taverna, J., Anane, S., & Singer, J. (2011). Developing public health clinical decision support systems (CDSS) for the outpatient community in New York City: Our experience. *BMC Public Health*, *11*(1), 753. doi:10.1186/1471-2458-11-753 PMID:21962009

Anshari, M., & Almunawar, M. N. (2016). Mobile Health (mHealth) Services and Online Health Educators. *Biomedical Informatics Insights*, 8, 19–27. doi:10.4137/BII.S35388 PMID:27257387

Bain, L. E., Awah, P. K., Geraldine, N., Kindong, N. P., Sigal, Y., Bernard, N., & Tanjeko, A. T. (2013). Malnutrition in Sub-Saharan Africa: Burden, causes and prospects. *The Pan African Medical Journal*, *15*, 120. doi:10.11604/pamj.2013.15.120.2535 PMID:24255726

Haslett, C., Chilvers, E. R., & Hunter, J. A. A. (1999). *Davidson's principles and practice of medicine.* Churchill Livingstone.

Lu, C., Hu, Y., Xie, J., Fu, Q., Leigh, I., Governor, S., & Wang, G. (2018). The Use of Mobile Health Applications to Improve Patient Experience: Cross-Sectional Study in Chinese Public Hospitals. *JMIR mHealth and uHealth, 6*(5), e126. doi:10.2196/mhealth.9145 PMID:29792290

Odekunle, F. F., Odekunle, R. O., & Shankar, S. (2017). Why sub-Saharan Africa lags in electronic health record adoption and possible strategies to increase its adoption in this region. *International Journal of Health Sciences, 11*(4), 59–64. PMID:29085270

Pantuvo, J. S., Naguib, R., & Wickramasinghe, N. (2011). Towards Implementing a Nationwide Electronic Health Record System in Nigeria. *International Journal of Healthcare Delivery Reform Initiatives, 3*(1), 39–55. doi:10.4018/jhdri.2011010104

Ra, H.-K., Yoon, H., Son, S., Stankovic, J., & Ko, J. (2018). HealthNode: Software Framework for Efficiently Designing and Developing Cloud-Based Healthcare Applications. *Mobile Information Systems., 2018*, 1–12. doi:10.1155/2018/6071580

Thamjamrassri, P., Song, Y., Tak, J., Kang, H., Kong, H. J., & Hong, J. (2018). Customer Discovery as the First Essential Step for Successful Health Information Technology System Development. *Healthcare Informatics Research, 24*(1), 79–85. doi:10.4258/hir.2018.24.1.79 PMID:29503756

UNICEF (United Nations Children's Fund). (2013). *Improving Child Nutrition: The Achievable Imperative for Global Progress.* UNICEF.

United Nations. (2015). *The Millennium Development Goals Report.* Author.

WHO. (n.d.). *Malnutrition World Health Organization, 2020* .https://www.who.int/news-room/fact-sheets/detail/malnutritionDate

Wickramasinghe, N., & Schaffer, J. (2010). *Realizing value driven eHealth solutions IBM Business of Government.* Retrieved from http://www.businessofgovernment.org/sites/default/files/Realizing%20Value%20Driven%20e-Health%20Solutions.pdf

Williams, F., & Boren, S. A. (2008, December). The role of electronic medical record in care delivery in developing countries. *International Journal of Information Management, 28*(6), 503–507. doi:10.1016/j.ijinfomgt.2008.01.016 PMID:30774175

Wyatt, J. C., & Sullivan, F. (2005). eHealth and the future: Promise or peril? *BMJ (Clinical Research Ed.), 331*(7529), 1391–1393. doi:10.1136/bmj.331.7529.1391 PMID:16339252

Chapter 18
Healthcare–Internet of Things and Its Components:
Technologies, Benefits, Algorithms, Security, and Challenges

Aman Tyagi

Gurukul Kangri University, Haridwar, India

ABSTRACT

Elderly population in the Asian countries is increasing at a very fast rate. Lack of healthcare resources and infrastructure in many countries makes the task of provding proper healthcare difficult. Internet of things (IoT) in healthcare can address the problem effectively. Patient care is possible at home using IoT devices. IoT devices are used to collect different types of data. Various algorithms may be used to analyse data. IoT devices are connected to the internet and all the data of the patients with various health reports are available online and hence security issues arise. IoT sensors, IoT communication technologies, IoT gadgets, components of IoT, IoT layers, cloud and fog computing, benefits of IoT, IoT-based algorithms, IoT security issues, and IoT challenges are discussed in the chapter. Nowadays global epidemic COVID19 has demolished the economy and health services of all the countries worldwide. Usefulness of IoT in COVID19-related issues is explained here.

INTRODUCTION

The Asian population is increasing at a very fast rate. The cities accommodating more population and it is increasing with time. Health facilities and resources are also growing but the growth rate is not enough to meet the requirements. Therefore, the health management in these cities is under tremendous pressure to provide medical facilities to cover the entirepopulation.In the year 2050 Asian population of elderly people will be too large to handle with present infrastructure. So there isneed to find new waysto provide thehealth care services to the large population.Use of IoT in Health careservices has capability to full-fill these needs. In some countriessufficient health care infrastructure is not available to full fill

DOI: 10.4018/978-1-5225-6067-8.ch018

medical needs of poor people population in particular. IoT is cost effective technology and it can be afforded by the developing and underdeveloped countries in Asia like Pakistan, Sri Lanka, Afghanistan, Nepal, Bangladesh etc. So it is required by their government to take initiatives and provide batter help for people living in rural and remote areas. As the population of the Asian countries will increase day by day, so the health care is out of reach ofthe most of the people or patients in developing countries. Moreover, poor citizencannot afford it. In some chronic diseases like heart failure, Asthma attack and diabetes, real-time monitoring via connected devices can savelife of the many patients.

According to the United Nations Population Fund (UNFPA, 2017) in the Asia the proportion of the elderly people is expected to grow from 10.5 percent to 22.4 percent during the years 2012–2050. Now in East Asia, the proportion of the elderly is expected to be increased34.5 percent by 2050. Japan (41.5 percent), South Korea (38.9 percent), China (34 percent) may be expected to report the highest proportions of the elderly population in that region by 2050.The S. R. Islam, D. Kwak, M. H. Kabir, M. Hossain, & K. S. Kwak (2015)conducted surveys on advances in IoT-based health care technologies and reviewed the state-of-the-art network architectures/ platforms, applications, and industrial trends in IoT-based health care solutions and analyzed distinct IoT security and privacy features, including security requirements, threat models, and attack taxonomies from the health care perspective.In their paper theNatarajan, Prasath, & Kokila(2016) discussed that the rapid development of Internet of things (IoT) technology makes it possible for connected various smart objects together through the Internet and provided more data interoperability methods for application purpose.*In the article Gnanaraj, Ranjana, & Thenmozhi (2019) explained that in hospitals it is very difficult for doctors to attend the patients, because doctors cannot be available all the time in the hospital because of their busy schedule. Hence there is a need for a solution to monitor the patients any time for the doctors from any place. With the development of Internet of Things (IoT) devices in the recent years a solution is proposed for this.* The Maksimović (2017) explained about enabling access to high-quality healthcare to anyone, from anywhere are the main advantages of the IoT-driven e-health systems and described as numbers of medical devicesand sensors and 24/7 monitoring of health parameters, consequently leaded to enormous quantities and varieties of data.In the article Routray and Anand (2017) explained the modern world where the quality of living has been degraded significantly IoT can certainly played a constructive role in providing better services.

IoT TECHNOLOGIES

In this section the different technologies used in IoT are discussed. IoT needs different sensors, connectivity and components. So all these technologies are discussed one by one.

IoT Sensors

There are many types of IoT sensor and each one has different purpose. So according to purpose and type sensors are described as follows in given Table 1 and Table 2.

There are different types of sensor used in patient body to collect the medical data. Some general sensors and their position in body are shown in Figure 1.

Table 1. Health care IoT Sensor

S.No.	IoT Sensor Name	Purpose
01	Body Position Sensor	Man current position. (e.g.: sit, lie down, stand, walk)
02	Accelerometer	Measure acceleration, Fall detection, Location and Posture
03	Gyroscopes	Measure orientation and Motion detection.
04	Snore Sensor	Snore noise measurement.
05	GPS	Location tracking and Motion detection
06	ECG	Watch cardiac activity
07	Spirometer	Measure the air capacity of the lungs.
08	EEG	Measure of brain waves
09	EOG	Watch eye movement
10	Glucometer Sensor	Use for approximate concentration of glucose in the blood.
11	EMG	Watch muscle activity
12	PPG	Blood velocity and Heart rate
13	GSR Sensor	Measure the electric conduction of skin.
14	Pulse Oximeter	Measure blood oxygen saturation
15	Blood Pressor	Measure blood pressure
16	SKT (Skin Temperature)	Measure skin temperature
17	Air Flow Sensor	Used for measure air movement quantity in lung.

IoT Communication Technologies

IoT devices, sensors and components are used to send and receive data. They communicate among themselveswirelessly. Hence, there is a need of wireless communication technologies. Some wireless technologies are described below:

1. **Bluetooth:** Bluetooth technology is short range, low power and used for wireless communication. It used public standard (IEEE 802.15.1). It may be used for connecting wireless sensors or other electronic devices.
2. **Wi-Fi:**Wi-Fi full form is Wireless Fidelity. It sends data through air with the help of radio frequencies. It allows many devices to exchange data. It is used to connect medical devices, mobile and laptop to internet.
3. **Infrared:** Infrared wavelies in the range of 300 GHz to 400 GHz. Infrared wavelengths are longer than visible light and shorter than microwaves. These waves can communicatewith various IoT sensors and devices.
4. **Nike+:**The Nike+ is a sport activity monitoring device. It is developed by Nike, Inc... It can monitor and store the distance and speed of the user. It is fitted inside the shoes. It can communicate with the Nike+ sports band, iPhone or iPods.
5. **ANT:**The ANT stands for Adaptive Network Topology. ANT is ultra-low power protocol. It is generally used for sports and fitness purposes. It sends data wirelessly from one device to other device.

Table 2. IoT Environment Sensors

S.No.	IoT Sensor Name	Purpose
01	Light Sensor	Measure light intensity
02	Smoke Sensor	Detects smoke and its level of attainment.
03	PIR	Detects the body heat and identify user location.
04	Temperature Sensor	To measure the temperature of close surface, like room and office.
05	Pressure Sensor	Measure the pressure of liquid and gas.
06	Switch Sensor	Detect open/close of door.
07	Proximity Sensor	Detects the presence of nearby objects.
08	Infrared Sensor	Senses certain characteristics of its surroundings. e.g.: heat, distance, flame monitor, moisture analysis and night vision.
09	RFID	Detect people and object location and identify them.
10	Ultrasonic	For location tracking.
11	Power Sensor	Calculates the power consumption.
12	Gas Sensor	Detect a gas leak in area.
13	Optical Sensor	Measure the physical quantity of light.
14	Humidity Sensor	Measure humidity of close room and office.
15	PDR	Used for real time localization and positioning.
16	Level Sensor	Detect the level of a substance.
17	pH Sensor	Measure the pH level in dissolve water.
18	Magnetometer	Use to measure the position of a patient or a person.
19	UWB	Tracking and detection of people.

Figure 1. Body sensors used in Human Body

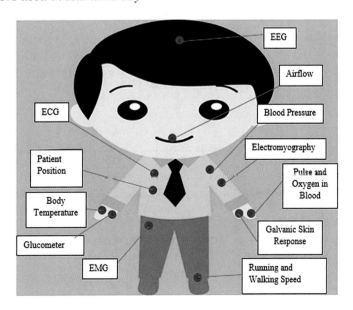

6. **Nearfield Communication**: It is a set of protocols for communication over a short distance up to 4 cmbetween two devices. It is a low speed communication. NFC greatly reduces the human error.

7. **WiMAX:** WiMAX is communication standard based on IEEE802.16. The extended form of WiMAX is Worldwide Interoperability for Microwave Access. It is used for wireless broadband communication.

8. **IrDA:**The Infrared Data Association (IrDA) is established in 1993 by a group of Industry-driven companies. It provides complete set of protocols along with specifications for infrared communication. It is used for data exchange among electronic and medical devices.

9. **Light Fidelity (Li-Fi):** Li-Fi has same application as that of Wi-Fi. The difference between two is that Li-Fi system is using optical waves in place of radio waves. In Li-Fi transceiver – fitted LED bulb is used for transmitting and receiving information. Li-Fi is a low cost high speed system. In Li-Fi it is not possible to transmit or receive data in the area where trees, walls or other obstacles are present. The Li-Fi was first introduced in the year 2011.

10. **Long Term Evolution (LTE):**LTE is a wireless broadband transmission standard. The LTE standard is developed by the Third Generation partnership project (3GPP). LTE is a communication standard used by mobile devices. It increases the communication and transmission capacity and speed.

11. **Long Term EvolutionAdvance (LTE-A):** LTE-A is a 4G mobile communication standard. As its name, LTE-A is used for enhancement and advancement of the LTE. LTE-A is an advance high speed network. LET-A promises to deliver 4G high speed standard. LTE-A is a state-of-the-art because of its speed and technology.

12. **ZigBee:** It is based on the IEEE 802.15.4 standard. It is a high level communication protocols. It is a low power, low data rate wireless networking standard. ZigBee range is short and it is used for communication purposes. Due to low power its transmission range is 10 to 100 meters.

13. **Bluetooth Low Energy (BLE):** It is designed by the Bluetooth Special Internet Group (Bluetooth SGI). It isused as a wireless personal area network. It is made for health care, fitness, security and home entertainment purposes. The main advantage of Bluetooth Low Energy (BLE) is that it consumes less power or energy. So application can run for long time.

14. **Z-Wave:** It is also a wireless communication protocol which is used locally. It can control wirelessly home appliances, IoT devices and security systems. The Z-Wave developed by Zensys in 1999. Its range is up to 100 meters. In Z-Wave technology, all devices are "mesh" with each other by transmitting signals. Z-Waves use low-energy radio waves to transmit and receive signals.

Gadgets of IoT

Rapid advancement in IoT, newer technologies and gadgets are introduced in the market. These IoT gadgets are useful for medical, physical fitness, sports and health care purposes. Some of the IoT gadgets are discussed below:

1. **Smart Phone:** Smart phones are the advanced mobile technologies which help in the health care services and technologies. Health care mobile apps can improve wellness of the patient. There are many mobile apps available in the market now. Smart phones arefrequently used in many areas of health care. Smart phones have various applications in the modern age. Some of them are discussed below:

a. **Applications of Smart Phone:** Technology based diagnosis support, remote diagnostics, telemedicine, GPS navigation, decentralized Health Management Information System (HMIS) and post visit patient surveillance etc.

b. Well known smart phones available in the market are: Samsung Galaxy J8, Straight Talk Apple iPhone XS, Google Pixel XL and Blackberry Z10.

2. **Smart Watches:** It is a digital type of watch different from ordinary watch. In smart watch many apps or features are provided. In modern smart watches, touchscreen interface is provided. Smart watch can also access smart phone apps. Smart watches are generally used for health and medical purposes. In the market smart watches are online available with lots of medical apps and applications. The smart watch is generally used for the purpose of activity tracking, heart rate monitoring, track and record outdoor activities, Blood pressure monitoring and sleep monitoring.

a. Some of smart watches are: Apple Watch (WatchOS), Samsung Gear (Android Wear) and LG Watch (Android Wear).

3. **Smart Bracelets (Smart wristband):** In the era of fast changing technology, life style of the person is also changing across the word. The demand of IoT gadgets related to physical fitness and healthcare is increasing day by day. The smart bracelets are generally used for medical and sports purposes. Many bracelets are available in the market. The cost of the bracelet depends upon the functions available. Some of the bracelet functions are listed below:

a. Sleep monitoring

b. Heart rate measurement

c. Blood pressure measurement

d. ECG

e. Step Count

f. Calorie burned

Bracelets available in the market are: Jawbone UP3, Fitbit Surge, Fitbit Charge, Lenovo Vibe Band VB10, Xiaomi Mi Band, Garmin Vivo smart and Samsung Galaxy Fit features etc.

4. **Smart Clothing:** Due to technology enhancement IoT gadgets are used in almost every walk of life including clothing. In smart clothing smart shirts are available in the market to keep an eye on heart rate, body temperature and physical movements. Smart pair of trousers also available in market to monitor the speed of the runner. Smart socks are used to monitor and watch running and walking activities. Smart clothing is also available in the form of smart dresses, smart blazers, smart cardigans and tailored pants.

Some of the smart clothing are: Lumo Run, NADI X Yoga Pants, Supa Powered Sports Bra, Hexoskin Smart Shirt and Athos Full Body Kit.

5. **Smart Clips:** The smart clip is new type of smart gadget. With the help of smart clips, slaps, punches, kicks and shakes type of effects can be detected. If smart clip found an emergency, it will trigger an alarm. Smart clip results may be used as evidence. Smart clips may be used as a hair clip by women. If her partner or non-partner does any violence or sexual violence smart clips record it. Smart clip is notavailable in market now. One can have them by ordering in advance (indiegogo. com).

6. **Smart Head Band:**There are different types of smart head bands available in the market according to their applications. They are used for the purpose of meditation, relaxation, EEG measurement, monitor brain waves, Enhances sleep, and daily sleep report and for plethysmography (PPG) signals. In the article Hachisu, Pan, Matsuda, Bourreau, & Suzuki(2018)used smart headband to monitor face to face state and also used smart headband for behavioral healthcare applications. The Kim, Ryoo, & Bae(2008) proposed a headbandto measure a photo-plethysmography (PPG) signal at the forehead. PPG signal is used for monitoring the heart rate and acceleration signals for steps counting.
   a. Smart headbands: Dream Smart Sleep Headband, Muse S, Philips Smart Sleep Headband and Viatom Checkme O2 Sleep Monitor.
7. **Smart Brush:**Smart toothbrush is needed because it removes more plaque in comparison to standard manual toothbrush. Sometime person does toothbrush very fast or in less time. There is an option of timer in smart toothbrush to fix the timing of brush as required by the user. A smart tooth brush can record brushing times, time taken by the brush at different parts of the human mouth, measure angle of hold the brush.

Smart Brush available in the market: Oral-B White Pro 1000 Power Rechargeable Electric Toothbrush, ara by kolibree, Philips Sonicare Flexcare Platinum connected Toothbrush, Oral-B Pro 7000 Smart Series Electric Toothbrush with Bluetooth and Philips sonicare HX 632/02 Kids Connected Electric Toothbrush.

8. **Smart Shoes:** Smart shoes are used by sports person who is regular in practice. It is used for performance monitoring of anathlete. Generally, accelerometer, a gyroscope, magnetometer, GPS and pressure sensors are used in smart shoes.
   a. Smart shoes: HyperAdapt 1.0, Under Armor HOVR Shoes, HOVR Sonic, HOVR Phantom, DigitSole Smart Shoes and Mi Jia Smart Shoes.
9. **Smart Goggles (Smart Glasses):** The goggles of the humans areenhanced in technology and become the smart goggles (smart glasses). Smart glasses are used to watch and record photos and video clips. Smart glasses can be used bya surgeon or dentist to improve, monitor and review his operation by seeking advice of experts in the relevant fields. It can be used by expert surgeon to demonstrate operation of a patient for beginners. It is also used in special military and spy operations. There is a special issue on smart glassesby Oppermann and Prinz (2016). Rzayev, Woźniak, Dingler, & Henze(2018) discussed about reading with the help of smart glasses.
   a. Smart Glasses are: Vuzix M300, Epson Moverio BT-300, Sony Smart Eye Glass, Jins Meme, HoloLens and Mira Prism.

Components of IoT

IoT have following components:

1. **IoT LAN:** LAN is a Local Area Network. IoT LAN is a local, short range communication network. It is not necessary that LAN is connected to internet. It may or may not be connected to internet. It connects deviceswithin a building or an organization.
2. **IoT WAN:** WAN is a Wide Area Network. IoT WAN is used to connect many network segments which are organizationally and geographically wide and connect them to the internet.

3. **IoT Node:** Nodes are the part of a network. Nodes are connected to each other inside a LAN or Node may be connected to the internet through a WAN directly.

4. **IoT Gateway:** The gateway is used to transmit data to the outside world called internet. A router is used to connect IoT LAN and IoT WAN to the internet. Prime function of IoT gate way is to forward packets between LAN and WAN on the IP layer. Address of the node is valid within gateway but outside gateway it is not valid. So it is also possible that address is repeated in other gateways.

5. **IoT Proxy:** Connection between devices like IoT sensors, computing devices and other IoT softwares and the internet are facilitated by proxy server. In many IoT problems these connections are necessarily required to collect data for analysis. Proxies may provide one a means to hide one's home IP address from the rest of the world.

IoT Component's Layer

Components of IoT in health care are organized in four layers:

1. **Sensing Layer:** It is used for sensing the patient or user current medical parameters. It consists of all sensors, RFIDs and Wireless Sensor Network (WSN). e.g.: ECG sensor, Spirometer, EEG, EOG, Glucometer Sensor, EMG etc.

2. **Grouping Layer:** This layer is used to collect all data and information and group them together. The data of groping layer is based on sensing layer.

3. **Processing Layer:** It consists of servers or group of servers for processing information and provides important results or information about patient conditions.

4. **Cloud Platform:** It is a very large platform used for storage of large amount of medical and health data of patients. Cloud stores all processed data from the processing layer. It can be used by many users via internet after data and results uploaded to the cloud.

Cloud Computing and Fog Computing for Health Data Storage

Cloud computing is the on-demand services where computer system resources, data storage and computing power are available without any investment by management and the staff of hospitals or organization. According to accessibility, cloud can be categorized as follows:

1. Public Cloud
2. Private Cloud
3. Hybrid Cloud

The resources of public cloud may be accessed by any person. In private cloud resources are accessed by organization or authorized person only. Hybrid cloud is a combination of public and private clouds. Data and resources available on demand via internet using following cloud services:

- Software as a Service (SaaS): In SaaS the software is available over the internet via a third party. Google Suite, Cisco WebEx, Citrix GoToMeeting and Workday may be used as SaaS.

- Infrastructure as a Service (IaaS): IaaS is a cloud based service. It is a paid service which provides services like storage and virtualization. Some IaaS areDigital Ocean, Rackspace, Amazon web services (AWS), Microsoft Azure and Google Compute Engine (GCE).
- Platform as a Service (PaaS): PaaS is one of the cloud computing services that provide a platform to the users to develop, run and manages the applications or software without bothering about complexity of maintaining or constructing infrastructure needed for an app. Examples of PaaS are: Window Aure, Google App Engine, Force.com and OpenShift.

Complexity in the cloud based services increases day by day due to increase of the large number of devices and data. Therefore, to store, access, analyze and collect large amount of data is a big problem. To address this issue the new technology called *fog computing*is introduced. Fog computing is also known as Edge computing or fogging. Fog computing started by CISCO in 2014. It gives faster response time than cloud computing in case of large and different varieties of complex data present. The fog computingmay be used to handle largeamount of data.

The Abuseta (2019)in his paper reviewed the fog computing paradigm particularly its impacts on the IoT applications. Bonomi, Milito, Zhu, & Addepalli(2012) suggested that fog computing characteristicsmake the Fog the appropriate platform for a number of critical Internet of Things (IoT) services and applications. Ashrafi, Hossain, Arefin, Das, & Chakrabarty(2018) in their work suggested that fog computing surpasses cloud computing. The Stergiou, Psannis, Kim,& Gupta(2018) presented survey of IoT and cloud computing in the article. The Pourqasem(2018) presented the cloud-based IoT platform.

BENEFITS OF SMART HEALTH CARE IoT

Some complex diseases need constant monitoring by the doctors so that doctors can act and change their treatment and care plan according to changes in patient condition. Some of the diseases which required constant monitoring are diabetes, blood pressure, sleeplessness and heart diseases. In these diseases the patient needs to take appointments, waiting in the clinic due to queue and traveling long distance if clinic is far away from home. Some time it is risky if there is a gap in checkup due to any reason.

Internet of Things (IoT) can address all the problems of the patients mentioned above. IoTsave the time and work load of the patients and doctors.IoT sensors can read and checkup patient's symptoms (blood pressure, glucose level, heart rate and ECG etc.) automatically. Patient symptoms and conditionsare continuously sensed by the IoT sensors. The IoT devices send daily checkup reports, symptoms and condition of the patient to the doctor via internet. On the basisofpatient checkup reports, symptoms and conditions doctors can priorities the appointment of the patient and make care plan of patient accordingly. Doctor can also improve quality of life of the patient and may change daily routine of the patient. Thereports and symptoms are added to the patient record automatically. If conditions of the patient monitored by IoT sensor is above a threshold (critical) value than hospital can arrange an ambulance to the patient immediately.

There are many benefits of IoT health care services. Some of these benefits are given below:

1. Doctor can monitor the response of his treatment given to the patient. If response of the patient is not satisfactory the treatment and care plan may be changedaccordingly by the doctor.
2. IoT healthcare services save lot of time of the patient who are extremely busy in their working.

3. It is useful for elderly people for disease monitoring and fall detection etc.

4. IoT healthcare is cost effective and efficient. It can be implemented even in developing and under-developed countries.

5. Using smart health IoT devices many diseases are diagnosed in early stages. Therefore, an easy control and treatment of the diseases is possible.

6. There are many problems in big and densely populated cities: like road blockage, traffic jam for a certain time period each day. Smart IoT health care devices can effectively handlethese situationsand timely help may be given to the patient.

7. In some remote areas there is no hospital and transportation problem is also there. With the help of smart IoT health care devices the infrastructure of IoT equipped hospitals can be used to overcome these problems from a large distance in remote areas.

8. Patients can get appointment, care plan and prescription on mobile or laptop.

9. The documents and medical reports are stored online and hence can be retrieved to see the history of the patient.

10. It is paper less and hence green technology.

11. Smart health care IoT can reduce the burden on the management.

12. Smart health care IoT is also useful in rural areas where good health facilities like doctors, hospitals, labs and staffs are not available.

13. Patient feelscomfortable; complete his daily works or duties without going to hospitals or labs for testing.

14. Patient enjoys his life with his family members at home.

15. Health care IoT devices help the hospital staff for searching drugs and track supplies of hospital requirements.

16. Hygiene of the hospital is improved and hospital is safe from infections.

17. All necessary medical reports, data and current real-time patient conditions are supervised by the doctor without moving from his office room.

INTRODUCTION TO SOME ALGORITHMS AND METHODOLOGY USED ON HEALTH CARE DATA

The algorithms and methodologies are used on collected data via sensors. The algorithms can detect the change in user/patient health data, behavior and condition. Accordingly care plan and treatment can be changed. The Tyagi and Singh(2014) diagnosed asthma and also found out level of control of asthmatic patient using decision tree and fuzzy inference system techniques and algorithms. According to Tyagi and Singh(2015) Case Base Reasoning (CBR) Technique is used to generate automatic care plan of asthmatic patient via knowledge of patient symptoms and reports. In the chapter Tyagi and Singh(2019) discussed about health information systems, tools and techniques used to develop the health information system and future research directions.The algorithms have many rules and conditions to judge the patient current situation. Some algorithms are discussed below:

1. **Activity Recognition:**All reports are sent daily to the doctor or related experts and stored in a re-cord also. The sensors collect the daily activity of a patient like "the patient wake up at 7 O' clock in the morning". User/patient can do multiple activities at a time. The activity recognition is also

used in the applications like smart city, smart home, smart office, and smart hospitals and also used in surveillance and security. Activity recognition involves multiple steps. The steps include gathering data from the body and with the help of sensors.This data is used to understand the users or patient activities.Activity recognition steps also include processing data, feature extraction, interpretation, prediction and classification. The smart mobile phones with sensors are used by userson daily basis. If the smart phone has all required sensors, then smart phone may be used for monitoring user's activities. Some of the technologies to observe activities of user are listed below in Table 3.

Table 3. Type of activities and technologies used

S. No.	Activities	Technologies
1.	Inside house or building	Bluetooth, PDR, RFID, Wi-Fi, Fingerprints, UWB, Switch Sensor and Infrared sensor.
2.	Outdoor	GPS, PDR, GSM, LTE, Wi-Fi, Bluetooth, Switch sensor and infrared sensor.
3.	Lying, Standing, Sitting, Walking, Sleeping, Wakeup and Exercise	Accelerometer, Body position sensor, RFID, Wi-Fi, Snore sensor, Magnetometer, Decision tree, Genetic algorithms, Neural network and Thresh-holding.
4.	Working place (Kitchen, Bathroom, Toilet, Bedroom, Office, Study timings and watching TV or mobile)	Wi-Fi, RFID, PDR, Bluetooth, Fingerprint, VWB, GPS, EOG, Accelerometer, Magnetometer, Proximity sensor, Neural networks and Thresh -holding.

Subasi, Radhwan, Kurdi, & Khateeb (2018) presented an intelligent m-healthcare system for human activity recognition by using data mining technologies. Rodriguez et al. (2017) presented an Internet of Things (IoT) approach to Human Activity Recognition (HAR) using remote monitoring of vital signs of heart patients. The Castro, Coral, Rodriguez, Cabra, & Colorado (2017) presented a novel system based on the Internet of Things (IoT) to Human Activity Recognition (HAR).Yao et al. (2018) presented WIS, an end-to-end web-based in-home monitoring system for convenient and efficient care delivery.

2. **Behavioral Pattern Detection:** The human behavior recognition can be done with the help of activity recognition. The human behavior can be classified as: normal, doubtful and hazardous. The normal activities are sitting and lying activities in bedroom of the person. The doubtful and hazardous activities are like longer walking or standing in the bedroom. With the help of behavioral pattern detection one can detect, the preference, habits and anomaly in human behavior. Many sensors are required to be installed in the house for collecting information about user's activities, environment and health conditions of user. Table 4 shows some behavioral conditions and technologies used.

Table 4. Classification and technologies for behavior detection

Behavior Classification	Technology and Algorithms
Normal Doubtful Hazardous	K-means algorithm, Gaussian Mixture Modal (GMM), Support Vector Machines (SVM), K-Nearest Neighborhood (KNN), Neural Network, Light sensor, Accelerometer, Surveillance cameras, RFID and Decision trees.

Fang, Ma, Wang, Qu, & Zhang (2016) have implemented a novel periodic frequent POI (points of interest) set mining methodology to discover the POI sets and find the efficiency and stability of the algorithm. Venkatesh, da Costa, Zou,& Ng (2017) in their research work proposed an engine that identifies the behavioral patterns of IoT device users.Ismail, Hassan, & Alsalamah (2019) presented a new model to explore the challenges associated with mining patterns from the body sensor data and their potential use in discovering normal human routines. TheKoutli, Theologou, Tryferidis, & Tzovaras (2019) introduced a non-intrusive, spatio-temporal abnormalbehavior detection approach. Rawassizadeh, Momeni, Dobbins, Gharibshah, & Pazzani (2016) in their work introduced a set of scalable algorithms to identify patterns of human daily behaviors.

3. **Anomaly Detection:**The goal ofanomaly detection is to detect abnormal or critical condition of user or patient. It is very important and crucial to find out anomaly detection with high level of accuracy because in critical condition patient need to be hospitalized as soon as possible. It increases the quality of life of elder persons. If the critical or emergency cases are found by anomaly detection algorithm than IoT devices send report to the relevant hospital and ringing the alarm. In anomaly emergency cases hospital sends an ambulance to the patient. Artificial Intelligence (AI) and Neural Network may be used in anomaly detection algorithm.

TheUkil, Bandyoapdhyay, Puri, & Pal (2016) discussed about proactive healthcare analytic specifically for cardiac disease. Sehatbakhsh, Alam, Nazari, Zajic, & Prvulovic (2018) proposed a new framework called SYNDROME for "externally" monitoring medical embedded devices. Carvalho, Teixeira, Dias, Meira, & Carvalho (2015) in theirarticle proposed a simple, intuitive and generic method for anomaly detection. The goal of the system proposed by Manashty, Light, & Yadav (2015) is to fill the gap between symptoms and diagnosis trend data in order to predict health anomalies accurately and quickly.

4. **Fall Detection:** Fall detection is very big problem in health care field. Mostly elderly persons are prone to fall. A good fall detection system would detect fall spontaneously and at same time ring an alarm to the hospital, relatives and nearby persons. In case of serious problems ambulance can be sent to the concerned person. The problem of falling of a person increases with his age. The accelerometer and gyroscope is used for measuring fall detection. There are naive bayes machine learning algorithm, Support Vector Machine (SVM), decision tree and KNN etc. algorithms are used for fall prediction. The fall detection can be classified according to Ajerla, Mahfuz, & Zulkernine (2019) into following four categories:

a. Fall forward from standing and use of hands to dampen fall
b. Fall forward from sanding: first impact on knees
c. Fall sideward from standing: bending legs
d. Fall backward while trying to sit on a chair.

Yacchirema, de Puga, Palau, & Esteve (2018) discussed fall detection system for elderly people using IoT and Big data. In the article Jannat & Haque (2019) an IoT based health monitoring and fall detection system for elderly people is discussed. Gutiérrez-Madroñal, La Blunda, Wagner, & Medina-Bulo (2019) presented a complete study of falls as relevant situations. Ngu, Tseng, Paliwal, Carpenter,

& Stipe (2018) proposed a system for using the streaming accelerometer data from commodity-based smart watch (IoT) devices to detect falls.

SECURITY AND CHALLENGES IN HEALTH CARE IoT

IoT is fast growing industry with interconnected devices and verity of IoT applications increasing at a very fast rate. As of now there are many challenges of security and privacy of IoT devices. Nowadays millions of connected devices and billions of sensors are used and these numbers are increasing fast. It is a big challenging task to provide privacy, security and reliable connectivity. IoT Threads are also growing day by day. By attacking, attacker gain physical access and in few cases full control of device can be taken. The strong password and encryption technology can protect our IoT devices and sensors. The attackers always take advantage of weaker passwords and lack of encryption.There are following security issues for physical objects:

1. **Physical attacks:** Most of the IoT devices are small in size and connected wirelessly to each other. Therefore, there is a possibility of security of information or data breach via physical attacks. Therefore, security of sensitive data in the IoT devices is essential. The more data in the transit, the more is the risk of physical attacks. The factors like identity, trust, privacy, reliability, responsibility and security must also be looked into to make the system foolproof.
2. **Integrating RFID into IoT:** RFID technology is used for tracking and tracing purposes. The RFID system is more prone to attacks. The data encryption can be used in RFID systems.
3. **Integrating WSNs into IoT:** The WSNs techniqueshave limited power and computational resources. Therefore, it is easy to be attacked. The attacker can damage the network by physical attack of the node. Critical information like security protocols, source code and other data may be leaked to the attackers.
4. **Denial of Service (DoS) attacks:** Through DoS and Distribute DoS (DDoS) attacks the data and resources may not be accessible to the users. If DoS is present in various nodes, then it is known as DDoS attack.
5. **Unauthorized access and control:** There are many types of persons accessingthe system for different applications. Therefore, we have to ensure that illegal users cannot enter in the system. For this proper, identification and authorization of its users is required. So that authorized persons or users are able to access the information.

IoT SECURITY REQUIREMENTS

1. *Confidentiality*: Information or data not accessed by unauthorized person or entity.
2. *Integrity*: Data and information has not been changed or destroyed in any unauthorized manner or way.
3. *Authentication*: In authentication the identity of person and entity is verified. The authentication is needed before establishing communication channel between entities for accessing information.
4. *Availability*: The system is operational, functional and free to use.
5. *Data Freshness*:IoThealth care network generally provides measurementvarying with time. The data should be new and fresh.

6. *Non-Repudiation*: In this situation one cannotdispute validity of concern contract successfully.
7. *Authorization*: It means only authorized nodes are able to access network services or resources.
8. *Resiliency*: If there is compromise among interconnected devices, then the network/information/ sensors/devices are still protected from any type of attack.
9. *Fault Tolerance*: If any fault occurs in the system, then respective security services are still working.
10. *Self-Healing*:Even if any medical device fails or run out of energy, then rest of the devices/ sensors work with minimum level of security.
11. *Secure Booting*: The authenticity and integrity of software must be verified via digital signatures, when device or system is bootedfirst time
12. *Interoperability*: The interoperability means everything must cooperate in a manner to provide the desired access control and service at a given point of time.
13. *Privacy*: The private data of any user is not leaked to any other network.
14. *Access Control*: The user is able to access those resources and services which are related to the users.
15. Notarization: In notarization the registration of data is done with the help of third party, so the accuracy and originality of data is assured.

SECURITY CHALLENGES

There are many challenges in security of IoT devices. Some challenges are discussed below:

- **Computational or Operational Limitations**: The Central Processing Unit(CPU) used in the IoT health devices is less powerful. IoT devices work on a low speed processor and devices are not able to solve large problems. It is very difficult to find security solutions because of less powerful processor and less resources.
- **Power and Energy Limitations**: The devices used in IoT health care are driven by small battery power becauseof small size of the devices. So when sensing is not required by the devices, the power of the devices is automatically off becauseof no longer use. That is power saving mode of devices is on and devices operate at low CPU speed to save energy. Therefore, security protocols cannot be run easily when power saving mode is on.
- **Memory Limitation**: IoT devices have very less memory, works on embedded operating system and use binary application. That's why there is no possibility to process complex security codes or protocols.
- **Scalability**: The number of IoT devices used is gradually increasing day by day. These increased numbers of devices are to be connected to the global network. It is really a challenging task to provide high security.
- **Mobility**:Almost all devices/sensors used in the IoT healthcare system are not static. These devices are connected to the internet. All the information is sent via internet and movability affects things like devices connectivity, data transfer rate and security etc. So to provide security is a big task.
- **Communication Technology**: The health care IoT devices are connected to both types of networks: the local network and global network. In local network different type of technologies are used such as Bluetooth, Bluetooth Low Energy, WiFi, LET, LET-A, Wi-Max and 4G etc. The

wireless channel characteristic of above networks makes wired technologies security scheme less suitable. It is toughto find out security scheme and protocols that can treat both wired and wireless channel characteristics with the same manner.

- **The Miscellaneous types of devices**:The IoT devicesand the IoT networks are connected with various types of devices like: Personal computer, sensors and smart phones. Each device has different energy, computation, memory and operating system capability etc. Therefore, it is difficult to design a security scheme and protocols that work on all kind of devices.
- **Data and Information Confidentiality**: The medical data of any person or patient is very sensitive and confidential. To protect and maintain confidentiality of data is to be ensured. For that purposes flow of control of data needs an authorization. If data is accessed by person or an entity the identity of the user must be verified.
- **A Multi-Protocol Network**: A protocol isneeded that can be used for local communication among various types of devices. For this, system needs a proprietary network protocol.
- **The Dynamic Topology**: The IoT based Network can be used at any place and at any time. Therefore, a new type of topology that has properties of existing topology and also have dynamic topology is needed.

In the articleMawgoud, Karadawy, & Tawfik (2019) proposed a new authentication approach through machine learning, to enhance the security level. Razzaq, Gill, Qureshi, & Ullah (2017) have done an extensive comprehensive study on security and privacy issues in IoT networks. The Mahmoud, Yousuf, Aloul, & Zualkernan (2015) presented an overview of security principles, technological and security challenges and proposed countermeasures and the future directions for securing the IoT framework. In the articleKumar, Vealey, & Srivastava (2016) reviewed security attacks from the perspective of layers that comprise IoT. Chokshi and Patel (2017) aimed at describing IoT architecture with security challenges in IoT and its usage in healthcare industry. TheBugeja, Jacobsson, & Davidsson (2016) presented an overview of the privacy breaches towards smart home domain. In their articleKim, Rathore, Ryu, J.H., Park & J.H., Park (2018) analyzed security issues, threats and solutions for IoT-CPS (IoT Cyber Physical System), and evaluated the existing researches. In their article Ziegeldorf, Morchon, & Wehrle(2014) presented privacy issues in the Internet of Things in details. In the article Lin, & Bergmann(2016) identified key for trusted smart Home systems. The Kai, Pang, & Cong(2013) proposed a novel security and privacy mechanism for health Internet of Things (Health-IoT) to solve the related problems.

CURRENT SCENARIO OF IoT

There are lots of applications of the IoT in health care. Some of them are shown in Figure 2.

Currently COVID19 virus spreads all over the world and becomes global epidemic. COVID19 patients can be treated more safely in the hospitals with the help of IoTdevices. In IoT devices the physical contact between patient and doctoris reduced to help in stopping the spread the dangerous disease. Due to COVID19 the hospitals are full in the affected cities.IoT home care treatment is definitely a better option to tackle the above problem. General patients are afraid to go to hospital nowadays due to global epidemic COVID19. Therefore, they will prefer the safer IoT health care option for treatment. It is easy to maintain social distancing with the help of IoT devices.

Figure 2. Applications of IoT in Health care

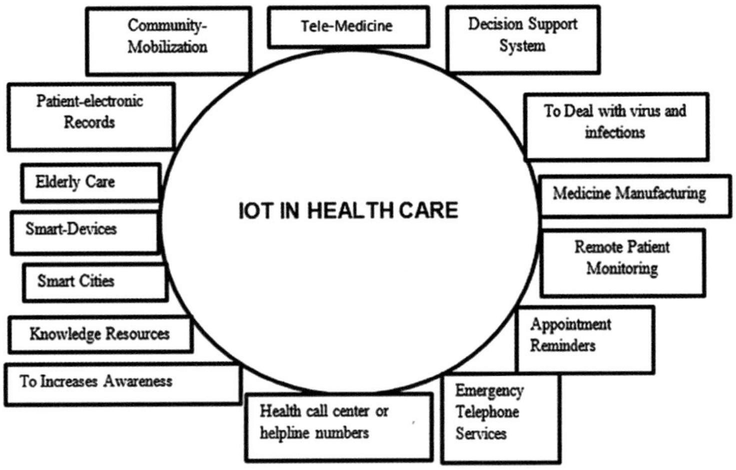

Currently Internet of Things (IoT) is a new trend in the health care field. In smart phone many sensors are present. In the current scenario lots of health apps are available in the market free of cost and some of them are available on payment basis. These apps are used for both health and fitness purposes. Users can monitor their health condition by using apps at their home place. These days India is using app Aarogya Setu for online tracking of COVID19 patients and alarming peoples if they are near to any COVID19 patient. For this purpose, IoT devices and sensors are also used. Arogya setu is proving an important step to fight global epidemic covid 19. It provides important information like Indian council of medical research approved laboratories with covid 19 testing facilities. The effectiveness of this app incresses with the number of users cicurity issues are addressed in this app.

REFERENCES

Abu seta, Y. (2019). *A Fog Computing Based Architecture for IoT Services and Applications Development.* arXiv preprint arXiv:1911.02403

Ajerla, D., Mahfuz, S., & Zulkernine, F. (2019). A real-time patient monitoring framework for fall detection. *Wireless Communications and Mobile Computing, 2019*, 1–13. doi:10.1155/2019/9507938

Ashrafi, T. H., Hossain, M. A., Arefin, S. E., Das, K. D., & Chakrabarty, A. (2018). Iot infrastructure: fog computing surpasses cloud computing. In *Intelligent Communication and Computational Technologies*. Springer. doi:10.1007/978-981-10-5523-2_5

Bonomi, F., Milito, R., Zhu, J., & Addepalli, S. (2012). Fog computing and its role in the internet of things. *Proceedings of the first edition of the MCC workshop on Mobile cloud computing.* 10.1145/2342509.2342513

Bugeja, J., Jacobsson, A., & Davidsson, P. (2016). On privacy and security challenges in smart connected homes. In *2016 European Intelligence and Security Informatics Conference (EISIC)*. IEEE. 10.1109/EISIC.2016.044

Carvalho, L. F., Teixeira, C., Dias, E. C., Meira, W., & Carvalho, O. (2015). A simple and effective method for anomaly detection in healthcare. *Proceedings of the SIAM International Conference on Data Mining Workshop.*

Castro, D., Coral, W., Rodriguez, C., Cabra, J., & Colorado, J. (2017). Wearable-based human activity recognition using an iot approach. *Journal of Sensor and Actuator Networks*, 6(4), 1–20.

Chokshi, A., & Patel, S. (2017). Internet of Things (IoT) IoT Architecture Security Challenges in IoT & Role of IoT in Healthcare Industry. *International Journal of Engineering Technology Science and Research*, 4(10), 822–825.

Fang, Z., Ma, C., Wang, X., Qu, J., & Zhang, S. (2016). Identify individuals behaviors based GPS trajectories in the Internet of Things. In *2016 First IEEE International Conference on Computer Communication and the Internet (ICCCI)*. IEEE. 10.1109/CCI.2016.7778948

Gnanaraj, V. V., Ranjana, P., & Thenmozhi, P.(2019). Patient Monitoring and Control System using Internet of Thing. *International Journal of Innovative Technology and Exploring Engineering*, 8(6S3), 120-123.

Gutiérrez-Madroñal, L., La Blunda, L., Wagner, M. F., & Medina-Bulo, I. (2019). Test event generation for a fall-detection IoT system. *IEEE Internet of Things Journal*, 6(4), 6642–6651. doi:10.1109/JIOT.2019.2909434

Hachisu, T., Pan, Y., Matsuda, S., Bourreau, B., & Suzuki, K. (2018). FaceLooks: A Smart Headband for Signaling Face-to-Face Behavior. *Sensors (Basel)*, 18(7), 1–20. doi:10.339018072066 PMID:29958435

Islam, S. R., Kwak, D., Kabir, M. H., Hossain, M., & Kwak, K. S. (2015). The internet of things for health care: A comprehensive survey. *IEEE Access: Practical Innovations, Open Solutions*, 3, 678–708. doi:10.1109/ACCESS.2015.2437951

Ismail, W. N., Hassan, M. M., & Alsalamah, H. A. (2019). Context-enriched regular human behavioral pattern detection from body sensors data. *IEEE Access: Practical Innovations, Open Solutions*, 7, 33834–33850. doi:10.1109/ACCESS.2019.2904122

Jannat, N., & Haque, M. T. R. (1587-1590). IoT Based Health Monitoring & Fall Detection System. *International Journal of Scientific & Engineering Research*, 10(6).

Kai, K. A. N. G., Pang, Z. B., & Cong, W. A. N. G. (2013). Security and privacy mechanism for health internet of things. *Journal of China Universities of Posts and Telecommunications*, 20(2), 64–68.

Kim, N. Y., Rathore, S., Ryu, J. H., Park, J. H., & Park, J. H. (2018). A Survey on Cyber Physical System Security for IoT: Issues, Challenges, Threats, Solutions. *Journal of Information Processing Systems*, 14(6), 1361–1384.

Kim, S., Ryoo, D., & Bae, C. (2008). Implementation of smart headband for the wearable healthcare. In *2008 Digest of Technical Papers-International Conference on Consumer Electronics*. IEEE.

Koutli, M., Theologou, N., Tryferidis, A., & Tzovaras, D. (2019). Abnormal Behavior Detection for elderly people living alone leveraging IoT sensors. In *2019 IEEE 19th International Conference on Bioinformatics and Bioengineering (BIBE)*. IEEE. 10.1109/BIBE.2019.00173

Kumar, S. A., Vealey, T., & Srivastava, H. (2016). Security in internet of things: Challenges, solutions and future directions. In *2016 49th Hawaii International Conference on System Sciences (HICSS)*. IEEE.

Lin, H., & Bergmann, N. W. (2016). IoT privacy and security challenges for smart home environments. *Information*, 7(3), 1–15. doi:10.3390/info7030044

Mahmoud, R., Yousuf, T., Aloul, F., & Zualkernan, I. (2015). Internet of things (IoT) security: Current status, challenges and prospective measures. In *2015 10th International Conference for Internet Technology and Secured Transactions (ICITST)*. IEEE.

Maksimović, M. (2017). Improving computing issues in internet of things driven e-health systems. *Proceedings of the International Conference for Young Researchers in Informatics, Mathematics and Engineering'17*.

Manashty, A., Light, J., & Yadav, U. (2015). Healthcare event aggregation lab (HEAL), a knowledge sharing platform for anomaly detection and prediction. In *2015 17th International Conference on E-health Networking, Application & Services (HealthCom)*. IEEE.

Mawgoud, A. A., Karadawy, A. I., & Tawfik, B. S. (2019). *A Secure Authentication Technique in Internet of Medical Things through Machine Learning.* arXiv preprint arXiv:1912.12143

Natarajan, K., Prasath, B., & Kokila, P. (2016). Smart health care system using internet of things. *Journal of Network Communications and Emerging Technologies*, 6(3), 37–42.

Ngu, A. H., Tseng, P. T., Paliwal, M., Carpenter, C., & Stipe, W. (2018). Smartwatch-based iot fall detection application. *Open Journal of Internet Of Things*, 4(1), 87–98.

Oppermann, L., & Prinz, W. (2016). Introduction to this Special Issue on Smart Glasses. *i-com, 15*(2), 123-132.

Pourqasem, J. (2018). Cloud-based IoT: Integration cloud computing with internet of things. *International Journal of Research in Industrial Engineering*, 7(4), 482–494.

Rawassizadeh, R., Momeni, E., Dobbins, C., Gharibshah, J., & Pazzani, M. (2016). Scalable daily human behavioral pattern mining from multivariate temporal data. *IEEE Transactions on Knowledge and Data Engineering*, 28(11), 3098–3112. doi:10.1109/TKDE.2016.2592527

Razzaq, M. A., Gill, S. H., Qureshi, M. A., & Ullah, S. (2017). Security issues in the Internet of Things (IoT): A comprehensive study. *International Journal of Advanced Computer Science and Applications*, 8(6), 383–388.

Rodriguez, C., Castro, D. M., Coral, W., Cabra, J. L., Velasquez, N., Colorado, J., Diego, M., & Trujillo, L. C. (2017). IoT system for human activity recognition using BioHarness 3 and smartphone. *Proceedings of the International Conference on Future Networks and Distributed Systems*. 10.1145/3102304.3105828

Routray, S. K., & Anand, S. (2017). Narrowband IoT for healthcare. In *2017 International Conference on Information Communication and Embedded Systems (ICICES)*. IEEE. 10.1109/ICICES.2017.8070747

Rzayev, R., Woźniak, P. W., Dingler, T., & Henze, N. (2018). Reading on smart glasses: The effect of text position, presentation type and walking. *Proceedings of the 2018 CHI Conference on Human Factors in Computing Systems*.

Sehatbakhsh, N., Alam, M., Nazari, A., Zajic, A., & Prvulovic, M. (2018). *Syndrome: Spectral analysis for anomaly detection on medical iot and embedded devices. In 2018 IEEE international symposium on hardware oriented security and trust (HOST)*. IEEE.

Stergiou, C., Psannis, K. E., Kim, B. G., & Gupta, B. (2018). Secure integration of IoT and cloud computing. *Future Generation Computer Systems*, *78*, 964–975. doi:10.1016/j.future.2016.11.031

Subasi, A., Radhwan, M., Kurdi, R., & Khateeb, K. (2018). IoT based mobile healthcare system for human activity recognition. In *2018 15th Learning and Technology Conference (L&T)*. IEEE. 10.1109/LT.2018.8368507

Tyagi, A., & Singh, P. (2014). Asthma diagnosis and level of control using decision tree and fuzzy system. *International Journal of Biomedical Engineering and Technology*, *16*(2), 169–181. doi:10.1504/IJBET.2014.065658

Tyagi, A., & Singh, P. (2015). ACS: Asthma care services with the help of case base reasoning technique. *Procedia Computer Science*, *48*, 561–567. doi:10.1016/j.procs.2015.04.136

Tyagi, A., & Singh, P. (2019). Health information system. In N. Wickramasinghe (Ed.), *Healthcare Policy and Reform: Concepts, Methodologies, Tools, and Applications* (pp. 1554–1564). IGI Global. doi:10.4018/978-1-5225-6915-2.ch070

Ukil, A., Bandyoapdhyay, S., Puri, C., & Pal, A. (2016). IoT healthcare analytics: The importance of anomaly detection. In *2016 IEEE 30th International Conference on Advanced Information Networking and Applications (AINA)*. IEEE.

United Nations Population Fund. (2017). Caring for Our Elders: Early Responses. United Nations Population Fund (UNFPA).

Venkatesh, P. K., da Costa, D. A., Zou, Y., & Ng, J. W. (2017). A framework to extract personalized behavioural patterns of user's IoT devices data. In *Proceedings of the 27th Annual International Conference on Computer Science and Software Engineering*. IBM Corp.

Yacchirema, D., de Puga, J. S., Palau, C., & Esteve, M. (2018). Fall detection system for elderly people using IoT and big data. *Procedia Computer Science*, *130*, 603–610. doi:10.1016/j.procs.2018.04.110

Yao, L., Sheng, Q. Z., Benatallah, B., Dustdar, S., Wang, X., Shemshadi, A., & Kanhere, S. S. (2018). WITS: An IoT-endowed computational framework for activity recognition in personalized smart homes. *Computing*, *100*(4), 369–385. doi:10.100700607-018-0603-z

Ziegeldorf, J. H., Morchon, O. G., & Wehrle, K. (2014). Privacy in the Internet of Things: Threats and challenges. *Security and Communication Networks*, *7*(12), 2728–2742. doi:10.1002ec.795

ADDITIONAL READING

Ahmed, M. U., Begum, S., & Fasquel, J. B. (Eds.). (2018). *Internet of Things (IoT) Technologies for HealthCare*. Springer International Publishing. doi:10.1007/978-3-319-76213-5

Borra, S., Thanki, R., & Dey, N. (2018). *Digital image watermarking: theoretical and computational advances*. CRC Press. doi:10.1201/9780429423291

Hassanien, A. E., Dey, N., & Borra, S. (Eds.). (2018). *Medical Big Data and internet of medical things: Advances, challenges and applications*. CRC Press. doi:10.1201/9781351030380

Krishna, P. V., Gurumoorthy, S., & Obaidat, M. S. (2019). *Internet of Things and Personalized Healthcare Systems*. Springer Singapore. doi:10.1007/978-981-13-0866-6

Kvedar, J. C., Colman, C., & Cella, G. (2015). *The internet of healthy things*. Partners Connected Health.

Raj, P., Chatterjee, J. M., Kumar, A., & Balamurugan, B. *Internet of Things Use Cases for the Healthcare Industry*. Springer International Publishing.

A. Ugon, B. Séroussi, & C. Lovis (Eds.). (2016). Transforming Healthcare with the Internet of Things: *Proceedings of the EFMI Special Topic Conference 2016* (Vol. 221). IOS Press.

Wickramasinghe, N., & Bodendorf, F. (2019). *Delivering Superior Health and Wellness Management with IoT and Analytics*. Springer Nature.

KEY TERMS AND DEFINITIONS

Decision Tree: A decision tree is a tree like model of decisions. In decision tree each branch represents the outcome of the test.

Gaussian Mixture Model (GMM): It is a probabilistic model in which, it is assumed that all the data points are generated from a miture of Gaussian distributions with unknown parameter.

Genetic Algorithm: Genatic algorithm is a metaheuristic which is inspired by the process of natural selection corresponding to the larger class of evolutionary algorithms.

K-Means Algorithm: It is an iterative algorithm that partition the hole data set into K non overlaping subsets (Clusters). Each data point belongs to only one subset.

K-Nearest Neighbourhood: K-nearest neighbourhood is a algorithum which stores all available cases and classifies new cases based on a similarity measure. It is used in statistical estimation and pattern recognition.

Neural Network: It is a network/circuit of artificial neurons or nodes.

RFID: It is called radio-frequency identification. It uses radio frequency electromagnetic waves to identify and track attached to an object automatically.

Support Vector Machines (SVM): Support vector machines are supervised learning models with related learning algorithms for analyising data to be used for classification and regression analysis.

Conclusion

In today's digital world the ability to consult with one's doctor and receive specific advice when and as needed should not be restricted by geography. Advances in Health 4.0 and telemedicine are making it possible to more readily consult with one's doctor when and as one needs. Clearly, there needs to be more work in this area and policies and regulations that enable more flexible health delivery models are essential.

As we enter the next decade of the 21st Century, we continue to witness the evolution of technological innovations which are impacting all aspects of life and industries across the globe. Healthcare has traditionally been slow to adopt technology solutions but over the last decade this trend has changed as healthcare organisations are rapidly trying to embrace leading analytic solutions, patient bed side solutions, EMRs and technology solutions to support hospital in the home initiatives (HIMSS, 2019). In conjunction with this increasing appetite in healthcare for technology solutions, healthcare professionals have become more efficient and productive, solely concentrating on the important aspects of the patients' health (Gillan et al., 2019). Today, these professionals worry less about client's data registrations and monitoring or other minor activities that consumed a significant amount of resources and more about the patient experience (Hooker, 2019).

Industrial advancements such as smartphones have spread their impact throughout healthcare. They have contributed to consultancy efficiency by replacing traditional and conventional consulting protocols. For example; patients only need a smartphone or similar device to book a session with a medical expert with an option to safeguard their privacy and have the sessions at their homes or there are over 300,000 Aps for diabetes management alone (Jimenez et al., 2019). Further, technology developments are not limited to improving convenience but also quality. Over the years, these advancements have improved the medical field by empowering the research of new drugs and treatments, thus boosting the general service quality (Phichitchaisopa, & Naenna, 2013). From magnetic resonance and scanners to more sophisticated antibiotics, all these would be impossible without a strong industrial-technological core (ibid). This innovative core has been the foundation of health 4.0, initially an industrial concept.

This need to embrace the advances in digital health and leverage the innovations in Health 4.0 to provide better access, higher quality and optimal value of care to all has never been more important than now as we begin to enter the post COVID-19 era. The 18 chapters in the preceding pages have served to highlight the critical areas we must focus on if we are to benefit and realise the full potential of wireless and mobile to deliver superior healthcare. Health 4.0 has evolved from the overall industry digitization. Moreover, it has borrowed and adapted several constructs and concepts. These concepts are founded on the basis of convenience, efficiency and quality service. Technologies such as cloud storage, artificial intelligence, IoT, 3D printing and others have been built to provide convenient and quality health care services. This has in turn enabled a shift from the traditional health service delivery process encompassed with rigidity and substandard quality to a more patient-centred approach. Today, health 4.0 is known for offering affordable, fast, accurate and patient convenient services. It has gone further and reinforced expert relationships, patient-doctor relationships presenting the sector as a collaborative professional environment. Patients have also been empowered and handed responsibility in their reactive and preventive health. Through smart gadgets, patients can take complete control of their health. All these developments have met some barriers and facilitators along the way. However, economic and social expectations have played a role in pushing these changes. Health product consumers need efficient and fast products, thus pushing the need for personalized body devices. These developments have just laid a foundation for future advancements. Coming technologies such as the Internet of systems and 5G technologies are expected to have massive impacts in the healthcare sector. Clearly the future is bright for wireless and mobile technology in healthcare but there are also many challenges along the road ahead and we must take care to ensure responsible design, development and deployment of these myriad of solutions if we are going to realise high value, high quality and high access healthcare delivery for all.

In closing, I hope this handbook will serve as a key resource to all healthcare stakeholders, researchers, health advocates, policy makers, regulators, payers, clinicians, consultants, patients and the community at large as we try to design, develop and deploy we have superior healthcare services.

Happy reading and good luck!

Nilmini Wickramasinghe
Swinburne University of Technology, Australia & Epworth HealthCare, Australia

REFERENCES

Gillan, C., Milne, E., Harnett, N., Purdie, T. G., Jaffray, D. A., & Hodges, B. (2019). Professional implications of introducing artificial intelligence in healthcare: An evaluation using radiation medicine as a testing ground. *Journal of Radiotherapy in Practice*, *18*(1), 5–9. doi:10.1017/S1460396918000468

HIMSS. (2019). *Digital Health Transformation: The Path Forward.* Available at https://www.himssconference.org/education/keynote-speakers

Hooker, K. (2019). *Enhancing the patient experience: a challenge for leadership in health care* (Master's Thesis). University of Pittsburgh.

Jimenez, G., Lum, E., & Car, J. (2019). 2019 Examining Diabetes Management Apps Recommended From a Google Search: Content Analysis. *JMIR mHealth and uHealth*, *7*(1), e11848. doi:10.2196/11848 PMID:30303485

Phichitchaisopa, N., & Naenna, T. (2013). Factors affecting the adoption of healthcare information technology. *EXCLI Journal*, *12*, 413. PMID:26417235

Compilation of References

8bit AVR Microcontrollers. (2016). http://www.atmel.com/Images/Atmel-42735-8-bit-AVR-Microcontroller-ATmega328-328P_Datasheet.pdf

Abbas, R., & Norris, A. C. (2018). *Inter-agency communication and information exchange in disaster healthcare.* Paper presented at the 15th Information Systems for Crisis Response and Management, Rochester, NY. http://idl.iscram.org/files/reemabbas/2018/2160_ReemAbbas+TonyNorris2018.pdf

Abbas, R., Norris, T., Madanian, S., & Parry, D. (2016). *Disaster e-health and interagency communication in disaster healthcare: A suggested road map.* Paper presented at the Health Informatics New Zealand (HiNZ), Auckland, New Zealand. https://www.researchgate.net/publication/311404397_Disaster_E-Health_and_Interagency_Communication_in_Disaster_Healthcare_A_Suggested_Road_Map

Abidi, S., Vallis, M., Piccinini-Vallis, H., Imran, S., & Abidi, S. (2018). Diabetes-related behavior change knowledge transfer to primary care practitioners and patients: Implementation and evaluation of a digital health platform. *JMIR Medical Informatics, 6*(2), e25. doi:10.2196/medinform.9629 PMID:29669705

Abu seta, Y. (2019). *A Fog Computing Based Architecture for IoT Services and Applications Development.* arXiv preprint arXiv:1911.02403

AbuKhousa, E., Mohamed, N., & Al-Jaroodi, J. (2012). e-Health cloud: Opportunities and challenges. *Future Internet, 4*(3), 621–645. doi:10.3390/fi4030621

ACCORD Study Group and ACCORD Eye Study Group. (2010). Effects of medical therapies on retinopathy progression in type 2 diabetes. *The New England Journal of Medicine, 363*(3), 233–244. doi:10.1056/NEJMoa1001288 PMID:20587587

Achananuparp, P., Lim, E.-P., Abhishek, V., & Yun, T. (2018). Eat & Tell: A Randomized Trial of Random-Loss Incentive to Increase Dietary Self-Tracking Compliance. *Proceedings of the 2018 International Conference on Digital Health,* 45–54. 10.1145/3194658.3194662

Action to Control Cardiovascular Risk in Diabetes (ACCORD) Study Group. (2008). Effects of intensive glucose lowering in type 2 diabetes. *The New England Journal of Medicine, 358*(24), 2545–2559. doi:10.1056/NEJMoa0802743 PMID:18539917

Agarwal, P., Mukerji, G., Desveaux, L., Ivers, N. M., Bhattacharyya, O., Hensel, J. M., Shaw, J., Bouck, Z., Jamieson, T., Onabajo, N., Cooper, M., Marani, H., Jeffs, L., & Bhatia, R. S. (2019). Mobile App for Improved Self-Management of Type 2 Diabetes: Multicenter Pragmatic Randomized Controlled Trial. *JMIR mHealth and uHealth, 7*(1), e10321. doi:10.2196/10321 PMID:30632972

Agerskov, M., Nielsen, A. M., Hansen, C. M., Hansen, M. B., Lippert, F. K., Wissenberg, M., Folke, F., & Rasmussen, L. S. (2015). Public access defibrillation: Great benefit and potential but infrequently used. *Resuscitation, 96*, 53–58. doi:10.1016/j.resuscitation.2015.07.021 PMID:26234893

Ahmed, A., & Sugianto, L. F. (2007). *A 3-tier architecture for the adoption of RFID in emergency management.* Paper presented at the Proceedings of the International Conference on Business and Information 2007, Tokyo, Japan.

Ahmed, A., & Sugianto, L. F. (2009). RFID in emergency management. In J. Symonds, J. Ayoade, & D. Parry (Eds.), *Auto-identification and ubiquitous computing applications* (pp. 137–155). IGI Global. doi:10.4018/978-1-60566-298-5.ch008

Aija, L. (2016). Mobile applications for chronic disease self-management: Building a bridge for behavior change. *Frontiers in Public Health, 4*. Advance online publication. doi:10.3389/conf.FPUBH.2016.01.00103

Ajerla, D., Mahfuz, S., & Zulkernine, F. (2019). A real-time patient monitoring framework for fall detection. *Wireless Communications and Mobile Computing, 2019*, 1–13. doi:10.1155/2019/9507938

Ajzen, H., & Fishbein, M. (1980). *Understanding attitudes and predicting social behavior.* Academic Press.

Ajzen, I., & Fishbein, M. (1980). *Understanding attitudes and predicting social behavior.* https://www.scienceopen.com/document?vid=c20c4174-d8dc-428d-b352-280b05eacdf7

Ajzen, I. (1985). From Intentions to Actions: A Theory of Planned Behavior. In J. Kuhl & J. Beckmann (Eds.), *Action Control: From Cognition to Behavior* (pp. 11–39). Springer., doi:10.1007/978-3-642-69746-3_2

Ajzen, I. (1991). The theory of planned behavior. *Organizational Behavior and Human Decision Processes, 50*(2), 179–211. doi:10.1016/0749-5978(91)90020-T

Akanbi, M. O., Ocheke, A. N., Agaba, P. A., Daniyam, C. A., Agaba, E. I., Okeke, E. N., & Ukoli, C. O. (2012). Use of Electronic Health Records in sub-Saharan Africa: Progress and challenges. *Journal of Medicine in the Tropics, 14*(1), 1–6. PMID:25243111

Akombi, B. J., Agho, K. E., Merom, D., Renzaho, A. M., & Hall, J. J. (2017). Child malnutrition in sub-Saharan Africa: A meta-analysis of demographic and health surveys (2006-2016). *PLoS One, 12*(5), e0177338. doi:10.1371/journal.pone.0177338 PMID:28494007

Akter, S., & Ray, P. (2010). *mHealth - an Ultimate Platform to Serve the Unserved.* IMIA Yearbook of Medical Informatics.

Akter, S., D'Ambra, J., & Ray, P. (2013). Development and validation of an instrument to measure user perceived service quality of mHealth. *Information & Management, 50*(4), 181–195. doi:10.1016/j.im.2013.03.001

Akyildiz, I. F., Su, W., Sankarasubramaniam, Y., & Cayirci, E. (2002). "A Survey on Sensor Networks," proc. *IEEE Communications Magazine, 40*(Aug), 102–114. doi:10.1109/MCOM.2002.1024422

Al-Durra, M., Torio, M.-B., & Cafazzo, J. A. (2015a). The Use of Behavior Change Theory in Internet-Based Asthma Self-Management Interventions: A Systematic Review. *Journal of Medical Internet Research, 17*(4), e89. doi:10.2196/jmir.4110 PMID:25835564

Allen, D. (1995). Hermeneutics: Philosophical traditions and nursing practice research. *Nursing Science Quarterly, 8*(4), 174–182. doi:10.1177/089431849500800408 PMID:8684726

Almashaqbeh, G., Hayajneh, T., & Vasilakos, A. V. (2014). A cloud-based interference-aware remote health observingsystem for non-hospitalized patients. *Proceedings of the IEEE 12th global communication conference (IEEE Globecom'14).*

Almashaqbeh, G., Hayajneh, T., Vasilakos, A. V., &Mohd, B. J. (2014). QoS-aware health observingsystem using cloud-based WBANs. *Journal of Medical Systems, 38*(121), 1–20. doi:10.1007/s10916-014-0121-2

Alnaeb, M., Alobaid, N., Seifalian, A., Mikhailidis, D., & Hamilton, G. (2007). Optical Techniques in the Assessment of Peripheral Arterial Disease. *Current Vascular Pharmacology*, *5*(1), 53–59. doi:10.2174/157016107779317242 PMID:17266613

Altay, N., & Green, W. G. III. (2006). OR/MS research in disaster operations management. *European Journal of Operational Research*, *175*(1), 475–493. doi:10.1016/j.ejor.2005.05.016

Ambulance Service Planning Office of Fire and Disaster Management Agency of Japan. (2016). *Effect of first aid for cardiopulmonary arrest*. Retrieved from http://www.fdma.go.jp/neuter/topics/fieldList9_3.html

American Diabetes Association (ADA). (2005). Clinical practice recommendations 2005. *Diabetes Care*, *28*, S1. PMID:15618109

American Heart Association. (2016). *Adult CPR and AED Skills Testing Checklist*. Retrieved from https://www.google. com/url?sa=t&rct=j&q=&esrc=s&source=web&cd=19&ved=2ahUKEwjKhcTfl5DpAhVRKuwKHdA_DS0QFjAS egQIARAB&url=https%3A%2F%2Fwww.cprconsultants.com%2Fwp-content%2Fuploads%2F2016%2F05%2FBLS-Adult-Skills-Checklist-2016.pdf&usg=AOvVaw1L4ObU_8YU-1h1SIlNpdEK

Aminian, M., & Naji, H. R. (2013). A Hospital Healthcare Monitoring System Using Wireless Sensor Networks. *J Health Med Inform*, *4*(121). doi:10.4172/2157-7420.1000121

Amirfar, S., Taverna, J., Anane, S., & Singer, J. (2011). Developing public health clinical decision support systems (CDSS) for the outpatient community in New York City: Our experience. *BMC Public Health*, *11*(1), 753. doi:10.1186/1471-2458-11-753 PMID:21962009

Ammenwerth, E., Iller, C., & Mahler, C. (2006, January 09). IT-adoption and the interaction of task, technology and individuals: A fit framework and a case study. *BMC Medical Informatics and Decision Making*, *6*(1), 3. doi:10.1186/1472-6947-6-3 PMID:16401336

Ammenweth, E., Graber, S., Herrmann, G., Burkle, T., & Konig, J. (2003). Evaluation of health information systems—Problems and challenges. *International Journal of Medical Informatics*, *71*(2-3), 125–135. doi:10.1016/S1386-5056(03)00131-X PMID:14519405

Amwell for Patients. (2020). *Amwell*. Retrieved from https://amwell.com/cm/

Analog devices Small, Low Power, 3-Axis ±3g Accelerometer. (2009). https://www.sparkfun.com/datasheets/Components/SMD/adxl335.pdf

Anosov, A. A., Isrefilov, M. G., & Pasechnik, V. I. (1995). Accuracy of solving an inverse problem of acoustothermography in non-correlation reception [in Russian]. *Radiotekhnika*, *9*, 49–57.

Anshari, M., & Almunawar, M. N. (2016). Mobile Health (mHealth) Services and Online Health Educators. *Biomedical Informatics Insights*, *8*, 19–27. doi:10.4137/BII.S35388 PMID:27257387

Archer, N., Fevrier-Thomas, U., Lokker, C., McKibbon, K. A., & Straus, S. E. (2011). Personal health records: A scoping review. *Journal of the American Medical Informatics Association*, *18*(4), 515–522. doi:10.1136/amiajnl-2011-000105 PMID:21672914

Ardalan, A., Masoomi, G., Goya, M., Ghaffari, M., Miadfar, J., Arvar, M., . . . Aghazadeh, M. (2009). Disaster health management: Iran's progress and challenges. *Iranian Journal of Public Health*, *38*(1), 93-97. Retrieved from http://ijph. tums.ac.ir/index.php/ijph/article/view/2860

Arnott, D., & Pervan, G. (2014). A Critical Analysis of Decision Support Systems Research Revisited: The Rise of Design Science. *Journal of Information Technology*, *29*(4), 269–293. doi:10.1057/jit.2014.16

Ashrafi, T. H., Hossain, M. A., Arefin, S. E., Das, K. D., & Chakrabarty, A. (2018). Iot infrastructure: fog computing surpasses cloud computing. In *Intelligent Communication and Computational Technologies*. Springer. doi:10.1007/978-981-10-5523-2_5

Aslani, N., Lazem, M., Mahdavi, S., & Garavand, A. (in press). A Review of Mobile Health Applications in Epidemic and Pandemic Outbreaks: Lessons Learned for COVID-19. *Archives of Clinical Infectious Diseases*. Advance online publication. doi:10.5812/archcid.103649

Atkins, L., Francis, J., Islam, R., O'Connor, D., Patey, A., Ivers, N., Foy, R., Duncan, E. M., Colquhoun, H., Grimshaw, J. M., Lawton, R., & Michie, S. (2017). A guide to using the Theoretical Domains Framework of behaviour change to investigate implementation problems. *Implementation Science; IS, 12*(1), 77. doi:10.1186/3012-017-0605-9 PMID:28637486

Atlas, D. (2015). *International diabetes federation*. IDF Diabetes Atlas.

Audet, A. M., Squires, D., & Doty, M. M. (2014). Where are we on the diffusion curve? Trends and drivers of primary care physicians' use of health information technology. *Health Services Research, 49*(1 Pt 2), 347–360. doi:10.1111/1475-6773.12139 PMID:24358958

Aufderheide, T., Hazinski, M. F., Nichol, G., Steffens, S. S., Buroker, A., McCune, R., ... Ramirez, R. R. (2006). Community lay rescuer automated external defibrillation programs: key state legislative components and implementation strategies: a summary of a decade of experience for healthcare providers, policymakers, legislators, employers, and community leaders from the American Heart Association Emergency Cardiovascular Care Committee, Council on Clinical Cardiology, and Office of State Advocacy. *Circulation, 113*(9), 1260–1270. doi:10.1161/CIRCULATIONAHA.106.172289 PMID:16415375

Australia's National Digital Health Strategy. (2018). *Australia's national digital health strategy: safe, seamless and secure: evolving health and care to meet the needs of modern Australia*. Australian Government and Australian Digital Health Agency. Retrieved from https://conversation.digitalhealth.gov.au/australias-national-digital-health-strategy

Australian Commission on Safety and Quality in Healthcare (ACSQII). (2010). *Patient-Centered Care: Improving Quality and Safety by Focusing Care on Patients and Consumers Discussion Paper*. Department of Health and Ageing, Sydney.

Australian Government, Department of Health. (2020, March 31). *Coronavirus Australia app*. Retrieved May 17, 2020, from https://www.health.gov.au/resources/apps-and-tools/coronavirus-australia-app

Australian Institute of Health and Welfare (AIHW). (2017). *Variation in hospital admission policies and practices: Australian hospital statistics*. Available at https://www.aihw.gov.au/reports/hospitals/variation-hospital-admission-policies-practices/contents/table-of-contents

Austrian Red Cross - Meet the STOPP CORONA App. (2020). *STOPP CORONA*. Retrieved from https://www.roteskreuz.at/site/meet-the-stopp-corona-app/

Baday, Calamak, Durmus, Davis, Steinmetz, & Demirci. (2015). Proposed Integrating Cell Phone Imaging with Magnetic Levitation (i-LEV) for Label-Free Blood Analysis at the Point-of-Living. *Small Nano Micro*. Doi:10.1002mll.201501845

Badescu, S. V., Tataru, C., Kobylinska, I.., Georgescu, E. L., Zahiu, D. M., Zăgrean, A. M., & Zăgrean, L. (2016). The association between diabetes mellitus and depression. *Journal of Medicine and Life, 9*(2), 120–125. PMID:27453739

Bai, J. W., Lovblom, L. E., Cardinez, M., Weisman, A., Farooqi, M. A., Halpern, E. M., ... Keenan, H. A. (2017). Neuropathy and presence of emotional distress and depression in longstanding diabetes: Results from the Canadian study of longevity in type 1 diabetes. *Journal of Diabetes and Its Complications, 31*(8), 1318–1324. doi:10.1016/j.jdiacomp.2017.05.002 PMID:28599823

Bain, L. E., Awah, P. K., Geraldine, N., Kindong, N. P., Sigal, Y., Bernard, N., & Tanjeko, A. T. (2013). Malnutrition in Sub-Saharan Africa: Burden, causes and prospects. *The Pan African Medical Journal, 15*, 120. doi:10.11604/pamj.2013.15.120.2535 PMID:24255726

Bala, H., Venkatesh, V., Venkatraman, S., Bates, J., & Brown, S. H. (2009). Disaster response in health care: A design extension for enterprise data warehouse. *Communications of the ACM, 52*(1), 136–140. doi:10.1145/1435417.1435448

Baldini, G., Braun, M., Hess, E., Oliveri, F., & Seuschek, H. (2009). *The use of secure RFID to support the resolution of emergency crises.* Paper presented at the 43rd Annual 2009 International Carnahan Conference on Security Technology, Zurich, Switzerland. 10.1109/CCST.2009.5335517

Bandura, A. (1986). Social foundations of thought and action. Academic Press.

Bandura, A. (1986). Social foundations of thought and action: A social cognitive theory. Prentice-Hall, Inc.

Bandura, A. (1991). Self-efficacy mechanism in physiological activation and health-promoting behavior. *Neurobiology of learning, emotion and affect*, 229-269.

Bandura, A. (1998). Health promotion from the perspective of social cognitive theory. *Psychology & Health, 13*(4), 623–649. doi:10.1080/08870449808407422

Bandura, A. (2004). Health Promotion by Social Cognitive Means. *Health Education & Behavior, 31*(2), 143–164. doi:10.1177/1090198104263660 PMID:15090118

Banka & Mary. (2014). Remote Monitoring of Heart Rate, Blood pressure and temperature of a person. *International Journal of Emerging Technology in Computer Science and Electronics, 8*(1).

Bardhan, I. R., & Thouin, M. F. (2012). *Health information technology and its impact on the quality and cost of healthcare delivery.* ScienceDirect.

Bardy, G. H., Lee, K. L., Mark, D. B., Poole, J. E., Toff, W. D., Tonkin, A. M., ... White, R. D. (2008). Home use of automated external defibrillators for sudden cardiac arrest. *The New England Journal of Medicine, 358*(17), 1793–1804. doi:10.1056/NEJMoa0801651 PMID:18381485

Barnett, K., Mercer, S. W., Norbury, M., Watt, G., Wyke, S., & Guthrie, B. (2012). Epidemiology of multimorbidity and implications for health care, research, and medical education: A cross-sectional study. *Lancet, 380*(9836), 37–43. doi:10.1016/S0140-6736(12)60240-2 PMID:22579043

Barteit, S., Neuhann, F., Bärnighausen, T., Bowa, A., Wolter, S., Siabwanta, H., & Jahn, A. (2019). Technology Acceptance and Information System Success of a Mobile Electronic Platform for Nonphysician Clinical Students in Zambia: Prospective, Nonrandomized Intervention Study. *Journal of Medical Internet Research, 21*(10), e14748. doi:10.2196/14748 PMID:31599731

Bartels, S. J., Pratt, S. I., Aschbrenner, K. A., Barre, L. K., Jue, K., Wolfe, R. S., Xie, H., McHugo, G., Santos, M., Williams, G. E., Naslund, J. A., & Mueser, K. T. (2013). Clinically significant improved fitness and weight loss among overweight persons with serious mental illness. *Psychiatric Services (Washington, D.C.), 64*(8), 729–736. doi:10.1176/appi.ps.003622012 PMID:23677386

Baskerville, N. B., Struik, L. L., Hammond, D., Guindon, G. E., Norman, C. D., Whittaker, R., Burns, C., Grindrod, K. A., & Brown, K. S. (2015). Effect of a Mobile Phone Intervention on Quitting Smoking in a Young Adult Population of Smokers: Randomized Controlled Trial Study Protocol. *Jmir Research Protocols, 4*(1). doi:10.2196/resprot.3823

Baskerville, N. B., Struik, L. L., & Dash, D. (2018). Crush the Crave: Development and Formative Evaluation of a Smartphone App for Smoking Cessation. *JMIR mHealth and uHealth, 6*(3), e52. doi:10.2196/mhealth.9011 PMID:29500157

Baskerville, N. B., Struik, L. L., Guindon, G. E., Norman, C. D., Whittaker, R., Burns, C., Hammond, D., Dash, D., & Brown, K. S. (2018). Effect of a Mobile Phone Intervention on Quitting Smoking in a Young Adult Population of Smokers: Randomized Controlled Trial. *JMIR mHealth and uHealth, 6*(10), e10893. doi:10.2196/10893 PMID:30355563

Bates, D. W., & Bitton, A. (2010). The Future Of Health Information Technology In The Patient-Centered Medical Home. *Health Affairs, 29*(4), 614–621. doi:10.1377/hlthaff.2010.0007 PMID:20368590

Bauer, A. M., Thielke, S. M., Katon, W., Unutzer, J., & Arean, P. (2014). Aligning health information technologies wiht effective service delivery models to improve chronic disease care. *Preventive Medicine, 66*, 167–172. doi:10.1016/j.ypmed.2014.06.017 PMID:24963895

Bauer, C. R. K. D., Ganslandt, T., Baum, B., Christoph, J., Engel, I., Löbe, M., ... Winter, A. (2016). Integrated data repository toolkit (IDRT). *Methods of Information in Medicine, 55*(2), 125–135. doi:10.3414/ME15-01-0082 PMID:26534843

Baumeister, R. F., Vohs, K. D., & Tice, D. M. (2007). The Strength Model of Self-Control. *Current Directions in Psychological Science, 16*(6), 351–355. doi:10.1111/j.1467-8721.2007.00534.x

BBC. (2020, February 11). *China launches coronavirus 'close contact detector' app.* Retrieved May 17, 2020, from https://www.bbc.com/news/technology-51439401

Becker, L., Eisenberg, M., Fahrenbruch, C., & Cobb, L. (1998). Public locations of cardiac arrest: Implications for public access defibrillation. *Circulation, 97*(21), 2106–2109. doi:10.1161/01.CIR.97.21.2106 PMID:9626169

Becker, M. H. (1974). The health belief model and personal health behavior. *Health Education Monographs, 2*(4), 324–473. doi:10.1177/109019817400200407

Belmon, L. S., Middelweerd, A., te Velde, S. J., & Brug, J. (2015). Dutch young adults ratings of behavior change techniques applied in mobile phone apps to promote physical activity: A cross-sectional survey. *JMIR mHealth and uHealth, 3*(4), e103. doi:10.2196/mhealth.4383 PMID:26563744

Ben Elhadj, H., Chaari, L., & Kamoun, L. (2012). A survey of routing protocols in wireless body area networks for healthcare applications. *Int. J. of E-Health and Medical Commun., 3*(2), 1–18.

Benes, J., Giglio, M., Brienza, N., & Michard, F. (2014). The effects of goal-directed fluid therapy based on dynamic parameters on post-surgical outcome: A meta-analysis of randomized controlled trials. *Critical Care (London, England), 18*(5), 584–594. doi:10.118613054-014-0584-z PMID:25348900

Bengio, Y., Janda, R., Yu, Y. W., Ippolito, D., Jarvie, M., Pilat, D., Struck, B., Krastev, S., & Sharma, A. (2020). The need for privacy with public digital contact tracing during the COVID-19 pandemic. *The Lancet Digital Health, 2*(7), e342–e344. doi:10.1016/S2589-7500(20)30133-3 PMID:32835192

Ben-Zeev, D., Kaiser, S. M., Christopher, J., Mark, B., & Duffecy, J. (2013, December). *Development and usability testing of FOCUS: A smartphone system for self-management of schizophrenia.* Academic Press.

Berman, A. H., Andersson, C., Gajecki, M., Rosendahl, I., Sinadinovic, K., & Blankers, M. (2019). Smartphone Apps Targeting Hazardous Drinking Patterns among University Students Show Differential Subgroup Effects over 20 Weeks: Results from a Randomized, Controlled Trial. *Journal of Clinical Medicine, 8*(11), 1807. doi:10.3390/jcm8111807 PMID:31661868

Berman, A. H., Gajecki, M., Fredriksson, M., Sinadinovic, K., & Andersson, C. (2015). Mobile Phone Apps for University Students With Hazardous Alcohol Use: Study Protocol for Two Consecutive Randomized Controlled Trials. *JMIR Research Protocols, 4*(4), e139. doi:10.2196/resprot.4894 PMID:26693967

Berrouiguet, S., Barrigón, M., Brandt, S., Nitzburg, G., Ovejero, S., Alvarez-Garcia, R., ... Lenca, P. (2017). Ecological assessment of clinicians' antipsychotic prescription habits in psychiatric inpatients: A novel web-and mobile phone–based prototype for a dynamic clinical decision support system. *Journal of Medical Internet Research, 19*(1), e25. doi:10.2196/jmir.5954 PMID:28126703

Bertoni, G., Daemen, J., Hoffert, S., Peeters, M., Van Assche, G., & Van Keer, R. (2020). Retrieved May 17, 2020, from Team Keccak: https://keccak.team/keccak_specs_summary.html

Bian, J., Weir, C., Unni, P., Borbolla, D., Reese, T., Wan, Y.-K., & Del Fiol, G. (2018). Interactive Visual Displays for Interpreting the Results of Clinical Trials: Formative Evaluation With Case Vignettes. *Journal of Medical Internet Research, 20*(6), e10507. doi:10.2196/10507 PMID:29941416

Bilham, R. (2010). Lessons from the Haiti earthquake. *Nature, 463*(7283), 878–879. doi:10.1038/463878a PMID:20164905

Binkley, P., Frontera, W., Standaert, D. G., & Stein, J. (2003). Predicting the potential of wearable technology. *IEEE Engineering in Medicine and Biology Magazine, 22*(3), 23–24. doi:10.1109/MEMB.2003.1213623 PMID:12845813

Bissell, R. A. (2005). Public health and medicine in emergency management. In D. McEntire (Ed.), *Disciplines, Disasters, and Emergency Management*. FEMA, Emergency Management Institute.

Blagec, K., Romagnoli, K. M., Boyce, R. D., & Samwald, M. (2016). Examining perceptions of the usefulness and usability of a mobile-based system for pharmacogenomics clinical decision support: A mixed methods study. *PeerJ, 1671*. Advance online publication. doi:10.7717/peerj.1671 PMID:26925317

Blaya, J. A., Fraser, H. S. F., & Holt, B. (2010). E-health technologies show promise in developing countries. *Health Affairs, 29*(2), 244–251. doi:10.1377/hlthaff.2009.0894 PMID:20348068

Bodenheimer, T. (2008). Coordinating Care - A Perilous Journey through the Health Care System. *The New England Journal of Medicine, 358*(10), 1064–1071. doi:10.1056/NEJMhpr0706165 PMID:18322289

Bogie, K., Zhang, G.-Q., Roggenkamp, S., Zeng, N., Seton, J., Tao, S., Bloostein, A. L., & Sun, J. (2018). Individualized Clinical Practice Guidelines for Pressure Injury Management: Development of an Integrated Multi-Modal Biomedical Information Resource. *JMIR Research Protocols, 7*(9), e10871. doi:10.2196/10871 PMID:30190252

Bogner, H. R., Morales, K. H., de Vries, H. F., & Cappola, A. R. (2012). Integrated management of type 2 diabetes mellitus and depression treatment to improve medication adherence: A randomized controlled trial. *Annals of Family Medicine, 10*(1), 15–22. doi:10.1370/afm.1344 PMID:22230826

Bollen, K. A., & Stine, R. A. (1992). Bootstrapping goodness-of-fit measures in structural equation models. *Sociological Methods & Research, 21*(2), 205–229. doi:10.1177/0049124192021002004

Bonomi, F., Milito, R., Zhu, J., & Addepalli, S. (2012). Fog computing and its role in the internet of things. *Proceedings of the first edition of the MCC workshop on Mobile cloud computing*. 10.1145/2342509.2342513

Borrelli, B., & Ritterband, L. M. (2015). Special Issue on eHealth and mHealth: Challenges and Future Directions for Assessment, Treatment, and Dissemination. *Health Psychology, 34*(Suppl), 1205–1208. doi:10.1037/hea0000323 PMID:26651461

Bradt, D. A., Abraham, K., & Franks, R. (2003). A strategic plan for disaster medicine in Australasia. *Emergency Medicine, 15*(3), 271–282. doi:10.1046/j.1442-2026.2003.00445.x PMID:12786649

Brammer, K., & Ziefling, G. (1982). *Kalman-Bewsy filter*. Nauka. (in Russian)

Braun, V., & Clarke, V. (2006). Using thematic analysis in psychology. *Qualitative Research in Psychology*, *3*(2), 77–101. doi:10.1191/1478088706qp063oa

Brindal, E., Hendrie, G. A., Freyne, J., & Noakes, M. (2018). Incorporating a Static Versus Supportive Mobile Phone App Into a Partial Meal Replacement Program With Face-to-Face Support: Randomized Controlled Trial. *JMIR mHealth and uHealth*, *6*(4), e41. doi:10.2196/mhealth.7796 PMID:29669704

Brindal, E., Hendrie, G., Taylor, P., Freyne, J., & Noakes, M. (2016). Cohort Analysis of a 24-Week Randomized Controlled Trial to Assess the Efficacy of a Novel, Partial Meal Replacement Program Targeting Weight Loss and Risk Factor Reduction in Overweight/Obese Adults. *Nutrients*, *8*(5), 265. doi:10.3390/nu8050265 PMID:27153085

British Heart Foundation. (2020). *Defibrillators*. Retrieved from https://www.bhf.org.uk/how-you-can-help/how-to-save-a-life/defibrillators

Brodersen, N. H., Steptoe, A., Boniface, D. R., Wardle, J., & Hillsdon, M. (2007). Trends in physical activity and sedentary behaviour in adolescence: Ethnic and socioeconomic differences. *British Journal of Sports Medicine*, *41*(3), 140–144. doi:10.1136/bjsm.2006.031138 PMID:17178773

Brooks, S. C., Hsu, J. H., Tang, S. K., Jeyakumar, R., & Chan, T. C. (2013). Determining risk for out-of-hospital cardiac arrest by location type in a Canadian urban setting to guide future public access defibrillator placement. *Annals of Emergency Medicine, 61*(5), 530-538. e532.

Brooks, B., Chan, S., Lander, P., Adamson, R., Hodgetts, G. A., & Deakin, C. D. (2015). Public knowledge and confidence in the use of public access defibrillation. *Heart (British Cardiac Society)*, *101*(12), 967–971. doi:10.1136/heartjnl-2015-307624 PMID:25926599

Brown, H., Terrence, J., Vasquez, P., Bates, D. W., & Zimlichman, E. (2014). Continuous Monitoring in an Inpatient Medical-Surgical Unit: A Controlled Clinical Trial. *The American Journal of Medicine*, *127*(3), 226–232. doi:10.1016/j.amjmed.2013.12.004 PMID:24342543

Brown, K. W., Ryan, R. M., & Creswell, J. D. (2007). Mindfulness: Theoretical Foundations and Evidence for its Salutary Effects. *Psychological Inquiry*, *18*(4), 211–237. doi:10.1080/10478400701598298

Brown, M. T., & Bussell, J. K. (2011). Medication Adherence: WHO Cares? *Mayo Clinic Proceedings*, *86*(4), 304–314. doi:10.4065/mcp.2010.0575 PMID:21389250

Brown, S. H., Fischetti, L. F., Graham, G., Bates, J., Lancaster, A. E., McDaniel, D., Gillon, J., Darbe, M., & Kolodner, R. M. (2007). Use of electronic health records in disaster response: The experience of Department of Veterans Affairs after Hurricane Katrina. *American Journal of Public Health*, *97*(Supplement_1), S136–S141. doi:10.2105/AJPH.2006.104943 PMID:17413082

Brownstein, J. S., Freifeld, C. C., & Madoff, L. C. (2009). Digital disease detection—Harnessing the Web for public health surveillance. *The New England Journal of Medicine*, *360*(21), 2153–2157. doi:10.1056/NEJMp0900702 PMID:19423867

Brunkard, J., Namulanda, G., & Ratard, R. (2008). Hurricane Katrina deaths, Louisiana, 2005. *Disaster Medicine and Public Health Preparedness*, *2*(4), 215–223. doi:10.1097/DMP.0b013e31818aaf55 PMID:18756175

Bruntin, M. B., Burke, M. F., Hoaglin, M. C., & Blumenthal, D. (2011). The Benefits Of Health Information Technology: A Review Of The Recent Literature Shows Predominantly Positive Results. *Health Affairs*. PMID:21383365

Buchan, P. G. (2020). *Australia Goes Hard and Goes Early on COVID-19*. Retrieved from https://www.csis.org/analysis/australia-goes-hard-and-goes-early-covid-19

Bugeja, J., Jacobsson, A., & Davidsson, P. (2016). On privacy and security challenges in smart connected homes. In *2016 European Intelligence and Security Informatics Conference (EISIC)*. IEEE. 10.1109/EISIC.2016.044

Caffrey, S. L., Willoughby, P. J., Pepe, P. E., & Becker, L. B. (2002). Public use of automated external defibrillators. *The New England Journal of Medicine*, *347*(16), 1242–1247. doi:10.1056/NEJMoa020932 PMID:12393821

Cai, H., Stott, M. A., Ozcelik, D., Parks, J. W., Hawkins, A. R., & Schmidt, H. (2016, November). On-chip wavelength multiplexed detection of cancer DNA biomarkers in blood. In *Biomicrofluidics*. AIP Publishing. . doi:10.1063/1.4968033

Callaway, D. W., Peabody, C. R., Hoffman, A., Cote, E., Moulton, S., Baez, A. A., & Nathanson, L. (2012). Disaster mobile health technology: Lessons from Haiti. *Prehospital and Disaster Medicine*, *27*(02), 148–152. doi:10.1017/S1049023X12000441 PMID:22588429

Camacho, J. Ch. A., Landis-Lewis, Z., Douglas, G., & Boyce, R. (2018). Comparing a Mobile Decision Support System Versus the Use of Printed Materials for the Implementation of an Evidence-Based Recommendation: Protocol for a Qualitative Evaluation. *JMIR Research Protocols*, *7*(4), e105. doi:10.2196/resprot.9827 PMID:29653921

Cameron, J. D., Ramaprasad, A., & Syn, T. (2017). An ontology of and roadmap for mHealth research. *International Journal of Medical Informatics*, *100*, 16–25. doi:10.1016/j.ijmedinf.2017.01.007 PMID:28241934

Campbell, T. (2014). *Clinical data repository versus a data warehouse — which do you need?* https://www.healthcatalyst.com/insights/clinical-data-repository-data-warehouse

Carrano, R., Passos, D., Magalhaes, L., & Albuquerque, C. (2013). Survey and taxonomy of duty cycling mechanisms in wireless sensor networks. IEEE Commun. Surveys Tutorials, 1–14.

Carrino, S., Caon, M., Khaled, O. A., Andreoni, G., & Mugellini, E. (2014, June). Pegaso: Towards a life companion. In *International Conference on Digital Human Modeling and Applications in Health, Safety, Ergonomics and Risk Management* (pp. 325-331). Springer.

Carrion, C., Caon, M., Carrino, S., Moliner, L. A., Lang, A., Atkinson, S., . . . Espallargues, M. (2015, September). Wearable lifestyle tracking devices: are they useful for teenagers? In *Adjunct Proceedings of the 2015 ACM International Joint Conference on Pervasive and Ubiquitous Computing and Proceedings of the 2015 ACM International Symposium on Wearable Computers* (pp. 669-674). Academic Press.

Carvalho, L. F., Teixeira, C., Dias, E. C., Meira, W., & Carvalho, O. (2015). A simple and effective method for anomaly detection in healthcare. *Proceedings of the SIAM International Conference on Data Mining Workshop*.

Carver, C. S., & Scheier, M. F. (1982). Control theory: A useful conceptual framework for personality–social, clinical, and health psychology. *Psychological Bulletin*, *92*(1), 111–135. doi:10.1037/0033-2909.92.1.111 PMID:7134324

Cascella, M., Rajnik, M., Cuomo, A., Dulebohn, S. C., & Di Napoli, R. (2020, April 6). Features, Evaluation and Treatment Coronavirus (COVID-19). *StatPearls*. Treasure Island, FL: StatPearls Publishing. Retrieved May 17, 2020, from https://www.ncbi.nlm.nih.gov/books/NBK554776/

Castro, D., Coral, W., Rodriguez, C., Cabra, J., & Colorado, J. (2017). Wearable-based human activity recognition using an iot approach. *Journal of Sensor and Actuator Networks*, *6*(4), 1–20.

Center for Disaster Philanthropy. (n.d.). *The disaster life cycle*. Retrieved from https://disasterphilanthropy.org/issue-insight/the-disaster-life-cycle/

Centers for Desease Control and Prevention. (2020, May 13). *Symptoms of Coronavirus*. Retrieved May 17, 2020, from https://www.cdc.gov/coronavirus/2019-ncov/symptoms-testing/symptoms.html

Central Disaster and Safety Countermeasures Headquarters (CDSCHQ). (2020, April 1). *Guide on the Installation of 'Self-quarantine Safety Protection App'.* Retrieved May 17, 2020, from http://ncov.mohw.go.kr/upload/ncov/file/202004/1585732793827_20200401181953.pdf

Centre for Research on the Epidemiology of Disasters. (n.d.). *The international disaster database.* Retrieved from http://www.emdat.be/

Chan, A. (2020). *COVID Symptom Study.* Retrieved from https://covid.joinzoe.com/us

Chang, H. (2020, March 26). *Taiwan's Epidemic Prevention Technology: An Inside Look.* Retrieved May 17, 2020, from https://english.cw.com.tw/article/article.action?id=2682

Chan, T. C., Killeen, J., Griswold, W., & Lenert, L. (2004). Information technology and emergency medical care during disasters. *Academic Emergency Medicine, 11*(11), 1229–1236. doi:10.1197/j.aem.2004.08.018 PMID:15528589

Chaundhry, B., Wang, J., Wu, S., Maglione, M., Mojica, W., Roth, E., ... Shekelle, P. G. (2006). Systematic Review: Impact of Health Information Technology on Quality, Efficiency, and Costs of Medical Care. *Annals of Internal Medicine.* PMID:16702590

Cheang, P., & Smith, P. (2003). *An overview of non-contact photoplethysmography.* Electronic Systems and Control Division Research, Dept Electron and Elect Eng.

Chen, C., Haddad, D., Selsky, J., Hoffman, J. E., Kravitz, R., Estrin, D. E., & Sim, I. (2012). Making Sense of Mobile Health Data: An Open Architecture to Improve Individual- and Population-Level Health. *Journal of Medical Internet Research, 14*(4), e112. doi:10.2196/jmir.2152 PMID:22875563

Chen, G., Chung, E., Meng, L., Alexander, B., Vu, T., Rinehart, J., & Cannesson, M. (2012, April). (212). Impact of non invasive and beat-to-beat arterial pressure monitoring on intraoperative hemodynamic management. *Journal of Clinical Monitoring and Computing, 26*(2), 133–140. doi:10.100710877-012-9344-2 PMID:22382920

Cheng, J., Kuai, D., Zhang, L., Yang, X., & Qiu, B. (2012). Psoriasis increased the risk of diabetes: A meta-analysis. *Archives of Dermatological Research, 304*(2), 119–125. doi:10.100700403-011-1200-6 PMID:22210176

Chen, L. M., & Ayanian, J. Z. (2014). Care Continuity and Care Coordination What Counts? *JAMA Internal Medicine, 174*(5), 749–750. doi:10.1001/jamainternmed.2013.14331 PMID:24638199

Chen, M., Gonzalez, S., Leung, V., Zhang, Q., & Li, M. (2010). A 2G-RFID-based e-healthcare system. *Wireless Communications, IEEE, 17*(1), 37–43. doi:10.1109/MWC.2010.5416348

Chin, W. W. (1998). The partial least squares approach to structural equation modeling. *Modern methods for business research, 295*(2), 295-336.

Chiti, F., Fantacci, R., & Lappoli, S. (2010). Contention delay minimization in wireless body sensor networks: A game theoretic perspective. *IEEE Global Telecommunications Conference,* 1-6. 10.1109/GLOCOM.2010.5683753

Cho, H., Ippolito, D., & Yu, Y. W. (2020). *Contact tracing mobile apps for COVID-19: Privacy considerations and related trade-offs.* Retrieved from https://arxiv.org/abs/2003.11511?utm_source=fccdburner&utm_medium=feed&utm_campaign=Feed%253A+arxiv%252FQSXk+%2528ExcitingAds%2521+cs+updates+on+arXiv.org%2529

Chokshi, A., & Patel, S. (2017). Internet of Things (IoT) IoT Architecture Security Challenges in IoT & Role of IoT in Healthcare Industry. *International Journal of Engineering Technology Science and Research, 4*(10), 822–825.

Chomutare, T., Fernandez-Luque, L., Årsand, E., & Hartvigsen, G. (2011). Features of mobile diabetes applications: Review of the literature and analysis of current applications compared against evidence-based guidelines. *Journal of Medical Internet Research, 13*(3), e65. doi:10.2196/jmir.1874 PMID:21979293

Cho, Y.-M., Lee, S., Islam, S. M. S., & Kim, S.-Y. (2018). Theories Applied to m-Health Interventions for Behavior Change in Low- and Middle-Income Countries: A Systematic Review. *Telemedicine Journal and e-Health, 24*(10), 727–741. doi:10.1089/tmj.2017.0249 PMID:29437546

Christensen, C. M., Bohmer, R. M., & Kenagy, J. (2000). Will Disruptive Innovations Cure Health Care>. *Harvard Business Review*. PMID:11143147

Cioca, M., & Cioca, L. I. (2010). Decision support systems used in disaster management. In C. S. Jao (Ed.), *Decision Support Systems*. INTECH. doi:10.5772/39452

Ciottone, G. R. (2006). *Disaster medicine*. Mosbey Elsevier.

Civaner, M. M., Vatansever, K., & Pala, K. (2017). Ethical problems in an era where disasters have become a part of daily life: A qualitative study of healthcare workers in Turkey. *PLoS One, 12*(3), e0174162. Advance online publication. doi:10.1371/journal.pone.0174162 PMID:28319151

Clancy, C. M., & Cronin, K. (2005). Evidence-based decision making: Global evidence, local decisions. *Health Affairs, 24*(1), 151–162. doi:10.1377/hlthaff.24.1.151 PMID:15647226

Claussen, J. (2012). Using Nanotechnology to Improve Lab on a Chip Devices. *Journal of Biochips & Tissue Chips*. . doi:10.4172/2153-0777.1000e117

Collen, M. F. (2015). *A history of medical informatics in the United States* (M. J. Ball, Ed.). Springer. doi:10.1007/978-1-4471-6732-7

Collins, L. M., Baker, T. B., Mermelstein, R. J., Piper, M. E., Jorenby, D. E., Smith, S. S., Christiansen, B. A., Schlam, T. R., Cook, J. W., & Fiore, M. C. (2011). The Multiphase Optimization Strategy for Engineering Effective Tobacco Use Interventions. *Annals of Behavioral Medicine : A Publication of the Society of Behavioral Medicine, 41*(2), 208–226. doi:10.100712160-010-9253-x

Con, D., & De Cruz, P. (2016). Mobile phone apps for inflammatory bowel disease self-management: A systematic assessment of content and tools. *JMIR mHealth and uHealth, 4*(1), e13. doi:10.2196/mhealth.4874 PMID:26831935

Conroy, L., Ó'Conaire, C., Coyle, S., Healy, G., Kelly, P., O'Connor, N., Caulfield, B., Connaghan, D., Smeaton, A., & Nixon, P. (2009). TennisSense: A Multi-Sensory Approach to Performance Analysis in Tennis. *Proceedings of the 27th International Society of Biomechanics in Sports Conference 2009*.

Contact Tracing Resources, C. D. C. (2020). *Guidelines for the Implementation and Use of Digital Tools to Augment Traditional Contact Tracing*. Retrieved from https://www.cdc.gov/coronavirus/2019-ncov/downloads/php/guidelines-digital-tools-contact-tracing.pdf

Coris, E. E., Miller, E., & Sahebzamani, F. (2005). Sudden cardiac death in Division I collegiate athletics: Analysis of automated external defibrillator utilization in National Collegiate Athletic Association Division I athletic programs. *Clinical Journal of Sport Medicine, 15*(2), 87–91. doi:10.1097/01.jsm.0000152715.12721.fa PMID:15782052

Cortez, N. G., Cohen, I. G., & Kesselheim, A. S. (2014). FDA regulation of mobile health technologies. *The New England Journal of Medicine, 371*(4), 372–379. doi:10.1056/NEJMhle1403384 PMID:25054722

Coto-Segura, P., Eiris-Salvado, N., González-Lara, L., Queiro-Silva, R., Martinez-Camblor, P., Maldonado-Seral, C., García-García, B., Palacios-García, L., Gomez-Bernal, S., Santos-Juanes, J., & Coto, E. (2013). Psoriasis, psoriatic arthritis and type 2 diabetes mellitus: A systematic review and meta-analysis. *British Journal of Dermatology, 169*(4), 783–793. doi:10.1111/bjd.12473 PMID:23772556

Courneya, K. S., & Friedenreich, C. M. (1999). Utility of the theory of planned behavior for understanding exercise during breast cancer treatment. Psycho-Oncology: Journal of the Psychological. *Social and Behavioral Dimensions of Cancer, 8*(2), 112–122. PMID:10335555

Craig, P., Dieppe, P., Macintyre, S., Michie, S., Nazareth, I., & Petticrew, M. (2008). Developing and evaluating complex interventions: The new Medical Research Council guidance. *BMJ (Clinical Research Ed.), 337.* Advance online publication. doi:10.1136/bmj.a1655 PMID:18824488

Craig, S., Goldberg, J., & Dietz, W. H. (1996). Psychosocial correlates of physical activity among fifth and eighth graders. *Preventive Medicine, 25*(5), 506–513. doi:10.1006/pmed.1996.0083 PMID:8888317

Cramer, J. A., Roy, A., Burrell, A., Fairchild, C. J., Fuldeore, M. J., Ollendorf, D. A., & Wong, P. K. (2008). Medication Compliance and Persistence: Terminology and Definitions. *Value in Health, 11*(1), 44–47. doi:10.1111/j.1524-4733.2007.00213.x PMID:18237359

Crane, D., Garnett, C., Michie, S., West, R., & Brown, J. (2018). A smartphone app to reduce excessive alcohol consumption: Identifying the effectiveness of intervention components in a factorial randomised control trial. *Scientific Reports, 8*(1), 4384. doi:10.103841598-018-22420-8 PMID:29531280

Cugelman, B. (2013). Gamification: What It Is and Why It Matters to Digital Health Behavior Change Developers. *JMIR Serious Games, 1*(1), e3. doi:10.2196/games.3139 PMID:25658754

Currie, C. J., Peyrot, M., Morgan, C. L., Poole, C. D., Jenkins-Jones, S., Rubin, R. R., Burton, C. M., & Evans, M. (2012). The Impact of Treatment Noncompliance on Mortality in People With Type 2 Diabetes. *Diabetes Care, 35*(6), 1279–1284. doi:10.2337/dc11-1277 PMID:22511257

Dafli, E., Antoniou, P., Ioannidis, L., Dombros, N., Topps, D., & Bamidis, P. (2015). Virtual patients on the semantic Web: A proof-of-application study. *Journal of Medical Internet Research, 17*(1), e16. doi:10.2196/jmir.3933 PMID:25616272

Daly, L. M., Horey, D., Middleton, P. F., Boyle, F. M., & Flenady, V. (2018). The Effect of Mobile App Interventions on Influencing Healthy Maternal Behavior and Improving Perinatal Health Outcomes: Systematic Review. *JMIR mHealth and uHealth, 6*(8), e10012. doi:10.2196/10012 PMID:30093368

Daneman, D. (2006). Type 1 diabetes. *Lancet, 367*(9513), 847–858. doi:10.1016/S0140-6736(06)68341-4 PMID:16530579

Daousi, C., MacFarlane, I. A., Woodward, A., Nurmikko, T. J., Bundred, P. E., & Benbow, S. J. (2004). Chronic painful peripheral neuropathy in an urban community: A controlled comparison of people with and without diabetes. *Diabetic Medicine, 21*(9), 976–982. doi:10.1111/j.1464-5491.2004.01271.x PMID:15317601

Darwish, L., Beroncal, E., Sison, M. V., & Swardfager, W. (2018). Depression in people with type 2 diabetes: Current perspectives. *Diabetes, Metabolic Syndrome and Obesity, 11,* 333–343. doi:10.2147/DMSO.S106797 PMID:30022843

Davenport, T., Eccles, R., & Prusak, L. (2009). Information politics. In D. A. Klein (Ed.), *The Strategic Management of Intellectual Capital.* Butterworth-Heinemann.

Davies, M., Brophy, S., Williams, R., & Taylor, A. (2006). The prevalence, severity, and impact of painful diabetic peripheral neuropathy in type 2 diabetes. *Diabetes Care, 29*(7), 1518–1522. doi:10.2337/dc05-2228 PMID:16801572

Davis, R., Campbell, R., Hildon, Z., Hobbs, L., & Michie, S. (2015). Theories of behaviour and behaviour change across the social and behavioural sciences: A scoping review. *Health Psychology Review*, *9*(3), 323–344. doi:10.1080/174371 99.2014.941722 PMID:25104107

de Almeida Lima, K. C., da Silva Borges, L., Hatanaka, E., Rolim, L. C., & de Freitas, P. B. (2017). Grip force control and hand dexterity are impaired in individuals with diabetic peripheral neuropathy. *Neuroscience Letters*, *659*, 54–59. doi:10.1016/j.neulet.2017.08.071 PMID:28867590

de Boer, J. (1995). An introduction to disaster medicine in Europe. *The Journal of Emergency Medicine*, *13*(2), 211–216. doi:10.1016/0736-4679(94)00147-2 PMID:7775793

De Freitas, P. B., & Lima, K. C. A. (2013). Grip force control during simple manipulation tasks in non-neuropathic diabetic individuals. *Clinical Neurophysiology*, *124*(9), 1904–1910. doi:10.1016/j.clinph.2013.04.002 PMID:23643574

de Vries, H., Dijkstra, M., & Kuhlman, P. (1988). Self-efficacy: The third factor besides attitude and subjective norm as a predictor of behavioural intentions. *Health Education Research*, *3*(3), 273–282. doi:10.1093/her/3.3.273

Deady, M., Choi, I., Calvo, R. A., Glozier, N., Christensen, H., & Harvey, S. B. (2017). eHealth interventions for the prevention of depression and anxiety in the general population: A systematic review and meta-analysis. *BMC Psychiatry*, *17*(1), 310. doi:10.118612888-017-1473-1 PMID:28851342

Deakin, C. D., Shewry, E., & Gray, H. H. (2014). Public access defibrillation remains out of reach for most victims of out-of-hospital sudden cardiac arrest. *Heart (British Cardiac Society)*, *100*(8), 619–623. doi:10.1136/heartjnl-2013-305030 PMID:24553390

Delic, A., & Zwitter, M. (2020). *Opaque Coronavirus Procurement Deal Hands Millions to Slovenian Gambling Mogul*. Retrieved from https://www.occrp.org/en/coronavirus/opaque-coronavirus-procurement-deal-hands-millions-to-slovenian-gambling-mogul

Demiris, G., & Kneale, L. (2015). Informatics Systems and Tools to Facilitate Patient-centered Care Coordination. *IMIA Yearbook of Medical Informatics*, 15-21.

den Bakker, C. M., Huirne, J. A., Schaafsma, F. G., de Geus, C., Bonjer, H. J., & Anema, J. R. (2019). Electronic Health Program to Empower Patients in Returning to Normal Activities After Colorectal Surgical Procedures: Mixed-Methods Process Evaluation Alongside a Randomized Controlled Trial. *Journal of Medical Internet Research*, *21*(1), e10674. doi:10.2196/10674 PMID:30694205

den Bakker, C. M., Schaafsma, F. G., van der Meij, E., Meijerink, W. J. H. J., van den Heuvel, B., Baan, A. H., Davids, P. H. P., Scholten, P. C., van der Meij, S., van Baal, W. M., van Dalsen, A. D., Lips, D. J., van der Steeg, J. W., Leclercq, W. K. G., Geomini, P. M. A. J., Consten, E. C. J., Koops, S. E. S., de Castro, S. M. M., van Kesteren, P. J. M., ... Anema, J. R. (2019). Electronic Health Program to Empower Patients in Returning to Normal Activities After General Surgical and Gynecological Procedures: Intervention Mapping as a Useful Method for Further Development. *Journal of Medical Internet Research*, *21*(2), e9938. doi:10.2196/jmir.9938 PMID:30724740

Desveaux, L., Agarwal, P., Shaw, J., Hensel, J. M., Mukerji, G., Onabajo, N., Marani, H., Jamieson, T., Bhattacharyya, O., Martin, D., Mamdani, M., Jeffs, L., Wodchis, W. P., Ivers, N. M., & Bhatia, R. S. (2016). A randomized wait-list control trial to evaluate the impact of a mobile application to improve self-management of individuals with type 2 diabetes: A study protocol. *BMC Medical Informatics and Decision Making*, *16*(1), 144. doi:10.118612911-016-0381-5 PMID:27842539

Devi, Winster, & Sasikumar. (2016). Patient health monitoring system (PHMS) using IoT devices. *International Journal of Computer Science & Engineering Technology, 7*(3).

Diabetes Control and Complications Trial Research Group. (1995). The effect of intensive diabetes treatment on the progression of diabetic retinopathy in insulin dependent diabetes mellitus. *Archives of Ophthalmology, 113*(1), 36–51. doi:10.1001/archopht.1995.01100010038019 PMID:7826293

Dicker, B., Todd, V. F., Tunnage, B., Swain, A., Smith, T., & Howie, G. (2019). Direct transport to PCI-capable hospitals after out-of-hospital cardiac arrest in New Zealand: Inequities and outcomes. *Resuscitation, 142,* 111–116. doi:10.1016/j.resuscitation.2019.06.283 PMID:31271727

Digital Health, C. R. C. (2020). Retrieved from digital health CRC: https://www.digitalhealthcrc.com/

Dijkstra, T. K., & Henseler, J. (2015). Consistent and asymptotically normal PLS estimators for linear structural equations. *Computational Statistics & Data Analysis, 81,* 10–23. doi:10.1016/j.csda.2014.07.008

Dijkstra, T. K., & Henseler, J. (2015). Consistent partial least squares path modeling. *Management Information Systems Quarterly, 39*(2), 297–316. doi:10.25300/MISQ/2015/39.2.02

Direito, A., Jiang, Y., Whittaker, R., & Maddison, R. (2015). Smartphone apps to improve fitness and increase physical activity among young people: Protocol of the Apps for IMproving FITness (AIMFIT) randomized controlled trial. *BMC Public Health, 15*(1), 635. doi:10.118612889-015-1968-y PMID:26159834

Dmitriev, V. N., Solntseva, L. V., & Gavrilov, L. R. (1987). An acoustic method for determining the temperature of locally heated biological tissues [in Russian]. *Meditsinskaya Radiologiya, 1,* 82–86.

Doam, C. R., Pruitt, S., Jacobs, J., Harris, Y., Bott, D. M., & Riley, W. L., & Oliver, A. (2014). Federal Efforts to Define and Advance Telehealth. *Work (Reading, Mass.).*

Dorsey, Chan, Feng. McConnell, Shaw, Trister, & Friend. (2017). The Use of Smartphones for Health Research. *Academic Medicine, 92*(2), 157-160. doi:10.1097/ACM.0000000000001205

Dos Santos, H., Bredehoft, M. D., Gonzalez, F. M., & Montgomery, S. (2016). Exercise video games and exercise self-efficacy in children. *Global pediatric health, 3,* 2333794X16644139.

Drechsler, A., & Hevner, A. (2016). A four-cycle model of IS design science research: capturing the dynamic nature of IS artifact design. Academic Press.

Drew, D. A., Nguyen, L. H., Steves, C. J., Menni, C., Freydin, M., Varsavsky, T., Sudre, C. H., Cardoso, M. J., Ourselin, S., Wolf, J., Spector, T. D., & Chan, A. T. (2020). Rapid Implementation of Mobile Technology for Real-time Epidemiology of COVID-19. *Science, 368*(6497), 1362–1367. Advance online publication. doi:10.1126cience.abc0473 PMID:32371477

Ducharme, J. (2013). Best practices in emergency medicine: What we have to consider if we wish to get it right. *Clinical Governance: An International Journal, 18*(4), 315–324. doi:10.1108/CGIJ-04-2012-0013

Dykes, P. C., Samal, L., Donahue, M., Greenberg, J. O., Hurley, A. A., Hasan, O., O'Malley, T. A., Venkatesh, A. K., Volk, L. A., & Bates, D. W. (2014). A patient-centered longitudinal care plan: Vision versus reality. *Journal of the American Medical Informatics Association, 21*(6), 1082–1090. doi:10.1136/amiajnl-2013-002454 PMID:24996874

Ebert, D. D., Van Daele, T., Nordgreen, T., Karekla, M., Compare, A., Zarbo, C., ... Kaehlke, F. (2018). Internet-and mobile-based psychological interventions: Applications, efficacy, and potential for improving mental health. *European Psychologist, 23*(3), 167–187. doi:10.1027/1016-9040/a000318

Edney, S. M., Olds, T. S., Ryan, J. C., Vandelanotte, C., Plotnikoff, R. C., Curtis, R. G., & Maher, C. A. (2020). A Social Networking and Gamified App to Increase Physical Activity: Cluster RCT. *American Journal of Preventive Medicine, 58*(2), e51–e62. doi:10.1016/j.amepre.2019.09.009 PMID:31959326

Edney, S., Plotnikoff, R., Vandelanotte, C., Olds, T., De Bourdeaudhuij, I., Ryan, J., & Maher, C. (2017). "Active Team" a social and gamified app-based physical activity intervention: Randomised controlled trial study protocol. *BMC Public Health*, *17*(1), 859. doi:10.118612889-017-4882-7 PMID:29096614

Edney, S., Ryan, J. C., Olds, T., Monroe, C., Fraysse, F., Vandelanotte, C., Plotnikoff, R., Curtis, R., & Maher, C. (2019). User Engagement and Attrition in an App-Based Physical Activity Intervention: Secondary Analysis of a Randomized Controlled Trial. *Journal of Medical Internet Research*, *21*(11), e14645. doi:10.2196/14645 PMID:31774402

Eisenman, D. P., Glik, D., Gonzalez, L., Maranon, R., Zhou, Q., Tseng, C. H., & Asch, S. M. (2009). Improving Latino disaster preparedness using social networks. *American Journal of Preventive Medicine*, *37*(6), 512–517. doi:10.1016/j.amepre.2009.07.022 PMID:19944917

Elbert, S. P., Dijkstra, A., & Oenema, A. (2016). A Mobile Phone App Intervention Targeting Fruit and Vegetable Consumption: The Efficacy of Textual and Auditory Tailored Health Information Tested in a Randomized Controlled Trial. *Journal of Medical Internet Research*, *18*(6), e147. doi:10.2196/jmir.5056 PMID:27287823

El-Gayar, O., Timsina, P., Nawar, N., & Eid, W. (2013). Mobile Applications for Diabetes Self-Management: Status and Potential. *Journal of Diabetes Science and Technology*, *7*(1), 247–262. doi:10.1177/193229681300700130 PMID:23439183

Elgendi, M. (2012, February). On the analysis of fingertip photoplethysmogram signals [Review]. *Current Cardiology Reviews*, *8*(1), 14–25. doi:10.2174/157340312801215782 PMID:22845812

Elhauge, E. (2010). *The Fragmentation of U.S. Health Care*. OXFORD Univeristy press. doi:10.1093/acprof:oso/9780195390131.001.0001

Elliott, R. (1993). Miller, W. R. and Rollnick, S. Motivational interviewing–preparing people to change addictive behaviour. New York: Guildford Press, 1991. Pp xviii + 348. £24.95. ISBN 0–89862–566–1. *Journal of Community & Applied Social Psychology*, *3*(2), 170–171. doi:10.1002/casp.2450030210

Emmanuel, D., Kola, S., & Mohana, J. (2014). A Survey on wireless Body Area Networks. International Journal of Scientific and Research Publications, 4(3), 1-7.

Endsley, M. R. (1988). Design and evaluation for situation awareness enhancement. *Proceedings of the Human Factors Society Annual Meeting*, *32*(2), 97-101. 10.1177/154193128803200221

Escoffery, C., McGee, R., Bidwell, J., Sims, C., Thropp, E. K., Frazier, C., & Mynatt, E. D. (2018). A review of mobile apps for epilepsy self-management. *Epilepsy & Behavior*, *81*, 62–69. doi:10.1016/j.yebeh.2017.12.010 PMID:29494935

European mHealthHub. (2020). *mHealth solutions for Managing the COVID-19 Outbreak*. Retrieved from https://mhealth-hub.org/mhealth-solutions-against-covid-19

Fadda, M., Galimberti, E., Fiordelli, M., Romano, L., Zanetti, A., & Schulz, P. J. (2017). Effectiveness of a smartphone app to increase parents' knowledge and empowerment in the MMR vaccination decision: A randomized controlled trial. *Human Vaccines & Immunotherapeutics*, *13*(11), 2512–2521. doi:10.1080/21645515.2017.1360456 PMID:29125783

Fajardo, J. T. B., & Oppus, C. M. (2010). A mobile disaster management system using the android technology. *WSEAS Transactions on Communications*, *9*(6), 343–353.

Falck, L., Zoller, M., Rosemann, T., Martínez-González, N. A., & Chmiel, C. (2019). Toward standardized monitoring of patients with chronic diseases in primary care using electronic medical records: Systematic review. *JMIR Medical Informatics*, *7*(2), e10879. doi:10.2196/10879 PMID:31127717

Fallahzadeh, R., Ma, Y., & Ghasemzadeh, H. (2016). Context-Aware System Design for Remote Health Monitoring: An Application to Continuous Edema Assessment. *IEEE Trans. Mob. Comput.*

Fang, Z., Ma, C., Wang, X., Qu, J., & Zhang, S. (2016). Identify individuals behaviors based GPS trajectories in the Internet of Things. In *2016 First IEEE International Conference on Computer Communication and the Internet (ICCCI)*. IEEE. 10.1109/CCI.2016.7778948

Fareeha. (2012). Review of Body Area Network technology and wireless medical monitoring. *International Journal of Information and Communication Technology Research, 2*(2).

FCC-Medical Body Area Networks - small entity compliance guide. (2013). http://www.fcc.gov/document/medical-body-area-networks

Fedele, D. A., Cushing, C. C., Fritz, A., Amaro, C. M., & Ortega, A. (2017). Mobile Health Interventions for Improving Health Outcomes in Youth A Meta-analysis. *JAMA Pediatrics, 171*(5), 461–469. doi:10.1001/jamapediatrics.2017.0042 PMID:28319239

Feltz, D. L., & Lirgg, C. D. (2001). Self-efficacy beliefs of athletes, teams, and coaches. Handbook of sport psychology, 2(2001), 340-361.

Fernandes, B., Afonso, J. A., & Simões, R. (2011). Vital signs monitoring and management using mobile devices. In *6th Iberian Conference on Information Systems and Technologies (CISTI 2011)* (pp. 1-6). IEEE.

Ferrara, G., Kim, J., Lin, S., Hua, J., & Seto, E. (2019). A Focused Review of Smartphone Diet-Tracking Apps: Usability, Functionality, Coherence With Behavior Change Theory, and Comparative Validity of Nutrient Intake and Energy Estimates. *JMIR mHealth and uHealth, 7*(5), e9232. doi:10.2196/mhealth.9232 PMID:31102369

Filipe, L., Fdez-Riverola, F., Costa, N., & Pereira, A. (2015). Wireless body area networks for healthcare applications: Protocol stack review. *International Journal of Distributed Sensor Networks, 11*(10), 1–23. doi:10.1155/2015/213705

Findlay, S., Palma, S., & Milne, R. (2020). *Coronavirus contact-tracing apps struggle to make an impact.* Retrieved from https://www.ft.com/content/21e438a6-32f2-43b9-b843-61b819a427aa

Fischer, P., Krueger, J. I., Greitemeyer, T., Vogrincic, C., Kastenmüller, A., Frey, D., Heene, M., Wicher, M., & Kainbacher, M. (2011). The bystander-effect: A meta-analytic review on bystander intervention in dangerous and non-dangerous emergencies. *Psychological Bulletin, 137*(4), 517–537. doi:10.1037/a0023304 PMID:21534650

Fishbein, M., & Ajzen, I. (1975). *Belief, attitude, intention, and behavior: An introduction to theory and research.* Addison-Wesley.

Fishbein, M., & Ajzen, I. (2010). *Predicting and Changing Behavior: The Reasoned Action Approach.* Taylor & Francis.

Fishbein, M., & Cappella, J. N. (2006). The role of theory in developing effective health communications. *Journal of Communication, 56*(suppl_1), 1–17. doi:10.1111/j.1460-2466.2006.00280.x

Fogg, B. J. (2009). A behavior model for persuasive design. *Proceedings of the 4th International Conference on Persuasive Technology - Persuasive '09*, 1. 10.1145/1541948.1541999

Fogg, B. J., & Hreha, J. (2010). Behavior Wizard: A Method for Matching Target Behaviors with Solutions. In T. Ploug, P. Hasle, & H. Oinas-Kukkonen (Eds.), *Persuasive Technology* (Vol. 6137, pp. 117–131). Springer Berlin Heidelberg. doi:10.1007/978-3-642-13226-1_13

Foley, L., Prapavessis, H., Maddison, R., Burke, S., McGowan, E., & Gillanders, L. (2008). Predicting physical activity intention and behavior in school-age children. *Pediatric Exercise Science, 20*(3), 342–356. doi:10.1123/pes.20.3.342 PMID:18714123

Folke, F., Lippert, F., Nielsen, S., Gislason, G. H., Hansen, M. L., Schramm, T. K., Sørensen, R., Fosbøl, E. L., Andersen, S. S., Rasmussen, S., Køber, L., & Torp-Pedersen, C. (2009). Location of Cardiac Arrest in a City Center: Strategic Placement of Automated External Defibrillators in Public Locations. *Circulation, 120*(6), 510–517. doi:10.1161/CIRCULATIONAHA.108.843755 PMID:19635969

Ford, P. (2020). *COVID-19 Pandemic Opens Up New Frontiers for Health Data Privacy.* Retrieved from https://www.healthcareitnews.com/news/europe/covid-19-pandemic-opens-new-frontiers-health-data-privacy

Forkan, A. R. M., Khalil, I., Ibaida, A., & Tari, Z. (2015). BDCaM: Big data for context-aware monitoring—A personalized knowledge discovery framework for assisted healthcare. *IEEE Transactions on Cloud Computing, 5*(4), 628-641.

Fornell, C., & Larcker, D. F. (1981). Evaluating structural equation models with unobservable variables and measurement error. *JMR, Journal of Marketing Research, 18*(1), 39–50. doi:10.1177/002224378101800104

Forrest, C. B., Glade, G. B., Baker, A. E., Bocian, A., Van Scharader, S., & Starfield, B. (2000). Coordination of Specialty Referrals and Physician Satisfaction With Referral Care. *Archives of Pediatrics & Adolescent Medicine, 154*(5), 499. doi:10.1001/archpedi.154.5.499 PMID:10807303

Foulonneau, A., Calvary, G., & Villain, E. (2016). Stop Procrastinating: TILT, Time is Life Time, a Persuasive Application. *Proceedings of the 28th Australian Conference on Computer-Human Interaction*, 508–516. 10.1145/3010915.3010947

Fraccaro, V., Balatsoukas, B., & Peek, V. D. V. (2017). Patient portal adoption rates: A systematic literature review and meta-analysis. *Studies in Health Technology and Informatics, 245*, 79–83. PMID:29295056

Frank, W. (2012, April). Lack of exercise is a major cause of chronic diseases. *Comprehensive Physiology, 2*(2), 1143–1211. PMID:23798298

Fry, E. A., & Lenert, L. A. (2005). *MASCAL: RFID tracking of patients, staff and equipment to enhance hospital response to mass casualty events.* Paper presented at the AMIA Annual Symposium Proceedings, Washington, DC.

Fuchs. (2015, November 23). *Detecting cancer cells before they form metastases.* ScienceDaily. Retrieved July 10, 2017, Karlsruhe Institute of Technology from www.sciencedaily.com/releases/2015/11/151123103326.htm

Furberg, R., Williams, P., Bagwell, J., & LaBresh, K. (2017). A mobile clinical decision support tool for pediatric cardiovascular risk-reduction clinical practice guidelines: Development and description. *JMIR mHealth and uHealth, 5*(3), e29. doi:10.2196/mhealth.6291 PMID:28270384

Gajecki, M., Andersson, C., Rosendahl, I., Sinadinovic, K., Fredriksson, M., & Berman, A. H. (2017). Skills Training via Smartphone App for University Students with Excessive Alcohol Consumption: A Randomized Controlled Trial. *International Journal of Behavioral Medicine, 24*(5), 778–788. doi:10.100712529-016-9629-9 PMID:28224445

Garnett, C. (2016). *Development and evaluation of a theory- and evidence-based smartphone app to help reduce excessive alcohol consumption.* Academic Press.

Garnett, C., Crane, D., Michie, S., West, R., & Brown, J. (2016). Evaluating the effectiveness of a smartphone app to reduce excessive alcohol consumption: Protocol for a factorial randomised control trial. *BMC Public Health, 16*(1), 536. doi:10.118612889-016-3140-8 PMID:27392430

Garth, Tirthankar, Renita, & Craig. (2012). Wireless Body Area Networks for Healthcare: A Survey. *International Journal of Ad hoc, Sensor & Ubiquitous Computing, 3*(3).

Gaudet, J., Gallant, F., & Bélanger, M. (2017). A bit of fit: Minimalist intervention in adolescents based on a physical activity tracker. *JMIR mHealth and uHealth, 5*(7), e92. doi:10.2196/mhealth.7647 PMID:28684384

GDPR. (2020). *What is GDPR, the EU's new data protection law?* Retrieved May 17, 2020, from https://gdpr.eu/what-is-gdpr/

Gefen, D., Straub, D., & Boudreau, M. C. (2000). Structural equation modeling and regression: Guidelines for research practice. *Communications of the Association for Information Systems, 4*(1), 7.

Gehlot, V., & Nigro, C. (2010). An Introduction to Systems Modeling and Simulation with Colored Petri Nets. *Proceedings of the 2010 Winter Simulation Conference*, 104-118. 10.1109/WSC.2010.5679170

Gerich, J. E. (2003, April). Contributions of insulin-resistance and insulin-secretory defects to the pathogenesis of type 2 diabetes mellitus. *Mayo Clinic Proceedings, 78*(4), 447–456. doi:10.4065/78.4.447 PMID:12683697

Global System for Mobile communication (GSM). (2001). *Requirements for GSM operation on railways, European Standard (Telecommunications series)*. http://www.etsi.org/deliver/etsi_en/301500_301599/301515/01.00.00_20/en_301515v010000c.pdf

Gnanaraj, V. V., Ranjana, P., & Thenmozhi, P.(2019). Patient Monitoring and Control System using Internet of Thing. *International Journal of Innovative Technology and Exploring Engineering, 8*(6S3), 120-123.

Godin, G. (1994). Theories of reasoned action and planned behavior: Usefulness for exercise promotion. *Medicine and Science in Sports and Exercise, 26*(11), 1391–1394. doi:10.1249/00005768-199411000-00014 PMID:7837960

Goff, D. C. Jr, Gerstein, H. C., Ginsberg, H. N., Cushman, W. C., Margolis, K. L., Byington, R. P., Buse, J. B., Genuth, S., Probstfield, J. L., & Simons-Morton, D. G.ACCORD Study Group. (2007). Prevention of cardiovascular disease in persons with type 2 diabetes mellitus: Current knowledge and rationale for the Action to Control Cardiovascular Risk in Diabetes (ACCORD) trial. *The American Journal of Cardiology, 99*(12), S4–S20. doi:10.1016/j.amjcard.2007.03.002 PMID:17599424

Gogia, S. B., Maeder, A., Mars, M., Hartvigsen, G., Basu, A., & Abbott, P. (2016). Unintended consequences of tele health and their possible solutions. *Yearbook of Medical Informatics, 25*(01), 41–46. doi:10.15265/IY-2016-012 PMID:27830229

Gonza'lez-Valenzuela, S., Liang, X., Cao, H., Chen, M., & Leung, V. C. (2013). *"Body area networks," in Autonomous Sensor Networks*. Springer.

Goodhue, D. (1995). Understanding user evaluations of information systems. *Management Science, 41*(12), 1827–1844. doi:10.1287/mnsc.41.12.1827

Goodhue, D. (1998). Development and measurement validity of a task-technology fit instrument for user evaluations of information systems. *Decision Sciences, 29*(1), 105–138. doi:10.1111/j.1540-5915.1998.tb01346.x

Government of Singapore. (2020, April 29). *SafeEntry*. Retrieved May 17, 2020, from https://safeentry.gov.sg/

Goyal, S., Lewis, G., Yu, C., Rotondi, M., Seto, E., & Cafazzo, J. A. (2016). Evaluation of a Behavioral Mobile Phone App Intervention for the Self-Management of Type 2 Diabetes: Randomized Controlled Trial Protocol. *JMIR Research Protocols, 5*(3), e174. doi:10.2196/resprot.5959 PMID:27542325

Goyal, S., Nunn, C. A., Rotondi, M., Couperthwaite, A. B., Reiser, S., Simone, A., Katzman, D. K., Cafazzo, J. A., & Palmert, M. R. (2017). A Mobile App for the Self-Management of Type 1 Diabetes Among Adolescents: A Randomized Controlled Trial. *JMIR mHealth and uHealth, 5*(6), e82. doi:10.2196/mhealth.7336 PMID:28630037

Goyen, M., & Debatin, J. F. (2009). Healthcare costs for new technologies. *European Journal of Nuclear Medicine and Molecular Imaging, 36*(S1), 139–143. doi:10.100700259-008-0975-y PMID:19104799

Gravina, R., Alinia, P., Ghasemzadeh, H., & Fortino, G. (2016). Multi-sensor fusion in body sensor networks: State-of-the-art and research challenges. *Information Fusion, 35*, 68–80. doi:10.1016/j.inffus.2016.09.005

Gregor, S., & Hevner, A. R. (2013). Positioning and Presenting Design Science Research for Maximum Impact. *MIS Quarterly, 37*(2), 337-355.

Grunau, B., Reynolds, J. C., Scheuermeyer, F. X., Stenstrom, R., Pennington, S., Cheung, C., ... Barbic, D. (2016). Comparing the prognosis of those with initial shockable and non-shockable rhythms with increasing durations of CPR: Informing minimum durations of resuscitation. *Resuscitation, 101*, 50–56. doi:10.1016/j.resuscitation.2016.01.021 PMID:26851705

Guest, G., MacQueen, K. M., & Namey, E. E. (2012). *Applied Thematic Analysis*. SAGE. doi:10.4135/9781483384436

Gutiérrez-Madroñal, L., La Blunda, L., Wagner, M. F., & Medina-Bulo, I. (2019). Test event generation for a fall-detection IoT system. *IEEE Internet of Things Journal, 6*(4), 6642–6651. doi:10.1109/JIOT.2019.2909434

Haarbrandt, B., Tute, E., & Marschollek, M. (2016). Automated population of an i2b2 clinical data warehouse from an open EHR-based data repository. *Journal of Biomedical Informatics, 63*, 277–294. doi:10.1016/j.jbi.2016.08.007 PMID:27507090

Hachisu, T., Pan, Y., Matsuda, S., Bourreau, B., & Suzuki, K. (2018). FaceLooks: A Smart Headband for Signaling Face-to-Face Behavior. *Sensors (Basel), 18*(7), 1–20. doi:10.339018072066 PMID:29958435

Hadda, E. B., Lamia, C., & Lotfi, K. (2012). A Survey of routing protocols in Wireless Body Area Networks for healthcare applications. International Journal of Ehealth and Medical Communications, 3(2), 1-18.

Hagger, M. S., Chatzisarantis, N., & Biddle, S. J. (2001). The influence of self-efficacy and past behaviour on the physical activity intentions of young people. *Journal of Sports Sciences, 19*(9), 711–725. doi:10.1080/02640410152475847 PMID:11522147

Hair, J. F. Jr, Hult, G. T. M., Ringle, C., & Sarstedt, M. (2016). *A primer on partial least squares structural equation modeling (PLS-SEM)*. Sage publications.

Hair, J., Hollingsworth, C. L., Randolph, A. B., & Chong, A. Y. L. (2017). An updated and expanded assessment of PLS-SEM in information systems research. *Industrial Management & Data Systems, 117*(3), 442–458. doi:10.1108/IMDS-04-2016-0130

Hajari, H., Salerno, J., Weiss, L. S., Menegazzi, J. J., Karimi, H., & Salcido, D. D. (2019). Simulating Public Buses as a Mobile Platform for Deployment of Publicly Accessible Automated External Defibrillators. *Prehospital Emergency Care*, 1–7. PMID:31124734

Hamilton, J. (2003). An internet-based bar code tracking system: Coordination of confusion at mass casualty incidents. *Disaster Management & Response, 1*(1), 25–28. doi:10.1016/S1540-2487(03)70007-8 PMID:12688307

Han, M., & Lee, E. (2018). Effectiveness of Mobile Health Application Use to Improve Health Behavior Changes: A Systematic Review of Randomized Controlled Trials. *Healthcare Informatics Research, 24*(3), 207. doi:10.4258/hir.2018.24.3.207 PMID:30109154

Hansen, C. M., Wissenberg, M., Weeke, P., Ruwald, M. H., Lamberts, M., Lippert, F. K., ... Torp-Pedersen, C. (2013). Automated external defibrillators inaccessible to more than half of nearby cardiac arrests in public locations during evening, nighttime, and weekends. *Circulation, 128*(20), 2224–2231. doi:10.1161/CIRCULATIONAHA.113.003066 PMID:24036607

Harrison, L. (2015). *Social media: indispensable during disasters*. Retrieved from https://www.medscape.com/view-article/847183

Hartin, P. J., Nugent, C. D., McClean, S. I., Cleland, I., Tschanz, J. T., Clark, C. J., & Norton, M. C. (2016). The Empowering Role of Mobile Apps in Behavior Change Interventions: The Gray Matters Randomized Controlled Trial. *JMIR mHealth and uHealth*, *4*(3), e93. doi:10.2196/mhealth.4878 PMID:27485822

Haskell, S. E., Post, M., Cram, P., & Atkins, D. L. (2009). Community public access sites: Compliance with American Heart Association recommendations. *Resuscitation*, *80*(8), 854–858. doi:10.1016/j.resuscitation.2009.04.033 PMID:19481852

Haslett, C., Chilvers, E. R., & Hunter, J. A. A. (1999). *Davidson's principles and practice of medicine*. Churchill Livingstone.

Hassandra, M., Lintunen, T., Hagger, M. S., Heikkinen, R., Vanhala, M., & Kettunen, T. (2017). An mHealth App for Supporting Quitters to Manage Cigarette Cravings With Short Bouts of Physical Activity: A Randomized Pilot Feasibility and Acceptability Study. *JMIR mHealth and uHealth*, *5*(5), e74. doi:10.2196/mhealth.6252 PMID:28550004

Hassandra, M., Lintunen, T., Kettunen, T., Vanhala, M., Toivonen, H.-M., Kinnunen, K., & Heikkinen, R. (2015). Effectiveness of a Mobile Phone App for Adults That Uses Physical Activity as a Tool to Manage Cigarette Craving After Smoking Cessation: A Study Protocol for a Randomized Controlled Trial. *JMIR Research Protocols*, *4*(4), e125. doi:10.2196/resprot.4600 PMID:26494256

Hausenblas, H. A., Carron, A. V., & Mack, D. E. (1997). Application of the theories of reasoned action and planned behavior to exercise behavior: A meta-analysis. *Journal of Sport & Exercise Psychology*, *19*(1), 36–51. doi:10.1123/jsep.19.1.36

Haynes, S., & Kim, K. K. (2016). A Mobile Care Coordination System for the Management of Complex Chronic Disease. *Nursing Informatics*. PMID:27332252

Heath, S. (2018). *Patient portal access use reaches 52% of healthcare consumers*. https://patientengagementhit.com/news/patient-portal-access-use-reach-52-of-healthcare-consumers

Hendershot, C. S., Witkiewitz, K., George, W. H., & Marlatt, G. A. (2011). Relapse prevention for addictive behaviors. *Substance Abuse Treatment, Prevention, and Policy*, *6*(1), 17. doi:10.1186/1747-597X-6-17 PMID:21771314

Henseler, J., Hubona, G., & Ray, P. A. (2016). Using PLS path modeling in new technology research: Updated guidelines. *Industrial Management & Data Systems*, *116*(1), 2–20. doi:10.1108/IMDS-09-2015-0382

Henseler, J., Ringle, C. M., & Sarstedt, M. (2016). Testing measurement invariance of composites using partial least squares. *International Marketing Review*, *33*(3), 405–431. doi:10.1108/IMR-09-2014-0304

Heraclides, A. M., Chandola, T., Witte, D. R., & Brunner, E. J. (2012). Work stress, obesity and the risk of Type 2 Diabetes: Gender-specific bidirectional effect in the Whitehall II study. *Obesity (Silver Spring, Md.)*, *20*(2), 428–433. doi:10.1038/oby.2011.95 PMID:21593804

Heraeus Medical. (n.d.). *How does the COVID-19 remote care solution work?* Retrieved from https://www.heraeus.com/us/hme/us_heraeuscare_covid19/us_covid_19_patient_monitoring

Herbec, A., Brown, J., Shahab, L., West, R., & Raupach, T. (2019). Pragmatic randomised trial of a smartphone app (NRT2Quit) to improve effectiveness of nicotine replacement therapy in a quit attempt by improving medication adherence: Results of a prematurely terminated study. *Trials*, *20*(1), 547. doi:10.118613063-019-3645-4 PMID:31477166

Hermanns, N., Caputo, S., Dzida, G., Khunti, K., Meneghini, L. F., & Snoek, F. (2013). Screening, evaluation, and management of depression in people with diabetes in primary care. *Primary Care Diabetes*, *7*(1), 1–10. doi:10.1016/j.pcd.2012.11.002 PMID:23280258

Hevner, A., March, S., Park, J., & Ram, S. (2004). Design science in information systems research. *Management Information Systems Quarterly*, *28*(1), 75–105. doi:10.2307/25148625

Hevner, A., & Wickramasinghe, N. (2017). *Design Science Research Opportunities in Healthcare*. Theories for Health Informatics Research.

Hibbard, J. H., & Greene, J. (2013). What the evidence shows about patient activation: Better health outcomes and care experiences; fewer data on costs. *Health Affairs*, *32*(2), 207–214. doi:10.1377/hlthaff.2012.1061 PMID:23381511

Hirshberg, A., Holcomb, J. B., & Mattox, K. L. (2001). Hospital trauma care in multiple-casualty incidents: Acritical view. *Annals of Emergency Medicine*, *37*(6), 647–652. doi:10.1067/mem.2001.115650 PMID:11385336

Holt, R. I., de Groot, M., & Golden, S. H. (2014). Diabetes and depression. *Current Diabetes Reports*, *14*(6), 491. doi:10.100711892-014-0491-3 PMID:24743941

Horne, R., Chapman, S. C. E., Parham, R., Freemantle, N., Forbes, A., & Cooper, V. (2013). Understanding Patients' Adherence-Related Beliefs about Medicines Prescribed for Long-Term Conditions: A Meta-Analytic Review of the Necessity-Concerns Framework. *PLoS One*, *8*(12), e80633. doi:10.1371/journal.pone.0080633 PMID:24312488

Huang, Z., Soljak, M., Boehm, B. O., & Car, J. (2018). Clinical relevance of smartphone apps for diabetes management: A global overview. *Diabetes/Metabolism Research and Reviews*, *34*(4), e2990. doi:10.1002/dmrr.2990 PMID:29431916

Hu, E. A., Pan, A., Malik, V., & Sun, Q. (2012). White rice consumption and risk of type 2 diabetes: Meta-analysis and systematic review. *BMJ (Clinical Research Ed.)*, *344*(3), e1454. doi:10.1136/bmj.e1454 PMID:22422870

Hung, K. K., Leung, C., Siu, A., & Graham, C. A. (2019). Good Samaritan Law and bystander cardiopulmonary resuscitation: Cross-sectional study of 1223 first-aid learners in Hong Kong. *Hong Kong Journal of Emergency Medicine*.

Hurling, R., Catt, M., De Boni, M., Fairley, B., Hurst, T., Murray, P., Richardson, A., & Sodhi, J. (2007). Using internet and mobile phone technology to deliver an automated physical activity program: Randomized controlled trial. *Journal of Medical Internet Research*, *9*(2), e7. doi:10.2196/jmir.9.2.e7 PMID:17478409

Husu, P., Paronen, O., Suni, J., & Vasankari, T. (2011). *Suomalaisten fyysinen aktiivisuus ja kunto 2010: terveyttä edistävän liikunnan nykytila ja muutokset* [The Physical Activity Levels of Finns, 2010]. Opetus ja Kulttuuriministeriön Julkaisuja.

Hutte. (1934), *Mannual (Handbook)*. Mashinistroenie. (in Russian)

Ienca, M., & Vayena, E. (2020). On the responsible use of digital data to tackle the COVID-19 pandemic. *Nature Medicine*, *26*(4), 463–464. doi:10.103841591-020-0832-5 PMID:32284619

IFRC. (2000). *Disaster preparedness training programme: Improving coordination*. Retrieved from https://www.ifrc.org/Global/Impcoor.pdf

Iglay, K., Hannachi, H., Joseph Howie, P., Xu, J., Li, X., Engel, S. S., Moore, L. M., & Rajpathak, S. (2016). Prevalence and co-prevalence of comorbidities among patients with type 2 diabetes mellitus. *Current Medical Research and Opinion*, *32*(7), 1243–1252. doi:10.1185/03007995.2016.1168291 PMID:26986190

Im, H., Castro, C. M., Shao, H., Liong, M., Song, J., & Pathania, D., … Lee, H. (2015, April 13). Digital diffraction analysis enables low-cost molecular diagnostics on a smartphone. Proceedings of the National Academy of Sciences. *Proceedings of the National Academy of Sciences*. 10.1073/pnas.1501815112

International Diabetes Federation. (2019). *IDF Diabetes Atlas* (9th ed.). Available at: https://www.diabetesatlas.org

International Telecommunication Union. (2019). *The State of Broadband: Broadband as a Foundation for Sustainable Development*. Retrieved from https://www.itu.int/dms_pub/itu-s/opb/pol/S-POL-BROADBAND.20-2019-PDF-E.pdf

Introduction to GPS - US Environmental protection agency. (2015). https://www.epa.gov/sites/production/files/2015-10/documents/global_positioning_system110_af.r4.pdf

Islam, S. R., Kwak, D., Kabir, M. H., Hossain, M., & Kwak, K. S. (2015). The internet of things for health care: A comprehensive survey. *IEEE Access: Practical Innovations, Open Solutions, 3*, 678–708. doi:10.1109/ACCESS.2015.2437951

Ismail, W. N., Hassan, M. M., & Alsalamah, H. A. (2019). Context-enriched regular human behavioral pattern detection from body sensors data. *IEEE Access: Practical Innovations, Open Solutions, 7*, 33834–33850. doi:10.1109/ACCESS.2019.2904122

Istepanian, R. S., Jovanov, E., & Zhang, Y. T. (2004). Introduction to the Special Section on M-Health: Beyond Seamless Mobility and Global Wireless Health-Care Connectivity. *IEEE Transactions on Information Technology in Biomedicine, 8*(4), 405–414. doi:10.1109/TITB.2004.840019 PMID:15615031

ITUNews Artificial Intelligence I Emerging Trends. (2020a). *COVID-19: How Korea is using innovative technology and AI to flatten the curve.* Retrieved from https://news.itu.int/covid-19-how-korea-is-using-innovative-technology-and-ai-to-flatten-the-curve/

ITUNews Artificial Intelligence I Emerging Trends. (2020b). *COVID-19: China's digital health strategies against the global pandemic.* Author. Retrieved from https://news.itu.int/covid-19-chinas-digital-health-strategies-against-the-global-pandemic/

Iwaya, L. H., Gomes, M. A., Simplício, M. A., Carvalho, T. C., Dominicini, C. K., Sakuragui, R. R., Rebelo, M. S., Gutierrez, M. A., Näslund, M., & Håkansson, P. (2013). Mobile health in emerging countries: A survey of research initiatives in Brazil. *International Journal of Medical Informatics, 82*(5), 283–298. doi:10.1016/j.ijmedinf.2013.01.003 PMID:23410658

Ja, B. (2006). What have we been priming all these years? On the development, mechanisms, and ecology of nonconscious social behavior. *European Journal of Social Psychology, 36*(2), 147–168. doi:10.1002/ejsp.336 PMID:19844598

Jacob, C., Sanchez-Vazquez, A., & Ivory, C. (2019). Clinicians' Role in the Adoption of an Oncology Decision Support App in Europe and Its Implications for Organizational Practices: Qualitative Case Study. *JMIR mHealth and uHealth, 7*(5), e13555. doi:10.2196/13555 PMID:31066710

James, J. J., Benjamin, G. C., Burkle, F. M. Jr, Gebbie, K. M., Kelen, G., & Subbarao, I. (2010). Disaster medicine and public health preparedness: A discipline for all health professionals. *Disaster Medicine and Public Health Preparedness, 4*(02), 102–107. doi:10.1001/dmp.v4n2.hed10005 PMID:20526129

James, J. J., & Walsh, L. (2011). E-health in preparedness and response. *Disaster Medicine and Public Health Preparedness, 5*(04), 257–258. doi:10.1001/dmp.2011.84 PMID:22146662

Jamil & Mehmet. (2010). Wireless Body Area Network (WBAN) for Medical Applications. *New Developments in Biomedical Engineering, 1*, 591-628.

Jannat, N., & Haque, M. T. R. (1587-1590). IoT Based Health Monitoring & Fall Detection System. *International Journal of Scientific & Engineering Research, 10*(6).

Javed, Y., & Norris, T. (2012). Measuring shared and team situation awareness of emergency decision makers. *International Journal of Information Systems for Crisis Response and Management, 4*(4), 1–15. doi:10.4018/jiscrm.2012100101

Jayaraman, P. P., Forkan, A. R. M., Morshed, A., Haghighi, P. D., & Kang, Y. B. (2020). Healthcare 4.0: A review of frontiers in digital health. *Wiley Interdisciplinary Reviews. Data Mining and Knowledge Discovery, 10*(2), e1350. doi:10.1002/widm.1350

Jensen, K., & Kristensen, L. M. (2009). *Coloured Petri Nets: Modelling and Validation of Concurrent Systems*. Springer-Verlag. doi:10.1007/b95112

Jimenez, G., Lum, E., & Car, J. (2019). Examining Diabetes Management Apps Recommended From a Google Search: Content Analysis. *JMIR mHealth and uHealth*, *7*(1), e11848. doi:10.2196/11848 PMID:30303485

John, B. M., Goh, D. H. L., Chua, A. Y. K., & Wickramasinghe, N. (2016). Graph-based Cluster Analysis to Identify Similar Questions: A Design Science Approach. *Journal of the Association for Information Systems*, *17*(9), 590.

Johns Hopkins University. (2020). *Coronavirus Resource Center*. Retrieved from https://coronavirus.jhu.edu/map.html

Jordan, S., McSwiggan, J., Parker, J., Halas, G., & Friesen, M. (2018). An mHealth App for decision-making support in wound dressing selection (wounDS): Protocol for a user-centered feasibility study. *JMIR Research Protocols*, *7*(4), e108. doi:10.2196/resprot.9116 PMID:29691213

Juutilainen, A., Lehto, S., Rönnemaa, T., Pyörälä, K., & Laakso, M. (2005). Type 2 diabetes as a "coronary heart disease equivalent": An 18-year prospective population-based study in Finnish subjects. *Diabetes Care*, *28*(12), 2901–2907. doi:10.2337/diacare.28.12.2901 PMID:16306552

Kahn, S. E. (2003). The relative contributions of insulin resistance and beta-cell dysfunction to the pathophysiology of type 2 diabetes. *Diabetologia*, *46*(1), 3–19. doi:10.100700125-002-1009-0 PMID:12637977

Kai, K. A. N. G., Pang, Z. B., & Cong, W. A. N. G. (2013). Security and privacy mechanism for health internet of things. *Journal of China Universities of Posts and Telecommunications*, *20*(2), 64–68.

Kaiser, A. B., Zhang, N., & Van der Pluijm, W. (2018). *Global prevalence of type 2 diabetes over the next ten years (2018-2028)*. American Diabetes Association. Available from https://diabetes.diabetesjournals.org/content/67/Supplement_1/202-LB

Kalman, R. Ye., & Bewsy, R. S. (1961). Now results in linear filtering and prediction theory, *Proc. of the American Society of mechanical engineers. Ser. D.*, *83*(1), 123–141.

Karami, A., Shah, V., Vaezi, R., & Bansal, A. (2019). Twitter speaks: A case of national disaster situational awareness. *Journal of Information Science*, *46*(3), 313–324. doi:10.1177/0165551519828620

Kari, T., & Makkonen, M. (2014). Explaining the usage intentions of exergames. *35th International Conference on Information Systems, Auckland 2014. Association for Information Systems (AIS)*.

Kari, T., Piippo, J., Frank, L., Makkonen, M., & Moilanen, P. (2016). To gamify or not to gamify? Gamification in exercise applications and its role in impacting exercise motivation. *BLED 2016: Proceedings of the 29th Bled eConference Digital Economy*.

Kari, J. T., Pehkonen, J., Hutri-Kähönen, N., Raitakari, O. T., & Tammelin, T. H. (2017). Longitudinal associations between physical activity and educational outcomes. *Medicine and Science in Sports and Exercise*, *49*(11), 2158–2166. doi:10.1249/MSS.0000000000001351 PMID:29045322

Kari, J. T., Tammelin, T. H., Viinikainen, J., Hutri-Kähönen, N., Raitakari, O. T., & Pehkonen, J. (2016). Childhood physical activity and adulthood earnings. *Medicine and Science in Sports and Exercise*, *48*(7), 1340–1346. doi:10.1249/MSS.0000000000000895 PMID:26871991

Kautzky-Willer, A., Harreiter, J., & Pacini, G. (2016). Sex and gender differences in risk, pathophysiology and complications of type 2 diabetes mellitus. *Endocrine Reviews*, *37*(3), 278–316. doi:10.1210/er.2015-1137 PMID:27159875

Kavitha, Balapriya, & Sundrarajan. (2016). A Survey of routing protocols in Wireless Body Area Networks. *South Asian Journal of Engineering and Technology, 2*(21), 44-51.

Kayyali, B., Knott, D., & Van Kuiken, S. (2013). The big-data revolution in US health care: Accelerating value and innovation. *McKinsey & Company, 2*(8), 1-13.

Keator, D. B., van Erp, T. G., Turner, J. A., Glover, G. H., Mueller, B. A., Liu, T. T., ... Toga, A. W. (2016). The function biomedical informatics research network data repository. *NeuroImage, 124*, 1074–1079. doi:10.1016/j.neuroimage.2015.09.003 PMID:26364863

Kebede, M. M., & Pischke, C. R. (2019). Popular diabetes apps and the impact of diabetes app use on self-care behaviour: A survey among the digital community of persons with diabetes on social media. *Frontiers in Endocrinology, 10*, 135. doi:10.3389/fendo.2019.00135 PMID:30881349

Keesara, S., Jonas, A., & Schulman, K. (2020). COVID-19 and health care's digital revolution. *The New England Journal of Medicine, 382*(23), e82. doi:10.1056/NEJMp2005835 PMID:32240581

Kennelly, M. A., Ainscough, K., Lindsay, K. L., O'Sullivan, E., Gibney, E. R., McCarthy, M., Segurado, R., DeVito, G., Maguire, O., Smith, T., Hatunic, M., & McAuliffe, F. M. (2018). Pregnancy Exercise and Nutrition With Smartphone Application Support: A Randomized Controlled Trial. *Obstetrics and Gynecology, 131*(5), 818–826. doi:10.1097/AOG.0000000000002582 PMID:29630009

Kennelly, M. A., Ainscough, K., Lindsay, K., Gibney, E., Mc Carthy, M., & McAuliffe, F. M. (2016). Pregnancy, exercise and nutrition research study with smart phone app support (Pears): Study protocol of a randomized controlled trial. *Contemporary Clinical Trials, 46*, 92–99. doi:10.1016/j.cct.2015.11.018 PMID:26625980

Kettunen, E., & Kari, T. (2018). Can Sport and Wellness Technology be My Personal Trainer?: Teenagers and Digital Coaching. In *Bled eConference*. University of Maribor Press. doi:10.18690/978-961-286-170-4.32

Khan, M., Chua, Z., Yang, Y., Liao, Z., & Zhao, Y. (2019). *From Pre-Diabetes to Diabetes: Diagnosis, Treatments and Translational Research*. Medicina. Available at https://www.mdpi.com/1010-660X/55/9/546

Khan, H., Vasilescu, L. G., & Khan, A. (2008). Disaster management cycle-a theoretical approach. *Journal of Management and Marketing, 6*(1), 43–50. http://www.mnmk.ro/documents/2008/2008-6.pdf

Khan, J. Y., & Yuce, M. R. (2010). Wireless body area network (WBAN) for medical applications. In C. Domenico (Ed.), *New Developments in Biomedical Engineering* (pp. 591–627). Intech Publishing.

Khankeh, H. R., Khorasani-Zavareh, D., Johanson, E., Mohammadi, R., Ahmadi, F., & Mohammadi, R. (2011). Disaster health-related challenges and requirements: A grounded theory study in Iran. *Prehospital and Disaster Medicine, 26*(3), 151–158. doi:10.1017/S1049023X11006200 PMID:21929828

Khan, Z. A., Sivakumar, S., Phillips, W., Robertson, B., & Javaid, N. (2015). QPRD: QoS-aware peering routing protocol for delay-sensitive data in hospital body area network. *Mobile Information Systems, 2015*, 16. doi:10.1155/2015/153232

Kharrazi, H., Gonzalez, C., Lowe, K., Huerta, T., & Ford, E. (2018). Forecasting the maturation of electronic health record functions among US hospitals: Retrospective analysis and predictive model. *Journal of Medical Internet Research, 20*(8), e10458. doi:10.2196/10458 PMID:30087090

Kharroubi, A. T., & Darwish, H. M. (2015). Diabetes mellitus: The epidemic of the century. *World Journal of Diabetes, 6*(6), 850–867. doi:10.4239/wjd.v6.i6.850 PMID:26131326

Khosravi, F., Trainor, P. J., Lambert, C., Kloecker, G., Wickstrom, E., Rai, S. N., & Panchapakesan, B. (2016, September 29). Static micro-array isolation, dynamic time series classification, capture and enumeration of spiked breast cancer cells in blood: the nanotube–CTC chip. In *Nanotechnology*. IOP Publishing. doi:10.1088/0957-4484/27/44/44lt03

Kim, S., Ryoo, D., & Bae, C. (2008). Implementation of smart headband for the wearable healthcare. In *2008 Digest of Technical Papers-International Conference on Consumer Electronics*. IEEE.

Kim, J., & Hastak, M. (2018a). Online human behaviors on social media during disaster responses. *The Journal of the NPS Center for Homeland Defense and Security*, *14*, 7–8. https://www.hsaj.org/articles/14135

Kim, J., & Hastak, M. (2018b). Social network analysis: Characteristics of online social networks after a disaster. *International Journal of Information Management*, *38*(1), 86–96. doi:10.1016/j.ijinfomgt.2017.08.003

Kim, M., Yune, S., Chang, S., Jung, Y., Sa, S. O., & Han, H. W. (2019). The Fever Coach Mobile App for Participatory Influenza Surveillance in Children: Usability Study. *JMIR mHealth and uHealth*, *7*(10), e14276. doi:10.2196/14276 PMID:31625946

Kim, N. Y., Rathore, S., Ryu, J. H., Park, J. H., & Park, J. H. (2018). A Survey on Cyber Physical System Security for IoT: Issues, Challenges, Threats, Solutions. *Journal of Information Processing Systems*, *14*(6), 1361–1384.

Kirsch, T. D., & Hsu, E. B. (2008). Disaster medicine: What's the reality? *Disaster Medicine and Public Health Preparedness*, *2*(1), 11–12. doi:10.1097/DMP.0b013e31816564ca PMID:18388650

Kirzinger, A., Munana, C., & Brodie, M. (2018). *Public Opinion on Chronic Illness in America*. Henry J. Kaiser Foundation.

Kishimori, T., Kiguchi, T., Kiyohara, K., Matsuyama, T., Shida, H., Nishiyama, C., ... Hayashida, S. (2020). Public-access automated external defibrillator pad application and favorable neurological outcome after out-of-hospital cardiac arrest in public locations: A prospective population-based propensity score-matched study. *International Journal of Cardiology*, *299*, 140–146. doi:10.1016/j.ijcard.2019.07.061 PMID:31400888

Kitamura, T., Iwami, T., Kawamura, T., Nagao, K., Tanaka, H., & Hiraide, A. (2010). Nationwide public-access defibrillation in Japan. *The New England Journal of Medicine*, *362*(11), 994–1004. doi:10.1056/NEJMoa0906644 PMID:20237345

Kitson, A., Marshall, A., Bassett, K., & Zeitz, K. (2013). What are the core elements of patient-centred care? A narrative review and synthesis of the literature from health policy, medicine and nursing. *Journal of Advanced Nursing*, *69*(1), 4–15. doi:10.1111/j.1365-2648.2012.06064.x PMID:22709336

Klochko, G. I., Logvinenko, A. I., & Sytnik, O. V. (2002). A signal processing algorithm for remote acoustic temperature meter [in Russian]. *Radiotekhnika*, *2*, 18–25.

Klonoff, D. C. (2019). Behavioral Theory: The Missing Ingredient for Digital Health Tools to Change Behavior and Increase Adherence. *Journal of Diabetes Science and Technology*, *13*(2), 276–281. doi:10.1177/1932296818820303 PMID:30678472

Knell, G., Durand, C. P., Kohl, H. W., Wu, I. H., & Gabriel, K. P. (2019). Prevalence and likelihood of meeting sleep, physical activity, and screen-time guidelines among US youth. *JAMA Pediatrics*, *173*(4), 387–389. doi:10.1001/jamapediatrics.2018.4847 PMID:30715096

Kobayashi, D., Sado, J., Kiyohara, K., Kitamura, T., Kiguchi, T., Nishiyama, C., ... Kawamura, T. (2020). Public location and survival from out-of-hospital cardiac arrest in the public-access defibrillation era in Japan. *Journal of Cardiology*, *75*(1), 97–104. doi:10.1016/j.jjcc.2019.06.005 PMID:31350130

Kok, J. L. A., Williams, A., & Zhao, L. (2015). Psychosocial interventions for people with diabetes and comorbid depression. A systematic review. *International Journal of Nursing Studies*, *52*(10), 1625–1639. doi:10.1016/j.ijnurstu.2015.05.012 PMID:26118440

Korinek, E. V., Phatak, S. S., Martin, C. A., Freigoun, M. T., Rivera, D. E., Adams, M. A., Klasnja, P., Buman, M. P., & Hekler, E. B. (2018). Adaptive step goals and rewards: A longitudinal growth model of daily steps for a smartphone-based walking intervention. *Journal of Behavioral Medicine*, *41*(1), 74–86. doi:10.100710865-017-9878-3 PMID:28918547

Kotabe, S., Sakano, T., Sebayashi, K., & Komukai, T. (2014). Rapidly deployable phone service to counter catastrophic loss of telecommunication facilities. *NTT Technical Review*, *12*(3), 1–11.

Koutli, M., Theologou, N., Tryferidis, A., & Tzovaras, D. (2019). Abnormal Behavior Detection for elderly people living alone leveraging IoT sensors. In *2019 IEEE 19th International Conference on Bioinformatics and Bioengineering (BIBE)*. IEEE. 10.1109/BIBE.2019.00173

Kramer, J.-N., Künzler, F., Mishra, V., Smith, S. N., Kotz, D., Scholz, U., Fleisch, E., & Kowatsch, T. (2020). Which Components of a Smartphone Walking App Help Users to Reach Personalized Step Goals? Results From an Optimization Trial. *Annals of Behavioral Medicine*. doi:10.1093/abm/kaaa002

Kramer, J.-N., Kunzler, F., Mishra, V., Presset, B., Kotz, D., Smith, S., Scholz, U., & Kowatsch, T. (2019). Investigating Intervention Components and Exploring States of Receptivity for a Smartphone App to Promote Physical Activity: Protocol of a Microrandomized Trial. *JMIR Research Protocols*, *8*(1), e11540. doi:10.2196/11540 PMID:30702430

Kravchenko, V. F. (2003). *Lectures on the theory of atomic functions an some of their application*. Radiotechnika. (in Russian)

Kravchenko, V. F., Labun'ko, O. S., & Lerer, A. M. (2009). *Calculation methods in present-day radiophysics*. Fizmatlit. (in Russian)

Kroll, T., Kehn, M., Ho, P. S., & Groah, S. (2007). The SCI exercise self-efficacy scale (ESES): Development and psychometric properties. *The International Journal of Behavioral Nutrition and Physical Activity*, *4*(1), 34. doi:10.1186/1479-5868-4-34 PMID:17760999

Kruglanski, A. W. (1996). Goals as knowledge structures. In *Linking cognition and motivation to behavior* (pp. 599–618). Guilford Press.

Kruglanski, A. W., Shah, J. Y., Fishbach, A., Friedman, R., Chun, W. Y., & Sleeth-Keppler, D. (2002). A theory of goal systems. In Advances in experimental social psychology (Vol. 34, pp. 331–378). Academic Press., doi:10.1016/S0065-2601(02)80008-9

Kumar, S. A., Vealey, T., & Srivastava, H. (2016). Security in internet of things: Challenges, solutions and future directions. In *2016 49th Hawaii International Conference on System Sciences (HICSS)*. IEEE.

Kumar, B., Robinson, R., & Till, S. (2015). Physical activity and health in adolescence. *Clinical Medicine*, *15*(3), 267–272. doi:10.7861/clinmedicine.15-3-267 PMID:26031978

Kyriacou, E. C., Pattichis, C. S., & Pattichis, M. S. (2009). *An overview of recent health care support systems for eEmergency and mHealth applications*. Paper presented at the Annual International Conference of the IEEE in Engineering in Medicine and Biology Society, Minneapolis, MN. 10.1109/IEMBS.2009.5333913

Kyriazis, D. (2013). Sustainable smart city IoT applications: Heat and electricity management & Eco-conscious cruise control for public transportation. *World of Wireless, Mobile and Multimedia Networks (WoWMoM), 2013 IEEE 14th International Symposium and Workshops on*, 1–5.

Laakso, M., & Kuusisto, J. (2007, August). Cerebrovascular disease in type 2 diabetes. In *International Congress Series* (Vol. 1303, pp. 65–69). Elsevier.

Laflamme, F. M., Pietraszek, W. E., & Rajadhyax, N. V. (2010). Reforming hospitals with IT investments. *The McKinsey Quarterly*, 27–33.

Lahtela, A. (2009). *A short overview of the RFID technology in healthcare.* Paper presented at the 4th International Conference on Systems and Networks Communications, Porto, Portugal. 10.1109/ICSNC.2009.77

Landi, H. (2016). *Study: 75% of adults will use personal health records by 2020, exceeding M.U. targets.* https://www.hcinnovationgroup.com/policy-value-based-care/news/13026586/study-75-of-adults-will-use-personal-health-records-by-2020-exceeding-mu-targets

Larimer, M. E., Palmer, R. S., & Marlatt, G. A. (1999). Relapse prevention. An overview of Marlatt's cognitive-behavioral model. *Alcohol Research & Health: The Journal of the National Institute on Alcohol Abuse and Alcoholism*, 23(2), 151–160. PMID:10890810

Larson, E. C., Saba, E., Kaiser, S., Goel, M., & Patel, S. N. (2017). Pulmonary monitoring using smartphones. In J. Rehg, S. Murphy, & S. Kumar (Eds.), *Mobile Health* (pp. 239–264). Springer. doi:10.1007/978-3-319-51394-2_13

Lee, H., Ghebre, R., Le, C., Jang, Y. J., Sharratt, M., & Yee, D. (2017). Mobile Phone Multilevel and Multimedia Messaging Intervention for Breast Cancer Screening: Pilot Randomized Controlled Trial. *JMIR mHealth and uHealth*, 5(11), e154. doi:10.2196/mhealth.7091 PMID:29113961

Lee, Y.-L., Cui, Y.-Y., Tu, M.-H., Chen, Y.-C., & Chang, P. (2018). Mobile health to maintain continuity of patient-centered care for chronic kidney disease: Content analysis of apps. *JMIR mHealth and uHealth*, 6(4), e10173. doi:10.2196/10173 PMID:29678805

Lehane, E., & McCarthy, G. (2007). Intentional and unintentional medication non-adherence: A comprehensive framework for clinical research and practice? A discussion paper. *International Journal of Nursing Studies*, 44(8), 1468–1477. doi:10.1016/j.ijnurstu.2006.07.010 PMID:16973166

Lenert, L. A., Palmer, D. A., Chan, T. C., & Rao, R. (2005). An intelligent 802.11 triage tag for medical response to disasters. *AMIA Aannual Symposium Proceedings*.

Lettieri, E., Masella, C., & Radaelli, G. (2009). Disaster management: Findings from a systematic review. *Disaster Prevention and Management: An International Journal*, 18(2), 117–136. doi:10.1108/09653560910953207

Levin, B. R. (1975). *Theoretical foundations of statistical radio engineering.* Sov. Radio. (in Russian)

Leviton, L. C. (1996). Integrating Psychology and Public Health. *The American Psychologist*, 10.

Levy, D. (2014). *Emerging mHealth: Paths for growth.* pwc.com.

Liang, T. P., & Wei, C. P. (2004). Introduction to the special issue: A framework for mobile commerce applications. *International Journal of Electronic Commerce*, 8(3), 7–17. doi:10.1080/10864415.2004.11044303

Liang, T.-P., Huang, C.-W., Yeh, Y.-H., & Lin, B. (2007). Adoption of mobile technology in business: A fit-viability model. *Industrial Management & Data Systems*, 107(8), 1154–1169. doi:10.1108/02635570710822796

Liberati, A., Altman, D. G., Tetzlaff, J., Mulrow, C., Gøtzsche, P. C., Ioannidis, J. P., Clarke, M., Devereaux, P. J., Kleijnen, J., & Moher, D. (2009). The PRISMA statement for reporting systematic reviews and meta-analyses of studies that evaluate health care interventions: Explanation and elaboration. *PLoS Medicine*, 6(7), e1000100. doi:10.1371/journal.pmed.1000100 PMID:19621070

Li, J., & Ray, P. (2010). Applications of eHealth for pandemic management. In *Proceedings of 12th International Conference on e-Health Networking, Applications and Services* (pp. 391-398). IEEE.

Lindfors, E., Somerkoski, B., Kärki, T., & Kokki, E. (2017). Perusopetuksen oppilaiden turvallisuusosaamisesta. In M. Kallio, R. Juvonen, & A. Kaasinen (Eds.), Jatkuvuus ja muutos opettajankoulutuksessa (pp. 109-120). Helsinki: Suomen ainedidaktinen tutkimusseura.

Lindstrøm, B., & Wells, L. (2002). Towards a Monitoring Framework for Discrete-Event System Simulations. In *Proceedings of the Sixth International Workshop on Discrete Event Systems (WODES'02)*, (pp. 127–134). IEEE Computer Society. 10.1109/WODES.2002.1167679

Lin, E. H., Katon, W., Rutter, C., Simon, G. E., Ludman, E. J., Von Korff, M., Young, B., Oliver, M., Ciechanowski, P. C., Kinder, L., & Walker, E. (2006). Effects of enhanced depression treatment on diabetes self-care. *Annals of Family Medicine*, *4*(1), 46–53. doi:10.1370/afm.423 PMID:16449396

Lin, F.-C., Wang, C.-Y., Shang, R., Hsiao, F.-Y., Lin, M.-S., Hung, K.-Y., ... Shen, L.-J. (2018). Identifying unmet treatment needs for patients with osteoporotic fracture: Feasibility study for an electronic clinical surveillance system. *Journal of Medical Internet Research*, *20*(4), e142. doi:10.2196/jmir.9477 PMID:29691201

Lin, H., & Bergmann, N. W. (2016). IoT privacy and security challenges for smart home environments. *Information*, *7*(3), 1–15. doi:10.3390/info7030044

Liu, Y., Liu, A., Hu, Y., Li, Z., Choi, Y.-J., Sekiya, H., & Li, J. (2016). FFSC: An Energy Efðciency Communications Approach for Delay Minimizing in Internet of Things. *IEEE Access, 4*, 3775–3793.

LM393. LM393E, LM293, LM2903, LM2903E, LM2903V, NCV2903 On semiconductor. (2016). https://www.onsemi.com/pub/Collateral/LM393-D.PDF

Lord, S. R., Menz, H. B., & Sherrington, C. (2006). Home environment risk factors for falls in older people and the efðcacy of home modiðcations. *Age and Ageing*, *35*(Suppl 2), ii55–ii59. doi:10.1093/ageing/afl088 PMID:16926207

LPC2148 Microcontroller. (2011). https://www.nxp.com/docs/en/data-sheet/LPC2141_42_44_46_48.pdf?

Lu, C., Hu, Y., Xie, J., Fu, Q., Leigh, I., Governor, S., & Wang, G. (2018). The Use of Mobile Health Applications to Improve Patient Experience: Cross-Sectional Study in Chinese Public Hospitals. *JMIR mHealth and uHealth*, *6*(5), e126. doi:10.2196/mhealth.9145 PMID:29792290

Luna, S., & Pennock, M. J. (2018). Social media applications and emergency management: A literature review and research agenda. *International Journal of Disaster Risk Reduction*, *28*, 565–577. doi:10.1016/j.ijdrr.2018.01.006

Lv, N., Xiao, L., Simmons, M., Rosas, L., Chan, A., & Entwistle, M. (2017). Personalized hypertension management using patient-generated health data integrated with electronic health records (EMPOWER-H): Six-month pre-post study. *Journal of Medical Internet Research*, *19*(9), e311. doi:10.2196/jmir.7831 PMID:28928111

Lwin, M. O., Yung, C. F., Yap, P., Jayasundar, K., Sheldenkar, A., Subasinghe, K., Foo, S., Gayantha, U., Xu, H., Chai, S. C., Kurlye, A., Chen, J., & Ang, B. S. P. (2017). FluMob: Enabling surveillance of acute respiratory infections in health-care workers via mobile phones. *Frontiers in Public Health*, *5*, 49. doi:10.3389/fpubh.2017.00049 PMID:28367433

Maar, M. A., Yeates, K., Perkins, N., Boesch, L., Hua-Stewart, D., Liu, P., Sleeth, J., & Tobe, S. W. (2017). A Framework for the Study of Complex mHealth Interventions in Diverse Cultural Settings. *JMIR mHealth and uHealth*, *5*(4), e47. doi:10.2196/mhealth.7044 PMID:28428165

MacPherson, M. M., Merry, K. J., Locke, S. R., & Jung, M. E. (2019). Effects of Mobile Health Prompts on Self-Monitoring and Exercise Behaviors Following a Diabetes Prevention Program: Secondary Analysis From a Randomized Controlled Trial. *JMIR mHealth and uHealth*, *7*(9), e12956. doi:10.2196/12956 PMID:31489842

Madanian, S., & Parry, D. (2019). IoT, cloud computing and big data: Integrated framework for healthcare in disasters. *Studies in Health Technology and Informatics*, *264*, 998–1002. doi:10.3233hti190374 PMID:31438074

Madapusi, A. (2008). *Post-Implementation Evaluation of Enterprise Resource Planning (ERP) Systems* (Doctoral Dissertation). University of North Texas.

Madden, G. J. (Ed.). (2012). *APA Handbook of Behavior Analysis*. American Psychological Association.

Madden, J. M., Lakoma, M. D., Rusinak, D., Lu, C. Y., & Soumerai, S. B. (2016). Missing clinical and behavioural health data in a large electronic health record (EHR) system. *Journal of the American Medical Informatics Association*, *23*(6), 1143–1149. doi:10.1093/jamia/ocw021 PMID:27079506

Mahmoud, R., Yousuf, T., Aloul, F., & Zualkernan, I. (2015). Internet of things (IoT) security: Current status, challenges and prospective measures. In *2015 10th International Conference for Internet Technology and Secured Transactions (ICITST)*. IEEE.

Maksimović, M. (2017). Improving computing issues in internet of things driven e-health systems. *Proceedings of the International Conference for Young Researchers in Informatics, Mathematics and Engineering'17*.

Malasanos, T., & Ramnitz, M. S. (2013). Diabetes clinic at a distance: Telemedicine bridges the gap. *Diabetes Spectrum*, *26*(4), 226–231. doi:10.2337/diaspect.26.4.226

Malvey, D., & Slovensky, D. J. (2014). mHealth Transforming Healthcare. Springer.

Manashty, A., Light, J., & Yadav, U. (2015). Healthcare event aggregation lab (HEAL), a knowledge sharing platform for anomaly detection and prediction. In *2015 17th International Conference on E-health Networking, Application & Services (HealthCom)*. IEEE.

Manusov, E. G., Diego, V. P., Smith, J., & Garza, J. R. (2019). UniMóvil: A Mobile Health Clinic Providing Primary Care to the Colonias of the Rio Grande Valley, South Texas. *Frontiers in Public Health*, *7*. PMID:31497586

Mao, R. D., & Ong, M. E. H. (2016). Public access defibrillation: Improving accessibility and outcomes. *British Medical Bulletin*, *118*(1), 25–32. doi:10.1093/bmb/ldw011 PMID:27034442

Markowitz, S. M., Gonzalez, J. S., Wilkinson, J. L., & Safren, S. A. (2011). A review of treating depression in diabetes: Emerging findings. *Psychosomatics*, *52*(1), 1–18. doi:10.1016/j.psym.2010.11.007 PMID:21300190

Mary & Sivakumar. (2012). A Reduced Order Transfer Function Models for Alstom Gasifier using Genetic Algorithm. *International Journal of Computer Applications, 46*(5), 1-6.

Mary. (2014). Modelling and control of MIMO Gasifier system during coal quality variations. *International Journal of Modelling. Identification and Control, 22*(4), 131–139.

Massey, C. N., Appel, S. J., Buchanan, K. L., & Cherrington, A. L. (2010). Improving diabetes care in rural communities: An overview of current initiatives and a call for renewed efforts. *Clinical Diabetes*, *28*(1), 20–27. doi:10.2337/diaclin.28.1.20

Masteller, B., Sirard, J., & Freedson, P. (2017). The Physical Activity Tracker Testing in Youth (PATTY) Study: Content Analysis and Children's Perceptions. *JMIR mHealth and uHealth*, *5*(4), e55. doi:10.2196/mhealth.6347 PMID:28455278

Maturana, C., Scott, R. E., & Palacios, M. (2012). e-Health and the haddon matrix: Identifying where and how e-health can assist in disaster managment. In M. J. F. Lievens (Ed.), Global Telemedicine and eHealth Updates: Knowledge Resources (Vol. 5, pp. 373-377). Grimbergen, Belgium: International Society for Telemedicine & eHealth (ISfTeH).

Maulin, P., & Wang, F. J. (2010). Applications, Challenges and Prospective In Emerging Body Area Networking Technologies. *IEEE Wireless Communications*, 1284–1536.

Mawgoud, A. A., Karadawy, A. I., & Tawfik, B. S. (2019). *A Secure Authentication Technique in Internet of Medical Things through Machine Learning.* arXiv preprint arXiv:1912.12143

McAuley, E., & Blissmer, B. (2000). Self-efficacy determinants and consequences of physical activity. *Exercise and Sport Sciences Reviews*, *28*(2), 85–88. PMID:10902091

McAuley, E., Szabo, A., Gothe, N., & Olson, E. A. (2011). Self-efficacy: Implications for physical activity, function, and functional limitations in older adults. *American Journal of Lifestyle Medicine*, *5*(4), 361–369. doi:10.1177/1559827610392704 PMID:24353482

McWilliams, j. (2016). Cost Containment and the Tale of Care Coordination. *The New England Journal of Medicine*, 2218–2219. PMID:27959672

Mehdy, M. M., Ng, P. Y., Shair, E. F., Saleh, N. I. M., & Gomes, C. (2017). Artificial Neural Networks in Image Processing for Early Detection of Breast Cancer. *Computational and Mathematical Methods in Medicine*, *2017*, 1–15. doi:10.1155/2017/2610628 PMID:28473865

Mehta, I. (2020, March 3). *China's coronavirus detection app is reportedly sharing citizen data with police.* Retrieved May 17, 2020, from https://thenextweb.com/china/2020/03/03/chinas-covid-19-app-reportedly-color-codes-people-and-shares-data-with-cops/

Melnick, E., Hess, E., Guo, G., Breslin, M., Lopez, K., Pavlo, A., Abujarad, F., Powsner, S. M., & Post, L. (2017). Patient-centered decision support: Formative usability evaluation of integrated clinical decision support with a patient decision aid for minor head injury in the emergency department. *Journal of Medical Internet Research*, *19*(5), e174. doi:10.2196/jmir.7846 PMID:28526667

Menezes, A. J., van Oorschot, P. C., & Vanstone, S. A. (2001). *Handbook of Applied Cryptography* (5th ed.). CRC Press.

Menezes, A., & Smart, N. (2004). Security of signature schemes in a multi-user setting. *Designs, Codes and Cryptography*, *33*(3), 261–274. doi:10.1023/B:DESI.0000036250.18062.3f

Merchant, R. M., & Asch, D. A. (2012). Can you find an automated external defibrillator if a life depends on it? *Circulation: Cardiovascular Quality and Outcomes*, *5*(2), 241–243. doi:10.1161/CIRCOUTCOMES.111.964825 PMID:22354936

Michard, F., Giglio, M. T., & Brienza, N. (2017). Perioperative goal-directed therapy with uncalibrated pulse contour methods: Impact on fluid management and postoperative outcome. *British Journal of Anaesthesia*, *119*(1), 22–30. doi:10.1093/bja/aex138 PMID:28605442

Michard, F., Mountford, W. K., Krukas, M. R., Ernst, F. R., & Fogel, S. L. (2015). Potential return on investment for implementation of perioperative goal-directed fluid therapy in major surgery: A nationwide database study. *Perioperative Medicine (London, England)*, *4*(1), 11. doi:10.118613741-015-0021-0 PMID:26500766

Michie, S., Atkins, L., & West, R. (2014). *The behaviour change wheel: a guide to designing interventions.* Silverback Publishing.

Michie, S., Richardson, M., Johnston, M., Abraham, C., Francis, J., Hardeman, W., Eccles, M. P., Cane, J., & Wood, C. E. (2013). The Behavior Change Technique Taxonomy (v1) of 93 Hierarchically Clustered Techniques: Building an International Consensus for the Reporting of Behavior Change Interventions. *Annals of Behavioral Medicine, 46*(1), 81–95. doi:10.100712160-013-9486-6 PMID:23512568

Michie, S., van Stralen, M. M., & West, R. (2011). The behaviour change wheel: A new method for characterising and designing behaviour change interventions. *Implementation Science; IS, 6*(1), 42. doi:10.1186/1748-5908-6-42 PMID:21513547

Michie, S., Wood, C. E., Johnston, M., Abraham, C., Francis, J. J., & Hardeman, W. (2015). Behaviour change techniques: The development and evaluation of a taxonomic method for reporting and describing behaviour change interventions (a suite of five studies involving consensus methods, randomised controlled trials and analysis of qualitative data). *Health Technology Assessment, 19*(99), 1–187. doi:10.3310/hta19990 PMID:26616119

Middleton, B., Bloomrosen, M., Dente, M. A., Hashmat, B., Koppel, R., Overhage, J. M., & Zhang, J. (2013). Enhancing patient safety and quality of care by improving the usability of electronic health record systems: Recommendations from AMIA. *Journal of the American Medical Informatics Association: JAMIA, 20*(e1), e2–e8. doi:10.1136/amiajnl-2012-001458 PMID:23355463

Middleton, S. E., Middleton, L., & Modafferi, S. (2014). Real-time crisis mapping of natural disasters using social media. *IEEE Intelligent Systems, 29*(2), 9–17. doi:10.1109/MIS.2013.126

Miljanovic, B., Glynn, R. J., Nathan, D. M., Manson, J. E., & Schaumberg, D. A. (2004). A prospective study of serum lipids and risk of diabetic macular edema in type 1 diabetes. *Diabetes, 53*(11), 2883–2892. doi:10.2337/diabetes.53.11.2883 PMID:15504969

Milne-Ives, M., Lam, C., De Cock, C., Van Velthoven, M. H., & Meinert, E. (2020). Mobile Apps for Health Behavior Change in Physical Activity, Diet, Drug and Alcohol Use, and Mental Health: Systematic Review. *JMIR mHealth and uHealth, 8*(3), e17046. doi:10.2196/17046 PMID:32186518

Ministry of Health and Welfare of South Korea. (2020). *Self-Check.* Apple App Store. Retrieved May 17, 2020, from https://apps.apple.com/us/app/self-diagnosis/id1501467779

Ministry of Health. Singapore. (2020). *TraceTogether.* Retrieved from https://www.healthhub.sg/apps/38/tracetogether-app

Misra, S., & Sarkar, S. (2015). Priority-based time-slot allocation in wireless body area networks during medical emergency situations: An evolutionary game-theoretic perspective. *IEEE Journal of Biomedical and Health Informatics, 19*(2), 541–548. doi:10.1109/JBHI.2014.2313374 PMID:24686307

Mitamura, H. (2008). Public access defibrillation: Advances from Japan. *Nature Clinical Practice. Cardiovascular Medicine, 5*(11), 690–692. doi:10.1038/ncpcardio1330 PMID:18779832

Mochari-Greenberger, H., Vue, L., Luka, A., Peters, A., & Pande, R. L. (2016). A tele-behavioural health intervention to reduce depression, anxiety, and stress and improve diabetes self-management. *Telemedicine Journal and e-Health, 22*(8), 624–630. doi:10.1089/tmj.2015.0231 PMID:26954880

Moghimi, F. H., De Steiger, R., Schaffer, J., & Wickramasinghe, N. (2013). The benefits of adopting e-performance management techniques and strategies to facilitate superior healthcare delivery: The proffering of a conceptual framework for the context of Hip and Knee Arthroplasty. *Health and technology, 3*(3), 237–247. doi:10.100712553-013-0057-4

Mohanty, B., Chughtai, A., & Rabhi, F. (2019). Use of mobile apps for epidemic surveillance and response–availability and gaps. *Global Biosecurity, 1*(2).

Moher, D., Liberati, A., Tetzlaff, J., & Altman, D. G. (2009). Preferred reporting items for systematic reviews and meta-analyses: The PRISMA statement. *PLoS Medicine, 6*(7), e1000097. doi:10.1371/journal.pmed.1000097 PMID:19621072

Mohseni, P., & Najafi, K. A. (2005). 1.48-mw low-phase-noise analog frequency modulator for wireless biotelemetry. *IEEE Transactions on Biomedical Engineering, 52*(5), 938–943. doi:10.1109/TBME.2005.845369 PMID:15887544

Morshed, A., Jayaraman, P. P., Sellis, T., Georgakopoulos, D., Villari, M., & Ranjan, R. (2017). Deep osmosis: Holistic distributed deep learning in osmotic computing. *IEEE Cloud Computing, 4*(6), 22–32. doi:10.1109/MCC.2018.1081070

Movassaghi, S., Abolhasan, M., Lipman, J., Smith, D., & Jamalipour, A. (2014). Wireless body area networks: A survey. *IEEE Communications Surveys and Tutorials, 16*(3), 1658–1686. doi:10.1109/SURV.2013.121313.00064

Mukhopadhyay. (2015). *Wearable Sensors for Human Activity Monitoring. IEEE Sensors Journal, 15(3)*.

Mummah, S. A., King, A. C., Gardner, C. D., & Sutton, S. (2016). Iterative development of Vegethon: A theory-based mobile app intervention to increase vegetable consumption. *The International Journal of Behavioral Nutrition and Physical Activity, 13*(1), 90. doi:10.118612966-016-0400-z PMID:27501724

Mummah, S. A., Mathur, M., King, A. C., Gardner, C. D., & Sutton, S. (2016). Mobile Technology for Vegetable Consumption: A Randomized Controlled Pilot Study in Overweight Adults. *JMIR mHealth and uHealth, 4*(2), e51. doi:10.2196/mhealth.5146 PMID:27193036

Mummah, S., Robinson, T. N., Mathur, M., Farzinkhou, S., Sutton, S., & Gardner, C. D. (2017). Effect of a mobile app intervention on vegetable consumption in overweight adults: A randomized controlled trial. *The International Journal of Behavioral Nutrition and Physical Activity, 14*(1), 125. doi:10.118612966-017-0563-2 PMID:28915825

Muraven, M., & Baumeister, R. F. (2000). Self-Regulation and Depletion of Limited Resources: Does Self-Control Resemble a Muscle? *Psychological Bulletin, 126*(2), 247–259. doi:10.1037/0033-2909.126.2.247 PMID:10748642

Murawski, B., Plotnikoff, R. C., Rayward, A. T., Oldmeadow, C., Vandelanotte, C., Brown, W. J., & Duncan, M. J. (2019). Efficacy of an m-Health Physical Activity and Sleep Health Intervention for Adults: A Randomized Waitlist-Controlled Trial. *American Journal of Preventive Medicine, 57*(4), 503–514. doi:10.1016/j.amepre.2019.05.009 PMID:31542128

Murawski, B., Plotnikoff, R. C., Rayward, A. T., Vandelanotte, C., Brown, W. J., & Duncan, M. J. (2018). Randomised controlled trial using a theory-based m-health intervention to improve physical activity and sleep health in adults: The Synergy Study protocol. *BMJ Open, 8*(2), e018997. doi:10.1136/bmjopen-2017-018997 PMID:29439005

Murphy, J. (2016). Engaging Nurses in the Design and Adoption of mHealth Tools for Care Coordination. *Nursing Informatics*. PMID:27332334

Myerburg, R. J., Velez, M., Rosenberg, D. G., Fenster, J., & Castellanos, A. (2003). Automatic External Defibrillators for Prevention of Out-of-Hospital Sudden Death: Effectiveness of the Automatic External Defibrillator. *Journal of Cardiovascular Electrophysiology, 14*(s9), S108–S116. doi:10.1046/j.1540-8167.14.s9.4.x PMID:12950531

Myers, M. D., & Venable, J. R. (2014). A set of ethical principles for design science research in information systems. *Information & Management, 51*(6), 801–809. doi:10.1016/j.im.2014.01.002

Natarajan, K., Prasath, B., & Kokila, P. (2016). Smart health care system using internet of things. *Journal of Network Communications and Emerging Technologies, 6*(3), 37–42.

National Association of Chronic Disease Directors Promoting Health. (n.d.). Why Public Health is Necessary to Improve Healthcare. *Preventing Disease*.

National Center for Chronic Disease Prevention and Health Promotion. (2009). *The Power of Prevention Chronic disease ... the public health challenge of the 21st cnetury*. Centers for Disease Control and Prevention.

National Diabetes Services Scheme. (2016). *Diabetes-related complication*. Available at: https://www.ndss.com.au/

Ng, K., Tynjälä, J., & Kokko, S. (2017). Ownership and use of commercial physical activity trackers among Finnish adolescents: Cross-sectional study. *JMIR mHealth and uHealth*, *5*(5), e61. doi:10.2196/mhealth.6940 PMID:28473304

Ngu, A. H., Tseng, P. T., Paliwal, M., Carpenter, C., & Stipe, W. (2018). Smartwatch-based iot fall detection application. *Open Journal of Internet Of Things*, *4*(1), 87–98.

Nguyen, L., & Wickramasinghe, N. (2017). An examination of the mediating role for a nursing information system. *AJIS. Australasian Journal of Information Systems*, *21*, 1–21. doi:10.3127/ajis.v21i0.1387

Nhavoto, J., Grönlund, Å., & Chaquilla, W. (2015). SMSaúde: Design, development, and implementation of a remote/mobile patient management system to improve retention in care for HIV/AIDS and tuberculosis patients. *JMIR mHealth and uHealth*, *3*(1), e26. doi:10.2196/mhealth.3854 PMID:25757551

NHS Near Me - Video Consulting with Near Me. (n.d.). *NearMe*. Retrieved from https://www.nearme.scot.

Nicaise, G. (2020). *Covid-19 and Donor Financing*. Retrieved from https://www.u4.no/publications/covid-19-and-donor-financing.pdf

Nichol, G., Thomas, E., Callaway, C. W., Hedges, J., Powell, J. L., Aufderheide, T. P., ... Dreyer, J. (2008). Regional variation in out-of-hospital cardiac arrest incidence and outcome. *Journal of the American Medical Association*, *300*(12), 1423–1431. doi:10.1001/jama.300.12.1423 PMID:18812533

Nihseniorhealth: About falls. (n.d.). Available online: http://nihseniorhealth.gov/falls/aboutfalls/01.html

Nikbakhsh, E., & Farahani, R. Z. (2011). Humanitarian logistics planning in disaster relief operations. *Logistics Operations and Management: Concepts and Models, 291*.

NIST. (2012, October 2). *NIST Selects Winner of Secure Hash Algorithm (SHA-3) Competition*. Retrieved May 17, 2020, from https://www.nist.gov/news-events/news/2012/10/nist-selects-winner-secure-hash-algorithm-sha-3-competition

Noordegraaf, A. V., Huirne, J. A. F., Pittens, C. A., van Mechelen, W., Broerse, J. E. W., Brölmann, H. A. M., & Anema, J. R. (2012). eHealth Program to Empower Patients in Returning to Normal Activities and Work After Gynecological Surgery: Intervention Mapping as a Useful Method for Development. *Journal of Medical Internet Research*, *14*(5), e124. doi:10.2196/jmir.1915 PMID:23086834

Norris, A. C., Martinez, S., Labaka, L., Madanian, S., Gonzalez, J. J., & Parry, D. (2015). *Disaster e-Health: A new paradigm for collaborative healthcare in disasters*. Paper presented at the The 12th International Conference on Information Systems for Crisis Response and Management, Kristiansand, Norway. http://idl.iscram.org/files/acnorris/2015/1252_ACNorris_etal2015.pdf

Nunnally, J. C. (1994). *Psychometric theory 3E*. Tata McGraw-Hill Education.

O'Keeffe, C., Nicholl, J., Turner, J., & Goodacre, S. (2011). Role of ambulance response times in the survival of patients with out-of-hospital cardiac arrest. *Emergency Medicine Journal*, *28*(8), 703–706. doi:10.1136/emj.2009.086363 PMID:20798090

Odekunle, F. F., Odekunle, R. O., & Shankar, S. (2017). Why sub-Saharan Africa lags in electronic health record adoption and possible strategies to increase its adoption in this region. *International Journal of Health Sciences*, *11*(4), 59–64. PMID:29085270

Oest, S. E., Hightower, M., & Krasowski, M. D. (2018). Activation and utilization of an electronic health record patient portal at an academic medical centre—Impact of patient demographics and geographic location. *Academic Pathology*, *5*, e2374289518797573. doi:10.1177/2374289518797573 PMID:30302394

Oinas-Kukkonen, H., & Harjumaa, M. (2009). Persuasive Systems Design: Key Issues, Process Model, and System Features. *Communications of the Association for Information Systems*, *24*. Advance online publication. doi:10.17705/1CAIS.02428

Oliver, D. (2017). David Oliver: Challenges for rural hospitals—the same but different. *BMJ (Clinical Research Ed.)*, *357*, 17–31. doi:10.1136/bmj.j17 PMID:28400387

Olson, C. A., & Thomas, J. F. (2017). Telehealth: No longer an idea for the future. *Advances in Pediatrics*, *64*(1), 347–370. doi:10.1016/j.yapd.2017.03.009 PMID:28688597

Omar, S., Adda, K., Youssef, Z., & Bernard, C. (2016). *ESR- Energy-aware and Stable routing protocol for WBAN Networks*. IEEE Publications.

Oppermann, L., & Prinz, W. (2016). Introduction to this Special Issue on Smart Glasses. *i-com*, *15*(2), 123-132.

Ose, D., Wensing, M., Szecsenyi, J., Joos, S., Hermann, K., & Miksch, A. (2009). Impact of primary care–based disease management on the health-related quality of life in patients with type 2 diabetes and comorbidity. *Diabetes Care*, *32*(9), 1594–1596. doi:10.2337/dc08-2223 PMID:19509007

Otto, C., Milenković, A., Sanders, C., & Jovanov, E. (2006). System Architecture of a Wireless Body Area Sensor Network For Ubiquitous Health Monitoring. *Journal of Mobile Multimedia*, *1*(4), 307–326.

Pan-European Privacy-Preserving Proximity Tracing. (n.d.). *PEPP-PT*. Retrieved from https://www.pepp-pt.org

Pantuvo, J. S., Naguib, R., & Wickramasinghe, N. (2011). Towards Implementing a Nationwide Electronic Health Record System in Nigeria. *International Journal of Healthcare Delivery Reform Initiatives*, *3*(1), 39–55. doi:10.4018/jhdri.2011010104

Paradis, M., Stiell, I., Atkinson, K., Guerinet, J., Sequeira, Y., Salter, L., Forster, A. J., Murphy, M. S. Q., & Wilson, K. (2018). Acceptability of a Mobile Clinical Decision Tool Among Emergency Department Clinicians: Development and Evaluation of The Ottawa Rules App. *JMIR mHealth and uHealth*, *6*(6), e10263. doi:10.2196/10263 PMID:29891469

Pardun, J. T. (1997). Good Samaritan laws: A global perspective. *Loy. LA Int'l & Comp. LJ*, *20*, 591.

Pasechnik, V. I. (1991). Acoustic tomography of biological object [in Russian]. *Radiotekhnika*, *8*, 65–72.

Patel, M. L., Hopkins, C. M., Brooks, T. L., & Bennett, G. G. (2019). Comparing Self-Monitoring Strategies for Weight Loss in a Smartphone App: Randomized Controlled Trial. *JMIR mHealth and uHealth*, *7*(2), e12209. doi:10.2196/12209 PMID:30816851

Patel, M. S., Asch, D. A., Rosin, R., Small, D. S., Bellamy, S. L., Heuer, J., Sproat, S., Hyson, C., Haff, N., Lee, S. M., Wesby, L., Hoffer, K., Shuttleworth, D., Taylor, D. H., Hilbert, V., Zhu, J., Yang, L., Wang, X., & Volpp, K. G. (2016). Framing Financial Incentives to Increase Physical Activity Among Overweight and Obese Adults: A Randomized, Controlled Trial. *Annals of Internal Medicine*, *164*(6), 385. doi:10.7326/M15-1635 PMID:26881417

Patel, V., Reed, M. E., & Grant, R. W. (2015). Electronic health records and the evolution of diabetes care: A narrative review. *Journal of Diabetes Science and Technology*, *9*(3), 676–680. doi:10.1177/1932296815572256 PMID:25711684

Pellegrini, C. A., Steglitz, J., Johnston, W., Warnick, J., Adams, T., McFadden, H. G., Siddique, J., Hedeker, D., & Spring, B. (2015). Design and protocol of a randomized multiple behavior change trial: Make Better Choices 2 (MBC2). *Contemporary Clinical Trials*, *41*, 85–92. doi:10.1016/j.cct.2015.01.009 PMID:25625810

Pell, J. P., Sirel, J. M., Marsden, A. K., Ford, I., Walker, N. L., & Cobbe, S. M. (2002). Potential impact of public access defibrillators on survival after out of hospital cardiopulmonary arrest: Retrospective cohort study. *BMJ (Clinical Research Ed.)*, *325*(7363), 515. doi:10.1136/bmj.325.7363.515 PMID:12217989

PEPP-PT e. V. i. Gr. (2020). *Pan-European Privacy-Preserving Proximity Tracing.* Retrieved May 17, 2020, from https://www.pepp-pt.org

Pervez, Hussain, & Kyung. (2009). Medical Applications of Wireless Body Area Networks. *International Journal of Digital Content Technology and Its Applications, 3*(3), 185-193.

Petersen, H., Baccelli, E., Wählisch, M., Schmidt, T. C., & Schiller, J. (2015). The role of the Internet of Things in network resilience. In R. Giaffreda, D. Cagáňová, Y. Li, R. Riggio, & A. Voisard (Eds.), *Internet of Things. IoT Infrastructures* (pp. 283–296). Springer International Publishing. doi:10.1007/978-3-319-19743-2_39

Pham, A., Bluett, E., Puthran, P., Sarkar, S., Kim, K., & Shankar, P. (2018). First 28: Design of a Mobile App for Neonatal Health Risk Assessment and Support for New Mothers. *Iproceedings*, *4*(2), e11740. doi:10.2196/11740

Pham, H. H., Schrag, D., O'Malley, A., Wu, B., & Bach, P. B. (2007). Care Patterns in Medicare and Their Implications for Pay for Performance. *The New England Journal of Medicine*, *356*(11), 1130–1139. doi:10.1056/NEJMsa063979 PMID:17360991

Pinsky, M. R., Clermont, G., & Hravnak, M. (2016). Predicting cardiorespiratory instability. *Critical Care (London, England)*, *20*(1), 70–77. doi:10.118613054-016-1223-7 PMID:26984263

Plotnikoff, R. C., Lubans, D. R., Costigan, S. A., Trinh, L., Spence, J. C., Downs, S., & McCargar, L. (2011). A test of the theory of planned behavior to explain physical activity in a large population sample of adolescents from Alberta, Canada. *The Journal of Adolescent Health*, *49*(5), 547–549. doi:10.1016/j.jadohealth.2011.03.006 PMID:22018572

Poncelet, A. N. (2003). Diabetic polyneuropathy. Risk factors, patterns of presentation, diagnosis, and treatment. *Geriatrics (Basel, Switzerland)*, *58*(6), 16–18. PMID:12813869

Portnov-Neeman, Y., & Amit, M. (2016). *The Effect of the Explicit Teaching Method on Learning the Working Backwards Strategy.* Academic Press.

Pourqasem, J. (2018). Cloud-based IoT: Integration cloud computing with internet of things. *International Journal of Research in Industrial Engineering*, *7*(4), 482–494.

Prochaska, J. O., & DiClemente, C. C. (2005). The Transtheoretical Approach. In J. C. Norcross & M. R. Goldfried (Eds.), *Handbook of psychotherapy integration* (2nd ed.). Oxford University Press. doi:10.1093/med:psych/9780195165791.003.0007

Public Access Defibrillation Trial Investigators. (2004). Public-access defibrillation and survival after out-of-hospital cardiac arrest. *The New England Journal of Medicine*, *351*(7), 637–646. doi:10.1056/NEJMoa040566 PMID:15306665

Puolitaival, M., & Lindfors, E. (2019). Turvallisuuskasvatuksen tavoitteiden tilannekuva perusopetuksessa–dokumenttiaineistoon perustuvaa pohdintaa. In Tutkimuksesta luokkahuoneisiin (Vol. 15, pp. 119-140). Suomen ainedidaktinen tutkimusseura. Ainedidaktisia tutkimuksia.

Qiu, Y., Haley, D., Chan, T., & Davis, L. (2016). Game theoretic framework for studying WBAN coexistence: 2-Player game analysis and n-player game estimation. *IEEE Australian Communications Theory Workshop*, 53-58. 10.1109/AusCTW.2016.7433609

Quan, A., Stiell, I., Perry, J., Paradis, M., Brown, E., Gignac, J., Wilson, L., & Wilson, K. (2020). Mobile Clinical Decision Tools Among Emergency Department Clinicians: Web-Based Survey and Analytic Data for Evaluation of The Ottawa Rules App. *JMIR mHealth and uHealth*, *8*(1), e15503. doi:10.2196/15503 PMID:32012095

Rabbi, M., Pfammatter, A., Zhang, M., Spring, B., & Choudhury, T. (2015). Automated personalized feedback for physical activity and dietary behavior change with mobile phones: A randomized controlled trial on adults. *JMIR mHealth and uHealth*, *3*(2), e42. doi:10.2196/mhealth.4160 PMID:25977197

Racine, T., & Kobinger, G. P. (2019). Challenges and perspectives on the use of mobile laboratories during outbreaks and their use for vaccine evaluation. *Human Vaccines & Immunotherapeutics*, *15*(10), 2264–2268. doi:10.1080/21645 515.2019.1597595 PMID:30893007

Raghupathi, W., & Raghupathi, V. (2018). An Empirical Study of Chronic Diseases in the United States: A Visual Analytics Approach to Public Health. *International Journal of Environmental Research and Public Health*, *15*(3), 431. doi:10.3390/ijerph15030431

Ra, H.-K., Yoon, H., Son, S., Stankovic, J., & Ko, J. (2018). HealthNode: Software Framework for Efficiently Designing and Developing Cloud-Based Healthcare Applications. *Mobile Information Systems.*, *2018*, 1–12. doi:10.1155/2018/6071580

Rajasekaran, Rekh, & Mary. (2015). *Non-Invasive Hemoglobin Measurement: A Great Blessing to the Rural Community*. Academic Press.

Rajasekaran, K. (2016). *Smart technologies for Non- invasive Biomedical Sensors to measure physiological parameters. In Handbook of Research on Healthcare Administration and Management*. IGI Global Publication.

Rajasekaran, K. (2016). *Smart technologies for Non-invasive Biomedical Sensors to measure physiological parameters. In Handbook of Research on Healthcare Administration and Management*. IGI Global Publication.

Ramaprasad, A., Syn, T., & Thirumalai, M. (2014). An Ontological Map for Meaningful Use of Healthcare Information Systems (MUHIS). *Proceedings of the International Conference on Health informatics*, 16-26.

Rana, J. S., Mittleman, M. A., Sheikh, J., Hu, F. B., Manson, J. E., Colditz, G. A., Speizer, F. E., Barr, R. G., & Camargo, C. A. (2004). Chronic obstructive pulmonary disease, asthma, and risk of type 2 diabetes in women. *Diabetes Care*, *27*(10), 2478–2484. doi:10.2337/diacare.27.10.2478 PMID:15451919

Rathbone, A. L., & Prescott, J. (2017). The use of mobile apps and SMS messaging as physical and mental health interventions: Systematic review. *Journal of Medical Internet Research*, *19*(8), e295. doi:10.2196/jmir.7740 PMID:28838887

Rawassizadeh, R., Momeni, E., Dobbins, C., Gharibshah, J., & Pazzani, M. (2016). Scalable daily human behavioral pattern mining from multivariate temporal data. *IEEE Transactions on Knowledge and Data Engineering*, *28*(11), 3098–3112. doi:10.1109/TKDE.2016.2592527

Rawat, J., Singh, A., Bhadauria, H. S., & Virmani, J. (2015). Computer Aided Diagnostic System for Detection of Leukemia Using Microscopic Images. *Procedia Computer Science*, *70*, 748–756. doi:10.1016/j.procs.2015.10.113

Razzaq, M. A., Gill, S. H., Qureshi, M. A., & Ullah, S. (2017). Security issues in the Internet of Things (IoT): A comprehensive study. *International Journal of Advanced Computer Science and Applications*, *8*(6), 383–388.

Rea, T. D., Olsufka, M., Bemis, B., White, L., Yin, L., Becker, L., Copass, M., Eisenberg, M., & Cobb, L. (2010). A population-based investigation of public access defibrillation: Role of emergency medical services care. *Resuscitation*, *81*(2), 163–167. doi:10.1016/j.resuscitation.2009.10.025 PMID:19962225

Reddy, G. P., Reddy, P. B., & Reddy, V. K. (2013). Body area networks. *J. of Telematics and Informatics*, *1*(1). Advance online publication. doi:10.12928/jti.v1i1.36-42

Reichard, P., Nilsson, B. Y., & Rosenqvist, U. (1993). The effect of long-term intensified insulin treatment on the development of microvascular complications of diabetes mellitus. *The New England Journal of Medicine*, *329*(5), 304–309. doi:10.1056/NEJM199307293290502 PMID:8147960

Reisig, W. (2013). *Understanding Petri Nets*. Springer-Verlag. doi:10.1007/978-3-642-33278-4

Rejintal, A., & Aswini, N. (2016). Image processing based leukemia cancer cell detection. In *2016 IEEE International Conference on Recent Trends in Electronics, Information & Communication Technology (RTEICT)*. IEEE. 10.1109/RTEICT.2016.7807865

Ricard-Gauthier, D., Wisniak, A., Catarino, R., van Rossum, A. F., Meyer-Hamme, U., Negulescu, R., … Petignat, P. (2015, October). Use of Smartphones as Adjuvant Tools for Cervical Cancer Screening in Low-Resource Settings. *Journal of Lower Genital Tract Disease*. . doi:10.1097/lgt.0000000000000136

Riccardo, C., Flavia, M., Ramona, R., Chiara, B., & Roberto, V. (2014). A Survey on Wireless Body Area Networks: Technologies and design challenges. IEEE Communications Surveys and Tutorials, 16(3), 1635-1657.

Ridgers, N. D., McNarry, M. A., & Mackintosh, K. A. (2016). Feasibility and effectiveness of using wearable activity trackers in youth: A systematic review. *JMIR mHealth and uHealth*, *4*(4), e129. doi:10.2196/mhealth.6540 PMID:27881359

Ringh, M., Herlitz, J., Hollenberg, J., Rosenqvist, M., & Svensson, L. (2009). Out of hospital cardiac arrest outside home in Sweden, change in characteristics, outcome and availability for public access defibrillation. *Scandinavian Journal of Trauma, Resuscitation and Emergency Medicine*, *17*(1), 18. doi:10.1186/1757-7241-17-18 PMID:19374752

Ringle, C. M., Wende, S., & Becker, J. M. (2015). *SmartPLS 3*. Boenningstedt: SmartPLS GmbH. Retrieved from http://www.smartpls.com

Rodriguez, C., Castro, D. M., Coral, W., Cabra, J. L., Velasquez, N., Colorado, J., Diego, M., & Trujillo, L. C. (2017). IoT system for human activity recognition using BioHarness 3 and smartphone. *Proceedings of the International Conference on Future Networks and Distributed Systems*. 10.1145/3102304.3105828

Roemer, E. (2016). A tutorial on the use of PLS path modeling in longitudinal studies. *Industrial Management & Data Systems*, *116*(9), 1901–1921. doi:10.1108/IMDS-07-2015-0317

Routray, S. K., & Anand, S. (2017). Narrowband IoT for healthcare. In *2017 International Conference on Information Communication and Embedded Systems (ICICES)*. IEEE. 10.1109/ICICES.2017.8070747

Rubin, S. (2012). The use of mhealth technology for pandemic preparedness. *Health Systems (Basingstoke, England)*, 21–24.

Rucigaj, S., Podobnik, B., Gradisek, P., & Sostaric, M. (2019). "AED Database of Slovenia"-an analysis of operation of Slovenian national public access defibrillators registry. *Resuscitation*, *142*, e47–e48. doi:10.1016/j.resuscitation.2019.06.113

Russo, C. (2011). *Emergency communication remains a challenge ten years after 9/11*. Retrieved from http://www.homelandsecuritynewswire.com/emergency-communication-remains-challenge-ten-years-after-911

Rüter, A. (2006). *Disaster medicine-performance indicators, information support and documentation: A study of an evaluation tool*. Linköping University. Retrieved from http://swepub.kb.se/bib/swepub:oai:DiVA.org:liu-7990?tab2=abs&language=

Rzayev, R., Woźniak, P. W., Dingler, T., & Henze, N. (2018). Reading on smart glasses: The effect of text position, presentation type and walking. *Proceedings of the 2018 CHI Conference on Human Factors in Computing Systems*.

Sabaté, E., & World Health Organization. (Eds.). (2003). *Adherence to long-term therapies: Evidence for action*. World Health Organization.

Salmasi, V., Maheshwari, K., Yang, D., Mascha, E. J., Singh, A., Sessler, D. I., & Kurz, A. (2017). Relationship between Intraoperative Hypotension, Defined by Either Reduction from Baseline or Absolute Thresholds, and Acute Kidney and Myocardial Injury after Noncardiac Surgery: A Retrospective Cohort Analysis. *Anesthesiology: The Journal of the American Society of Anesthesiologists*, *126*(1), 47–65. doi:10.1097/ALN.0000000000001432 PMID:27792044

Samaneh, M., Mehran, A., Justin, L., David, S., & Abbas, J. (2014). Wireless Body Area Networks: A Survey. IEEE Communications Surveys and Tutorials, 16(3), 1658-1686.

Sandal, L., Stochkendahl, M., Svendsen, M., Wood, K., Øverås, C., Nordstoga, A., ... Cooper, K. (2019). An App-Delivered Self-Management Program for People With Low Back Pain: Protocol for the selfBACK Randomized Controlled Trial. *JMIR Research Protocols*, *8*(12), e14720. doi:10.2196/14720 PMID:31793897

Sander, M., & Lemcke, A. (2020, April 19). Radius erlaubt: wie Taiwans Handy-Überwachung funktioniert. *Neue Zürcher Zeitung*. Retrieved May 17, 2020, from https://www.nzz.ch/technologie/wie-taiwans-handy-ueberwachung-funktioniert-ld.1551839

Sankaran, S., Dendale, P., & Coninx, K. (2019). Evaluating the Impact of the HeartHab App on Motivation, Physical Activity, Quality of Life, and Risk Factors of Coronary Artery Disease Patients: Multidisciplinary Crossover Study. *JMIR mHealth and uHealth*, *7*(4), e10874. doi:10.2196/10874 PMID:30946021

Sankaran, S., Frederix, I., Haesen, M., Dendale, P., Luyten, K., & Coninx, K. (2016). A Grounded Approach for Applying Behavior Change Techniques in Mobile Cardiac Tele-Rehabilitation. *Proceedings of the 9th ACM International Conference on PErvasive Technologies Related to Assistive Environments*. 10.1145/2910674.2910680

Sapirie, S. (2000). *Assessing health information systems. In Design and implementation of health information systems*. World Health Organization.

Sargent, R. D. (2011). Verification and validation of simulation models. *Proceedings of the 2011 Winter Simulation Conference*, 183–198. 10.1109/WSC.2011.6147750

Sarstedt, M., Henseler, J., & Ringle, C. M. (2011). Multigroup analysis in partial least squares (PLS) path modeling: Alternative methods and empirical results. *Adv Int Mark*, *22*, 195–218. doi:10.1108/S1474-7979(2011)0000022012

Satoh-Asahara, N., Ito, H., Akashi, T., Yamakage, H., Kotani, K., Nagata, D., Nakagome, K., & Noda, M. (2016). A patient-held medical record integrating depression care into diabetes care. *Japanese Clinical Medicine*, *7*, 19–22. doi:10.4137/JCM.S39766 PMID:27478395

Schaefer, S. E., Ching, C. C., Breen, H., & German, J. B. (2016). Wearing, thinking, and moving: Testing the feasibility of fitness tracking with urban youth. *American Journal of Health Education*, *47*(1), 8–16. doi:10.1080/19325037.2015.1111174

Scheerman, J. F. M., Meijel, B., Empelen, P., Verrips, G. H. W., Loveren, C., Twisk, J. W. R., Pakpour, A. H., Braak, M. C. T., & Kramer, G. J. C. (2020). The effect of using a mobile application ("WhiteTeeth") on improving oral hygiene: A randomized controlled trial. *International Journal of Dental Hygiene*, *18*(1), 73–83. doi:10.1111/idh.12415 PMID:31291683

Scheerman, J. F. M., van Empelen, P., van Loveren, C., & van Meijel, B. (2018). A Mobile App (WhiteTeeth) to Promote Good Oral Health Behavior Among Dutch Adolescents with Fixed Orthodontic Appliances: Intervention Mapping Approach. *JMIR mHealth and uHealth*, *6*(8), e163. doi:10.2196/mhealth.9626 PMID:30120085

Scheerman, J. F. M., van Meijel, B., van Empelen, P., Kramer, G. J. C., Verrips, G. H. W., Pakpour, A. H., Van den Braak, M. C. T., & van Loveren, C. (2018). Study protocol of a randomized controlled trial to test the effect of a smartphone application on oral-health behavior and oral hygiene in adolescents with fixed orthodontic appliances. *BMC Oral Health*, *18*(1), 19. doi:10.118612903-018-0475-9 PMID:29415697

Schneier, B. (1995). *Applied Cryptography: Protocols, Algorithms and Source Code in C* (2nd ed.). John Wiley & Sons.

Schwarzer, R., & Renner, B. (2000). Social-cognitive predictors of health behavior: Action self-efficacy and coping self-efficacy. *Health Psychology: Official Journal of the Division of Health Psychology, American Psychological Association*, *19*(5), 487–495. doi:10.1037/0278-6133.19.5.487 PMID:11007157

Sehatbakhsh, N., Alam, M., Nazari, A., Zajic, A., & Prvulovic, M. (2018). *Syndrome: Spectral analysis for anomaly detection on medical iot and embedded devices. In 2018 IEEE international symposium on hardware oriented security and trust (HOST)*. IEEE.

Selvin, E., Marinopoulos, S., Berkenblit, G., Rami, T., Brancati, F. L., Powe, N. R., & Golden, S. H. (2004). Meta-analysis: Glycosylated hemoglobin and cardiovascular disease in diabetes mellitus. *Annals of Internal Medicine*, *141*(6), 421–431. doi:10.7326/0003-4819-141-6-200409210-00007 PMID:15381515

Seto, E., Ware, P., Logan, A., Cafazzo, J., Chapman, K., Segal, P., & Ross, H. (2017). Self-management and clinical decision support for patients with complex chronic conditions through the use of smartphone-based telemonitoring: Randomized controlled trial protocol. *JMIR Research Protocols*, *6*(11), e229. doi:10.2196/resprot.8367 PMID:29162557

Seyedi, Kibret, Lai, & Faulkner. (2013). *A survey on intrabody communications for body area network applications*. Academic Press.

Shamdani, A., & Nicolai, B. (2012). *Applications of RFID in incident management*. Paper presented at the The 7th International Multi-Conference on Computing in the Global Information Technology, Venice, Italy.

Shan, S. (2020, March 25). Virus Outbreak: CHT working alone on tracking system: agency. *Taipei Times*, 3. Retrieved May 17, 2020, from https://www.taipeitimes.com/News/taiwan/archives/2020/03/25/2003733339

Shaw, J., & Tanamas, S. (2012) *Diabetes the silent pandemic and its impacts on Australia*. Available at: https://static.diabetesaustralia.com.au/s/fileassets/diabetes-australia/e7282521-472b-4313-b18e-be84c3d5d907.pdf

Shaw, J., Rudzicz, F., Jamieson, T., & Goldfarb, A. (2019). Artificial Intelligence and the Implementation Challenge. *Journal of Medical Internet Research*, *21*(7), e13659. doi:10.2196/13659 PMID:31293245

Shelley, K. (2007). Photoplethysmography: Beyond the Calculation of Arterial Oxygen Saturation and Heart Rate. *Anesthesia and Analgesia*, 105. PMID:18048895

Shelukhin, O. I., & Alyabiev, S. P. (1984). Preliminary filtering in a Kalman filter under the a priori uncertainty conditions [in Russian]. *Radiotekhnika*, *8*, 53–57.

Shi, S. G. (1992). Accurate and efficient double-bootstrap confidence limit method. *Computational Statistics & Data Analysis*, *13*(1), 21–32. doi:10.1016/0167-9473(92)90151-5

Sieben, C., Scott, R. E., & Palacios, M. (2012). e-Health and disaster management cycle. In M. Jordanova & F. Lievens (Eds.), Global Telemed eHealth Updates: Knowl Resources (pp. 368-372). Academic Press.

Simons, D., De Bourdeaudhuij, I., Clarys, P., De Cocker, K., Vandelanotte, C., & Deforche, B. (2018a). A Smartphone App to Promote an Active Lifestyle in Lower-Educated Working Young Adults: Development, Usability, Acceptability, and Feasibility Study. *JMIR mHealth and uHealth*, *6*(2), e44. doi:10.2196/mhealth.8287 PMID:29463491

Simons, D., De Bourdeaudhuij, I., Clarys, P., De Cocker, K., Vandelanotte, C., & Deforche, B. (2018b). Effect and Process Evaluation of a Smartphone App to Promote an Active Lifestyle in Lower Educated Working Young Adults: Cluster Randomized Controlled Trial. *JMIR mHealth and uHealth*, *6*(8), e10003. doi:10.2196/10003 PMID:30143477

Singh, B., & Kaur, M. (2010). IT applications in healthcare. *Proceedings of the International Conference and Workshop on Emerging Trends in Technology.* 10.1145/1741906.1741940

Singh, D. A., & Shi, L. (2019). *Essentials of The U.S. Health Care System.* Jones & Bartlett Learning.

Singh, N., Hess, E., Guo, G., Sharp, A., Huang, B., Breslin, M., & Melnick, E. (2017). Tablet-based patient-centered decision support for minor head injury in the emergency department: Pilot study. *JMIR mHealth and uHealth, 5*(9), e144. doi:10.2196/mhealth.8732 PMID:28958987

Singh, S. P., Urooj, S., & Lay-Ekuakille, A. (2016). Breast Cancer Detection Using PCPCET and ADEWNN: A Geometric Invariant Approach to Medical X-Ray Image Sensors. *IEEE Sensors Journal, 16*(12), 4847–4855. doi:10.1109/JSEN.2016.2533440

Sirard, J. R., & Pate, R. R. (2001). Physical activity assessment in children and adolescents. *Sports Medicine (Auckland, N.Z.), 31*(6), 439–454. doi:10.2165/00007256-200131060-00004 PMID:11394563

Sloane, E. B., & Gehlot, V. (2007). Use of Coloured Petri Net models in planning, design, and simulation of intelligent wireless medical device networks for safe and flexible hospital capacity management. *International Journal of Networking and Virtual Organisations, 4*(2), 118–129. doi:10.1504/IJNVO.2007.013538

Soh, C., Kien, S. S., & Tay-Yap, J. (2000). Cultural fi t and misfi t: Is ERP a universal solution? *Communications of the ACM, 43*(4), 47–51. doi:10.1145/332051.332070

Solomon, D. H., Massarotti, E., Garg, R., Liu, J., Canning, C., & Schneeweiss, S. (2011). Association between disease-modifying antirheumatic drugs and diabetes risk in patients with rheumatoid arthritis and psoriasis. *Journal of the American Medical Association, 305*(24), 2525–2531. doi:10.1001/jama.2011.878 PMID:21693740

Song, Y., Klevak, A., Manson, J. E., Buring, J. E., & Liu, S. (2010). Asthma, chronic obstructive pulmonary disease, and type 2 diabetes in the Women's Health Study. *Diabetes Research and Clinical Practice, 90*(3), 365–371. doi:10.1016/j.diabres.2010.09.010 PMID:20926152

Sotskov, B. M., & Shcherbakov, V. Yu. (1985). Theory and technology of Kalman filtering in the presence of interfering parameters [in Russian]. *Zarubezhnaya Radioelektronika, 2,* 3–29.

Spring, B., Pellegrini, C., McFadden, H. G., Pfammatter, A. F., Stump, T. K., Siddique, J., King, A. C., & Hedeker, D. (2018). Multicomponent mHealth Intervention for Large, Sustained Change in Multiple Diet and Activity Risk Behaviors: The Make Better Choices 2 Randomized Controlled Trial. *Journal of Medical Internet Research, 20*(6), e10528. doi:10.2196/10528 PMID:29921561

Statista. (2020). *Number of smartphone users worldwide from 2016 to 2021.* Retrieved from https://www.statista.com/statistics/330695/number-of-smartphone-users-worldwide/

Stergiou, C., Psannis, K. E., Kim, B. G., & Gupta, B. (2018). Secure integration of IoT and cloud computing. *Future Generation Computer Systems, 78,* 964–975. doi:10.1016/j.future.2016.11.031

Subasi, A., Radhwan, M., Kurdi, R., & Khateeb, K. (2018). IoT based mobile healthcare system for human activity recognition. In *2018 15th Learning and Technology Conference (L&T).* IEEE. 10.1109/LT.2018.8368507

Subbe, C. P., Duller, B., & Bellomo, R. (2017). Effect of an automated notification system for deteriorating ward patients on clinical outcomes. *Critical Care (London, England), 21*(1), 52–60. doi:10.118613054-017-1635-z PMID:28288655

Sullivan, A. N., & Lachman, M. E. (2016). Behavior Change with Fitness Technology in Sedentary Adults: A Review of the Evidence for Increasing Physical Activity. *Frontiers in Public Health, 4,* 289. doi:10.3389/fpubh.2016.00289 PMID:28123997

Sun, C. L., Karlsson, L., Torp-Pedersen, C., Morrison, L. J., Brooks, S. C., Folke, F., & Chan, T. C. (2019). In Silico Trial of Optimized Versus Actual Public Defibrillator Locations. *Journal of the American College of Cardiology, 74*(12), 1557–1567. doi:10.1016/j.jacc.2019.06.075 PMID:31537265

Sundberg, K., Wengström, Y., Blomberg, K., Hälleberg-Nyman, M., Frank, C., & Langius-Eklöf, A. (2017, February 24). Early detection and management of symptoms using an interactive smartphone application (Interaktor) during radiotherapy for prostate cancer. In *Supportive Care in Cancer*. Springer Nature. . doi:10.100700520-017-3625-8

Sunio, V., & Schmocker, J.-D. (2017). Can we promote sustainable travel behavior through mobile apps? Evaluation and review of evidence. *International Journal of Sustainable Transportation, 11*(8), 553–566. doi:10.1080/15568318.2017.1300716

Su, T., Han, X., Chen, F., Du, Y., Zhang, H., Yin, J., Tan, X., Chang, W., Ding, Y., Han, Y., & Cao, G. (2013). Knowledge levels and training needs of disaster medicine among health professionals, medical students, and local residents in Shanghai, China. *PLoS One, 8*(6), e67041. doi:10.1371/journal.pone.0067041 PMID:23826190

Sutjiredjeki, E., Soegijoko, S., Mengko, T. L. R., Tjondronegoro, S., Astami, K., & Muhammad, H. U. (2009). *Application of a mobile telemedicine system with multi communication links for disaster reliefs in indonesia.* Paper presented at the World Congress on Medical Physics and Biomedical Engineering, Munich, Germany. 10.1007/978-3-642-03904-1_96

Taenzer, A. H., Pyke, J. B., McGrath, S. P., & Blike, G. T. (2010). Impact of Pulse Oximetry Surveillance on Rescue Events and Intensive Care Unit Transfers: A Before-and-After Concurrence Study. *Anesthesiology, 112*(2), 282–287. doi:10.1097/ALN.0b013e3181ca7a9b PMID:20098128

Tang, Q., Tummala, N., Gupta, S., & Schwiebert, L. (2005). Communication scheduling to minimize thermal effects of implanted biosensor networks in homogeneous tissue. *IEEE Transactions on Biomedical Engineering, 52*(7), 1285–1294. doi:10.1109/TBME.2005.847527 PMID:16041992

Tan, M. L., Prasanna, R., Stock, K., Hudson-Doyle, E., Leonard, G., & Johnston, D. (2017). Mobile applications in crisis informatics literature: A systematic review. *International Journal of Disaster Risk Reduction, 24*, 297–311. doi:10.1016/j.ijdrr.2017.06.009

Telford, J., & Cosgrave, J. (2007). The international humanitarian system and the 2004 Indian Ocean earthquake and tsunamis. *Disasters, 31*(1), 1–28. doi:10.1111/j.1467-7717.2007.00337.x PMID:17367371

Terry, D. J., & O'Leary, J. E. (1995). The theory of planned behaviour: The effects of perceived behavioural control and self-efficacy. *British Journal of Social Psychology, 34*(2), 199–220. doi:10.1111/j.2044-8309.1995.tb01058.x PMID:7620846

Thacker, J. K. M., Mountford, W. K., Ernst, F. R., Krukas, M. R., & Mythen, M. G. (2016). Perioperative Fluid Utilization Variability and Association with Outcomes: Considerations for Enhanced Recovery Efforts in Sample US Surgical Populations. *Annals of Surgery, 263*(3), 502–510. doi:10.1097/SLA.0000000000001402 PMID:26565138

Thamjamrassri, P., Song, Y., Tak, J., Kang, H., Kong, H. J., & Hong, J. (2018). Customer Discovery as the First Essential Step for Successful Health Information Technology System Development. *Healthcare Informatics Research, 24*(1), 79–85. doi:10.4258/hir.2018.24.1.79 PMID:29503756

The Guardian. (2020). *Coronavirus app: will Australians trust a government with a history of tech fails and data breaches?* Available at: https://www.theguardian.com/australia-news/2020/apr/26/coronavirus-app-will-australians-trust-a-government-with-a-history-of-tech-fails-and-data-breaches

The Hindu. (2020, May 8). Watch | How does the Aarogya Setu app work? *The Hindu.* Retrieved May 17, 2020, from https://www.thehindu.com/news/national/how-does-the-aarogya-setu-appwork/

Thompson, S., Altay, N., Green, W. G. III, & Lapetina, J. (2006). Improving disaster response efforts with decision support systems. *International Journal of Emergency Management, 3*(4), 250–263. doi:10.1504/IJEM.2006.011295

Tinetti, M. E., Fried, T. R., & Boyd, C. M. (2012). *Designing Health Care for the Most Common Chronic Condition - Multimorbidity.* JAMA Network. doi:10.1001/jama.2012.5265

Ting, D. S. W., Carin, L., Dzau, V., & Wong, T. Y. (2020). Digital technology and COVID-19. *Nature Medicine, 26*(4), 459–461. doi:10.103841591-020-0824-5 PMID:32284618

Tjan, A. (2001). Finally, a way to put your internet portfolio in order. *Harvard Business Review, 79*(2), 76–85. PMID:11213700

Tombor, I., Beard, E., Brown, J., Shahab, L., Michie, S., & West, R. (2018). Randomized factorial experiment of components of the SmokeFree Baby smartphone application to aid smoking cessation in pregnancy. *Translational Behavioral Medicine, 9*(4), 583–593. doi:10.1093/tbm/iby073 PMID:30011020

Tombor, I., Shahab, L., Brown, J., Crane, D., Michie, S., & West, R. (2016). Development of SmokeFree Baby: A smoking cessation smartphone app for pregnant smokers. *Translational Behavioral Medicine, 6*(4), 533–545. doi:10.100713142-016-0438-0 PMID:27699682

TrackerS. (n.d.). Retrieved from: https://www.sports-tracker.com

Tran, C., Dicker, A., Leiby, B., Gressen, E., Williams, N., & Jim, H. (2020). Utilizing Digital Health to Collect Electronic Patient-Reported Outcomes in Prostate Cancer: Single-Arm Pilot Trial. *Journal of Medical Internet Research, 22*(3), e12689. doi:10.2196/12689 PMID:32209536

Trepte, S., Reinecke, L., Ellison, N. B., Quiring, O., Yao, M. Z., & Ziegele, M. (2017, January-March). A Cross-Cultural Perspective on the Privacy Calculus. *Social Media + Society,* 1-13. doi:10.1177/2056305116688035

Trzeciak, S., & Rivers, E. P. (2003). Emergency department overcrowding in the United States: An emerging threat to patient safety and public health. *Emergency Medicine Journal, 20*(5), 402–405. doi:10.1136/emj.20.5.402 PMID:12954674

Tun, S. Y. Y., Madanian, S., & Mirza, F. (2020). Internet of things (IoT) applications for elderly care: A reflective review. *Aging Clinical and Experimental Research.* Advance online publication. doi:10.100740520-020-01545-9 PMID:32277435

Turcu, C., & Popa, V. (2009). *An RFID-based system for emergency health care services.* Paper presented at the International Conference on Advanced Information Networking and Applications Workshops, Bradford, UK. 10.1109/WAINA.2009.107

TVNZ. (2020). *World Health Organisation praises New Zealand for its 'very systematic' response to Covid-19 pandemic.* Retrieved from https://www.tvnz.co.nz/one-news/new-zealand/world-health-organisation-praises-new-zealand-its-very-systematic-response-covid-19-pandemic

Tyagi, A., & Singh, P. (2014). Asthma diagnosis and level of control using decision tree and fuzzy system. *International Journal of Biomedical Engineering and Technology, 16*(2), 169–181. doi:10.1504/IJBET.2014.065658

Tyagi, A., & Singh, P. (2015). ACS: Asthma care services with the help of case base reasoning technique. *Procedia Computer Science, 48,* 561–567. doi:10.1016/j.procs.2015.04.136

Tyagi, A., & Singh, P. (2019). Health information system. In N. Wickramasinghe (Ed.), *Healthcare Policy and Reform: Concepts, Methodologies, Tools, and Applications* (pp. 1554–1564). IGI Global. doi:10.4018/978-1-5225-6915-2.ch070

Ubbink, T. (2004). Toe Blood Pressure Measurements in Patients Suspected of Leg Ischaemia: A New Laser Doppler Device Compared with Photoplethysmography. *European Journal of Vascular and Endovascular Surgery, 27*(6), 629–634. doi:10.1016/j.ejvs.2004.01.031 PMID:15121114

UK Prospective Diabetes Study Group (UPDSG). (1998). Tight blood pressure control and risk of macrovascular and microvascular complications in type 2 diabetes: UKPDS 38. *British Medical Journal, 317*(7160), p.703.

Ukil, A., Bandyoapdhyay, S., Puri, C., & Pal, A. (2016). IoT healthcare analytics: The importance of anomaly detection. In *2016 IEEE 30th International Conference on Advanced Information Networking and Applications (AINA)*. IEEE.

Ulku, E. E., & Camurcu, A. Y. (2013). Computer aided brain tumor detection with histogram equalization and morphological image processing techniques. In *2013 International Conference on Electronics, Computer and Computation (ICECCO)*. IEEE. 10.1109/ICECCO.2013.6718225

Umble, E., Haft, R., & Umble, M. (2003). Enterprise Resource Planning: Implementation Procedures and Critical Success Factors. *European Journal of Operational Research, 146*(2), 241-257.

UN Department of Global Communications. (2020). *UN mobilizes global cooperation in science-based COVID-19 responses*. Retrieved from https://www.un.org/en/un-coronavirus-communications-team/un-mobilizes-global-cooperation-science-based-covid-19-responses

Underwood, S. (2010). Improving disaster management. *Communications of the ACM, 53*(2), 18–20. doi:10.1145/1646353.1646362

Ungku, F. (2020, March 20). Singapore launches contact tracing mobile app to track coronavirus infections. *Technology News*. Retrieved May 17, 2020, from https://www.reuters.com/article/us-health-coronavirus-singapore-technolo-idUSKBN2171ZQ

UNICEF (United Nations Children's Fund). (2013). *Improving Child Nutrition: The Achievable Imperative for Global Progress*. UNICEF.

United Nations Population Fund. (2017). Caring for Our Elders: Early Responses. United Nations Population Fund (UNFPA).

United Nations. (2007). *Hyogo framework for action 2005-2015: Building the resilience of nations and communities to disasters*. Retrieved from https://www.unisdr.org/files/1037_hyogoframeworkforactionenglish.pdf

United Nations. (2015). *Sendai framework for disaster risk reduction 2015-2030*. Retrieved from https://www.unisdr.org/files/43291_sendaiframeworkfordrren.pdf

United Nations. (2015). *The Millennium Development Goals Report*. Author.

Unno, N., Inuzuka, K., Mitsuoka, H., Ishimaru, K., Sagara, D., & Konno, H. (2006). Automated Bedside Measurement of Penile Blood Flow Using Pulse-Volume Plethysmography. *Surgery Today, 36*(3), 257–261. doi:10.100700595-005-3139-8 PMID:16493536

Uscher-Pines, L., Bouskill, K., Sousa, J., Shen, M., & Fischer, S. H. (2019). *Experiences of Medicaid programs and health centres in implementing telehealth*. RAND. doi:10.7249/RR2564

Uwaoma, C., Mansingh, G., Pepper, W., Lu, W., & Xiang, S. (2019). Estimation of Physical Activity Level and Ambient Condition Thresholds for Respiratory Health using Smartphone Sensors. In PECCS (pp. 113-120). SCITEPRESS. doi:10.5220/0008170001130120

Uwaoma, C., & Mansingh, G. (2018). Certainty Modeling of a Decision Support System for Mobile Monitoring of Exercise-induced Respiratory Conditions. In *Proceedings of the 51st Hawaii International Conference on System Sciences* (pp. 2957-2966). HICSS. 10.24251/HICSS.2018.375

Van Acker, K., Bouhassira, D., De Bacquer, D., Weiss, S., Matthys, K., Raemen, H., Mathieu, C., & Colin, I. M. (2009). Prevalence and impact on quality of life of peripheral neuropathy with or without neuropathic pain in type 1 and type 2 diabetic patients attending hospital outpatients clinics. *Diabetes & Metabolism, 35*(3), 206–213. doi:10.1016/j.diabet.2008.11.004 PMID:19297223

van Beurden, S. B., Smith, J. R., Lawrence, N. S., Abraham, C., & Greaves, C. J. (2019). Feasibility Randomized Controlled Trial of ImpulsePal: Smartphone App-Based Weight Management Intervention to Reduce Impulsive Eating in Overweight Adults. *JMIR Formative Research, 3*(2), e11586. doi:10.2196/11586 PMID:31038464

van Heerden, A., Sen, D., Desmond, C., Louw, J., & Richter, L. (2017). App-supported promotion of child growth and development by community health workers in Kenya: Feasibility and acceptability study. *JMIR mHealth and uHealth, 5*(12), e182. doi:10.2196/mhealth.6911 PMID:29208588

van Kollenburg, R., de Bruin, D., & Wijkstra, H. (2019). Validation of the Electronic Version of the International Index of Erectile Function (IIEF-5 and IIEF-15): A Crossover Study. *Journal of Medical Internet Research, 21*(7), e13490. doi:10.2196/13490 PMID:31267983

Venkatesh, P. K., da Costa, D. A., Zou, Y., & Ng, J. W. (2017). A framework to extract personalized behavioural patterns of user's IoT devices data. In *Proceedings of the 27th Annual International Conference on Computer Science and Software Engineering*. IBM Corp.

Verbiest, M., Borrell, S., Dalhousie, S., Tupa'i-Firestone, R., Funaki, T., Goodwin, D., Grey, J., Henry, A., Hughes, E., Humphrey, G., Jiang, Y., Jull, A., Pekepo, C., Schumacher, J., Te Morenga, L., Tunks, M., Vano, M., Whittaker, R., & Ni Mhurchu, C. (2018). A Co-Designed, Culturally-Tailored mHealth Tool to Support Healthy Lifestyles in Maori and Pasifika Communities in New Zealand: Protocol for a Cluster Randomized Controlled Trial. *JMIR Research Protocols, 7*(8), e10789. doi:10.2196/10789 PMID:30135054

Verbruggen, F., Best, M., Bowditch, W. A., Stevens, T., & McLaren, I. P. L. (2014). The inhibitory control reflex. *Neuropsychologia, 65*, 263–278. doi:10.1016/j.neuropsychologia.2014.08.014 PMID:25149820

Vileikyte, L., Rubin, R. R., & Leventhal, H. (2004). Psychological aspects of diabetic neuropathic foot complications: An overview. *Diabetes/Metabolism Research and Reviews, 20*(S1), S13–S18. doi:10.1002/dmrr.437 PMID:15150807

Villalba-Mora, E., Peinado, I., & Guerrero, D. P. F. (2017). eHealth and diabetes: Designing a novel system for remotely monitoring older adults with type 2 diabetes. Diabetes in Old Age, Fourth Edition. doi:10.1002/9781118954621.ch14

Vo, A. H., Brooks, G. B., Bourdeau, M., Farr, R., & Raimer, B. G. (2010). University of Texas Medical Branch telemedicine disaster response and recovery: Lessons learned from hurricane Ike. *Telemedicine Journal and e-Health, 16*(5), 627–633. doi:10.1089/tmj.2009.0162 PMID:20575732

Wadoum, R. G., Samin, A., Mafopa, N. G., Giovanetti, M., Russo, G., Turay, P., Tura, J., Kargbo, M., Kanu, M. T., Kargbo, B., Akpablie, J., Cain, C. J., Pasin, P., Batwala, V., Sobze, M. S., Potesta, M., Minutolo, A., Colizzi, V., & Montesano, C. (2017). Mobile health clinic for the medical management of clinical sequelae experienced by survivors of the 2013–2016 Ebola virus disease outbreak in Sierra Leone, West Africa. *European Journal of Clinical Microbiology & Infectious Diseases, 36*(11), 2193–2200. doi:10.100710096-017-3045-1 PMID:28695354

Waeckerle, J. F., Lillibridge, S. R., Burkle, F. M. Jr, & Noji, E. K. (1994). Disaster medicine: Challenges for today. *Annals of Emergency Medicine, 23*(4), 715–718. doi:10.1016/S0196-0644(94)70304-3 PMID:8161037

Walker, A., Sirel, J. M., Marsden, A. K., Cobbe, S. M., & Pell, J. P. (2003). Cost effectiveness and cost utility model of public place defibrillators in improving survival after prehospital cardiopulmonary arrest. *BMJ (Clinical Research Ed.), 327*(7427), 1316. doi:10.1136/bmj.327.7427.1316 PMID:14656838

Walsh, L., Subbarao, I., Gebbie, K., Schor, K. W., Lyznicki, J., Strauss-Riggs, K., ... James, J. J. (2012). Core competencies for disaster medicine and public health. *Disaster Medicine and Public Health Preparedness*, 6(1), 44–52. doi:10.1001/dmp.2012.4 PMID:22490936

Ware, P., Ross, H., Cafazzo, J., Boodoo, C., Munnery, M., & Seto, E. (2020). Outcomes of a Heart Failure Telemonitoring Program Implemented as the Standard of Care in an Outpatient Heart Function Clinic: Pretest-Posttest Pragmatic Study. *Journal of Medical Internet Research*, 22(2), e16538. doi:10.2196/16538 PMID:32027309

Wartella, E., Rideout, V., Montague, H., Beaudoin-Ryan, L., & Lauricella, A. (2016). Teens, health and technology: A national survey. *Media and communication, 4*(3), 13-23.

Watson. (2014). A novel time–frequency-based 3D Lissajous figure method and its application to the determination of oxygen saturation from the photoplethysmogram. *Measurement Science & Technology*.

Weisfeldt, M. L., Everson-Stewart, S., Sitlani, C., Rea, T., Aufderheide, T. P., Atkins, D. L., ... Gray, R. (2011). Ventricular tachyarrhythmias after cardiac arrest in public versus at home. *The New England Journal of Medicine, 364*(4), 313–321. doi:10.1056/NEJMoa1010663 PMID:21268723

Weisfeldt, M. L., Sitlani, C. M., Ornato, J. P., Rea, T., Aufderheide, T. P., Davis, D., ... Maloney, J. (2010). Survival after application of automatic external defibrillators before arrival of the emergency medical system: Evaluation in the resuscitation outcomes consortium population of 21 million. *Journal of the American College of Cardiology, 55*(16), 1713–1720. doi:10.1016/j.jacc.2009.11.077 PMID:20394876

West, R. (2007). The PRIME Theory of motivation as a possible foundation for addiction treatment. *Drug Addiction Treatment in the 21st Century: Science and Policy Issues.*

White, C., Plotnick, L., Kushma, J., Hiltz, S. R., & Turoff, M. (2009). An online social network for emergency management. *International Journal of Emergency Management, 6*(3), 369–382. doi:10.1504/IJEM.2009.031572

Whitfield, R., Colquhoun, M., Chamberlain, D., Newcombe, R., Davies, C. S., & Boyle, R. (2005). The Department of Health National Defibrillator Programme: Analysis of downloads from 250 deployments of public access defibrillators. *Resuscitation, 64*(3), 269–277. doi:10.1016/j.resuscitation.2005.01.003 PMID:15733753

WHO. (2010). *Hospitals must be protected during natural disasters*. Retrieved from https://www.who.int/news-room/detail/11-12-2010-hospitals-must-be-protected-during-natural-disasters

WHO. (n.d.). *Malnutrition World Health Organization, 2020* .https://www.who.int/news-room/fact-sheets/detail/malnutritionDate

WHO/FAO Expert Consultation. (2003). *WHO Technical Report Series 916 Diet, Nutrition, and the Prevention of Chronic Diseases*. Geneva: WHO. Available from http://health.euroafrica.org/books/dietnutritionwho.pdf

Wicklund, E. (2020a). *Experts Weigh in on Post-COVID-19 Telehealth Rules and Policies*. Retrieved from https://mhealthintelligence.com/news/experts-weigh-in-on-post-covid-19-telehealth-rules-and-policies

Wicklund, E. (2020b). *Using Telehealth in a Pandemic: Focus on Flexibility and Scalability*. Retrieved from https://mhealthintelligence.com/news/using-telehealth-in-a-pandemic-focus-on-flexibility-scalability

Wickramasinghe, N., & Schaffer, J. (2010). *Realizing value driven eHealth solutions IBM Business of Government*. Retrieved from http://www.businessofgovernment.org/sites/default/files/Realizing%20Value%20Driven%20e-Health%20Solutions.pdf

Wickramasinghe, N. (2019). *Handbook of Research on Optimizing Healthcare Management Techniques*. IGI.

Wickramasinghe, N., John, B., George, J., & Vogel, D. (2019). Achieving Value-Based Care in Chronic Disease Management: The DiaMonD (diabetes monitoring device) Solution. *JMIR Diabetes*, *4*(2), e10368. doi:10.2196/10368 PMID:31066699

Wickramasinghe, N., & von Lubitz, D. (2007). *Knowledge-Based Enterprise: Theories and Fundamentals*. IGI Global. doi:10.4018/978-1-59904-237-4

Wildevuur, S. E., & Simonse, L. W. (2015). Information and communication technology–enabled person-centered care for the "big five" chronic conditions: Scoping review. *Journal of Medical Internet Research*, *17*(3), e77. doi:10.2196/jmir.3687 PMID:25831199

Williams, F., & Boren, S. A. (2008, December). The role of electronic medical record in care delivery in developing countries. *International Journal of Information Management*, *28*(6), 503–507. doi:10.1016/j.ijinfomgt.2008.01.016 PMID:30774175

Wilson, E. V., Wang, W., & Sheetz, S. D. (2014). Underpinning a guiding theory of patient-centered e-health. communications of the association for information systems. *Communications of the Association for Information Systems*, *34*. Advance online publication. doi:10.17705/1CAIS.03416

Woldaregay, A., Årsand, E., Botsis, T., Albers, D., Mamykina, L., & Hartvigsen, G. (2019). Data-driven blood glucose pattern classification and anomalies detection: Machine-learning applications in type 1 diabetes. *Journal of Medical Internet Research*, *21*(5), e11030. doi:10.2196/11030 PMID:31042157

World Food Programme. (2016). *Mobile vulnerability analysis and mapping (mVAM)*. Retrieved from https://www.wfp.org/publications/2016-mobile-vulnerability-analysis-mapping-mvam

World Health Organisation. (2020). *Cardiovascular diseases (CVDs)*. Retrieved from https://www.who.int/news-room/fact-sheets/detail/cardiovascular-diseases-(cvds)

World Health Organization (WHO). (2016). *Global report on diabetes: executive summary* (No. WHO/NMH/NVI/16.3). World Health Organization. Available from https://apps.who.int/iris/bitstream/handle/10665/204871/9789241565257 eng.pdf?sequence=1

World Health Organization. (2018). *Physical Activity Fact Sheet*. Retrieved from http://www.who.int/ mediacentre/factsheet

World Health Organization. (2020, March 11). *WHO Director-General's opening remarks at the media briefing on CO-VID-19 - 11 March 2020*. Retrieved May 17, 2020, from https://www.who.int/dg/speeches/detail/who-director-generals-opening-remarks-at-the-media-briefing-on-covid-19---11-march-2020

World Health Organization. (2020, March 26). *Virus origin / Reducing animal-human transmission of emerging pathogens*. Retrieved May 17, 2020, from https://www.who.int/health-topics/coronavirus/who-recommendations-to-reduce-risk-of-transmission-of-emerging-pathogens-from-animals-to-humans-in-live-animal-markets

World Health Organization. (Ed.). (2009). *Global health risks: Mortality and burden of disease attributable to selected major risks*. World Health Organization.

Wu, Y., Ding, Y., Tanaka, Y., & Zhang, W. (2014). Risk factors contributing to type 2 diabetes and recent advances in the treatment and prevention. *International Journal of Medical Sciences*, *11*(11), 1185–1200. doi:10.7150/ijms.10001 PMID:25249787

Wu, Y., Yao, X., Vespasiani, G., Nicolucci, A., Dong, Y., Kwong, J., Li, L., Sun, X., Tian, H., & Li, S. (2017). Mobile app-based interventions to support diabetes self-management: A systematic review of randomized controlled trials to identify functions associated with glycemic efficacy. *JMIR mHealth and uHealth*, *5*(3), e35. doi:10.2196/mhealth.6522 PMID:28292740

Wyatt, J. C., & Sullivan, F. (2005). eHealth and the future: Promise or peril? *BMJ (Clinical Research Ed.)*, *331*(7529), 1391–1393. doi:10.1136/bmj.331.7529.1391 PMID:16339252

Xie, J., & Deng, W. (2017). Psychosocial intervention for patients with type 2 diabetes mellitus and comorbid depression: A meta-analysis of randomized controlled trials. *Neuropsychiatric Disease and Treatment*, *13*, 2681–2690. doi:10.2147/NDT.S116465 PMID:29123401

Xie, L. J., & Cheng, M. H. (2012). Body adipose distribution among patients with type 2 diabetes mellitus. *Obesity Research & Clinical Practice*, *6*(4), e270–e279. doi:10.1016/j.orcp.2012.09.003 PMID:24331587

Xu, J., Wang, G. A., Li, J., & Chau, M. (2007). Complex problem solving: Identity matching based on social contextual information. *Journal of the Association for Information Systems*, *8*(10), 525-545.

Yacchirema, D., de Puga, J. S., Palau, C., & Esteve, M. (2018). Fall detection system for elderly people using IoT and big data. *Procedia Computer Science*, *130*, 603–610. doi:10.1016/j.procs.2018.04.110

Yang, J., Lee, J., Rao, A., & Touqan, N. (2009). Interorganizational communications in disaster management. In V. Weerakkody, M. Janssen, & Y. Dwivedi (Eds.), *Handbook of Research on ICT-Enabled Transformational Government: A Global Perspective* (pp. 240–257). IGI Global. doi:10.4018/978-1-60566-390-6.ch013

Yao, L., Sheng, Q. Z., Benatallah, B., Dustdar, S., Wang, X., Shemshadi, A., & Kanhere, S. S. (2018). WITS: An IoT-endowed computational framework for activity recognition in personalized smart homes. *Computing*, *100*(4), 369–385. doi:10.100700607-018-0603-z

Yasmin, F., Banu, B., Zakir, S. M., Sauerborn, R., Ali, L., & Souares, A. (2016). Positive influence of short message service and voice call interventions on adherence and health outcomes in case of chronic disease care: A systematic review. *BMC Medical Informatics and Decision Making*, *16*(1), 46. doi:10.118612911-016-0286-3 PMID:27106263

Ye, C., Wang, O., Liu, M., Zheng, L., Xia, M., Hao, S., ... Huang, C. (2019). A Real-Time Early Warning System for Monitoring Inpatient Mortality Risk: Prospective Study Using Electronic Medical Record Data. *Journal of Medical Internet Research*, *21*(7), e13719. doi:10.2196/13719 PMID:31278734

Ye, Q., Khan, U., Boren, S. A., Simoes, E. J., & Kim, M. S. (2018). An analysis of diabetes mobile application features compared to AADE7™: Addressing self-management behaviors in people with diabetes. *Journal of Diabetes Science and Technology*, *12*(4), 808–816. doi:10.1177/1932296818754907 PMID:29390917

Yin, J., Karimi, S., Lampert, A., Cameron, M., Robinson, B., & Power, R. (2015). *Using social media to enhance emergency situation awareness.* Paper presented at the 24th International Joint Conference on Artificial Intelligence, Buenos Aires, Argentina.

Yoo, T. (2018). *4 ways technology can help us respond to disasters.* Retrieved from https://www.weforum.org/agenda/2018/01/4-ways-technology-can-play-a-critical-role-in-disaster-response/

Zakaria, N. D., Ong, M. E. H., Gan, H. N., Foo, D., Doctor, N., Leong, B. S. H., ... Charles, R. (2014). Implications for public access defibrillation placement by non-traumatic out-of-hospital cardiac arrest occurrence in S ingapore. *Emergency Medicine Australasia*, *26*(3), 229–236. doi:10.1111/1742-6723.12174 PMID:24712826

Zarinabad, N., Meeus, E. M., Manias, K., Foster, K., & Peet, A. (2018). Automated Modular Magnetic Resonance Imaging Clinical Decision Support System (MIROR): An Application in Pediatric Cancer Diagnosis. *JMIR Medical Informatics*, *6*(2), e30. doi:10.2196/medinform.9171 PMID:29720361

Zhang, J., Chen, K., & Fan, Z. H. (2016). *Circulating Tumor Cell Isolation and Analysis. Advances in Clinical Chemistry.* Elsevier. doi:10.1016/bs.acc.2016.03.003

Zhao, J., Freeman, B., & Li, M. (2016). Can Mobile Phone Apps Influence People's Health Behavior Change? An Evidence Review. *Journal of Medical Internet Research*, *18*(11), e287. doi:10.2196/jmir.5692 PMID:27806926

Zhong, S., Clark, M., Hou, X.-Y., Zang, Y., & FitzGerald, G. (2014). Progress and challenges of disaster health management in China: A scoping review. *Global Health Action*, *7*(1), 24986. doi:10.3402/gha.v7.24986 PMID:25215910

Ziegeldorf, J. H., Morchon, O. G., & Wehrle, K. (2014). Privacy in the Internet of Things: Threats and challenges. *Security and Communication Networks*, *7*(12), 2728–2742. doi:10.1002ec.795

Zimmerman, B. J. (2000). Self-efficacy: An essential motive to learn. *Contemporary Educational Psychology*, *25*(1), 82–91. doi:10.1006/ceps.1999.1016 PMID:10620383

Ziober, B. L., Mauk, M. G., Falls, E. M., Chen, Z., Ziober, A. F., & Bau, H. H. (2007). *Lab-on-a-chip for oral cancer screening and diagnosis. Head & Neck*. Wiley-Blackwell. doi:10.1002/hed.20680

Zou, L., Liu, B., Chen, C., & Chen, C. W. (2014). Bayesian game based power control scheme for interWBAN interference mitigation. *IEEE Global Communications Conference*, 240-245.

About the Contributors

Nilmini Wickramasinghe completed five degrees at the University of Melbourne, Australia, and then accepted a full scholarship to undertake PhD studies at Case Western Reserve University's Weatherhead School of Management in Cleveland, Ohio USA in health informatics management. She later completed an executive program in value-based healthcare at Harvard Business School. For over 20 years she has been actively, researching and teaching within various aspects of digital health in both US and Australia Professor Wickramasinghe collaborates with leading scholars at various premier healthcare organizations and universities throughout Australasia, US and Europe. Professor Wickramasinghe is well published with more than 400 referred scholarly articles, more than 15 books, numerous book chapters, an encyclopaedia and a well established funded research track record. She holds a patent around analytics solution for managing healthcare data and is the editor-in-chief of two scholarly journals. In recognition of her outstanding contribution to her scientific discipline of Digital Health, Professor Wickramasinghe was awarded the 2020 Alexander von Humboldt Research Award.

* * *

Kodieswari A., Assistant Professor, Bannari Amman Institute of Technology. She is pursuing Doctoral Degree in the field of Image processing and SoC. She is interested in designing of medical diagnosing tools with the latest technology.Her area of expertise is Medical image processing, Machine learning, System on Chip and Artificial Intelligent.She was previously worked in leading Multi National Company.

Reem Abbas is a PhD candidate at Auckland University of Technology (AUT). She is interested in eHealth and is looking into finding new ways of improving healthcare delivery during natural and man-made disasters. Abbas research on cross-agency collaboration and information exchange addresses the communication challenges between clinical and emergency management personnel during disasters, and how these two groups can make effective use of the available e-health tools that are currently revolutionizing mainstream healthcare. Her research also aims at developing a curriculum that could be standardised for enhancing communication during disasters. Abbas has been influenced to the line of eHealth because it combines her technical background with her experience in international humanitarian organizations including the UN and ICRC. She is very much interested in using her technical background in impacting healthcare during disastrous situations. She is part of a team aiming to define a new discipline that combines disaster medicine, disaster management, and eHealth with the aim of revolutionizing healthcare during disasters.

Clement Chimezie Aladi (Rev. Fr.) was born in Imo state, Nigeria, in 1983. He holds a Bachelor's Degree in Philosophy and Theology from the Pontifical Urban University Rome Italy, a Bachelor's Degree in Arts from Imo State University Owerri, Nigeria, and a Master's Degree in Systems Engineering from Loyola Marymount University Los Angeles USA. He is a certified Microsoft technician and have been into IT for 11 years. He is currently a Ph.D student in Information Systems and Technology at Claremont Graduate University, Claremont, California.

Will Critchley, M.Sc. (sport sciences), MBA (International Sport Management), is a graduate student from the University of Jyväskylä (Finland) and a sport technology specialist. He has previously done research with endurance athletes. He is also working in the field of sport and exercise psychology and is therefore interested in combining psychology and the use of technology in order to promote healthier and more physically active lifestyle to various populations.

Omar El-Gayar, Ph.D., is a Professor of Information Systems at Dakota State University. Dr. El-Gayar has an extensive administrative experience at the college and university levels as the Dean for the College of Information Technology, United Arab Emirates University (UAEU) and the Founding Dean of Graduate Studies and Research, Dakota State University. His research interests include: analytics, business intelligence, and decision support with applications in problem domain areas such as healthcare, environmental management, and security planning and management. His inter-disciplinary educational background and training is in information technology, computer science, economics, and operations research. Dr. El-Gayar's industry experience includes working as an analyst, modeler, and programmer. His numerous publications appear in various information technology related fields. He is a member of AIS, ACM, INFORMS, and DSI.

C. Suganthi Evangeline is currently working as Assistant Professor, Department of Electrical Technology at Karunya University, Coimbatore, India. She is pursuing her Ph.D. as part time researcher in Vehicular Communication at School of Electronics Engineering, VIT University, Vellore. Her main research areas are Vehicular Communication Networks and Embedded Systems. She received her Masters in Communication Engineering at Coimbatore Institute of Technology.

Abdur Forkan received his PhD degree in Computer Science from RMIT University. He is an early career researcher working in the area of digital health and data analytics. He is currently a Senior Research Engineer (Software and Data Analytics) in Digital Innovation Lab of Swinburne University of Technology. His research interests include health informatics, applied machine learning, data science, ubiquitous computing and cloud computing. He has published in top-ranked journals and conferences. He received RMIT CSIT publication award in 2015. He also worked as Software Engineer in Relisoruce Technologies Ltd, a leading USA-based software outsourcing company in Dhaka, Bangladesh from 2007 to 2012. There he worked in different software projects for world-renown companies such as Warner Brother's, MEI Group, and Electronic Arts.

Rima Artonian Gibbings has worked as an application developer in healthcare systems and she is an assistant professor at the University of North Georgia and an associate teacher at the University of Illinois in Chicago. As a health informatics researcher, she offers a technical approach that links her background in application development with public health topics, addressing current technical requirements.

Prem Prakash Jayaraman is the Head of Digital Innovation Lab at Department at Swinburne University of Technology. Previously he was a Post Doctoral Research Scientist in the Digital Productivity and Services Flagship of Commonwealth Scientific and Industrial Research Organization (CSIRO – Australian Government's Premier Research Agency). He is broadly interested in the research areas of Internet of Things, Mobile and Cloud Computing, Health Informatics and application of Data Science techniques and methodologies in real-world settings. He was a key contributors and one of the architects of the Open Source Internet of Things project (OpenIoT) that has won the prestigious Black Duck Rookie of the Year Award in 2013 (https://github.com/OpenIotOrg/openiot). He is recipient of Swinburne's Vice Chancellor's Team Award for Digital Innovation in 2018 and is the recipient of 2 best paper awards (IEA-AIE 2010 and HICSS 2016) and several hackathon challenges including, Unearthed Mining Hackathon 2015, Melbourne, The 4th International Conference on IoT (2014) at MIT media lab, Cambridge, MA and IoT Week 2014, London.

R. Jegan completed his B.Tech in Electronics and Communication Engineering from Anna University, Chennai M.Tech in Embedded Systems from Karunya University, Coimbatore. He received PhD in biomedical research area from Anna University, Chennai, India. Currently he is working as assistant professor in the Programme of Electronics and Instrumentation/ Biomedical Engineering, Karunya University, Coimbatore. He has 8 years of teaching experience. He has published 35 papers in international journals and Conferences. He has guided more than 30 M.Tech research scholars. He has received best researcher award in the year 2013-2014 in the field of biomedical engineering.

Shane Joachim is a Master of Information and Communication Technologies (Research - Computer Science) student at Swinburne University of Technology. Apart of his thesis, he is currently researching in the area of digital health. Shane is currently a Product Developer at a Microsoft associate company. Over his time there, Shane has produced software solutions for clients such as Bhpbilliton (BHB), Metro, Reece, Telstra, and United Nations High Commissioner for Refugees (UNHCR). He is also a part of the Digital Innovation Lab at Swinburne University of Technology. Shane's research interests range from a number of topics, such as health informatics, Internet of Things, health 4.0 and data science.

Tuomas Kari, D.Sc. (Econ. and Bus.Adm.), is a Postdoctoral Researcher (Information Systems Science) at the Institute for Advanced Management Systems Research (Turku, Finland). He also acts as a research fellow at the University of Jyväskylä, Finland. His dissertation was about the usage of exergames. His research interest is the use of technology in everyday life, especially in the context of health and wellness. His topics of research include exergaming, sports-, health-, and wellness technology, self-tracking, information systems usage, user behavior, adoption and diffusion, gamification, and e-sports among others. He has published, for example, in Information Systems Journal, International Conference on Information Systems (ICIS), CHI Play, International Journal of Networking and Virtual Organizations, Journal of Virtual Worlds Research, and International Journal of Gaming and Computer-Mediated Simulations

Eeva Kettunen, M.Sc. (Sport Sciences), MBA (International Business), is a Doctoral student researcher (Information Systems, Sport Sciences) at the University of Jyväskylä (Finland). Her dissertation topic is related to sport and wellness technology and what how can it be used to motivate people towards more physically active lifestyle. Her studies are focused especially on digital coaching as well as on physical activity of teenagers. Due to her sport and exercise psychology background her research interest is combining psychology and the use of technology in order to promote healthier and more physically active lifestyle to various populations.

Eila Lindfors, Professor in Craft, Design and Technology Education since 2013, works at the University of Turku in the Faculty of Education, Finland. One of her main research interests is safety and security in education. She has published over 100 research articles in refereed journals and chaired several Safety and Security in Education symposia.

Samaneh Madanian is a lecturer at the Department of Computer Science with a multi-disciplinary background and profile. She graduated from Staffordshire University with a Master's in IT Management (2010) in which she worked on the application of Radio Frequency Identification (RFID) in supply chains. After obtaining her Master's, she worked in the industry for several years as a business analyst and project manager, focusing specifically on requirement analysis, integrated system analysis and design. Her PhD, in Disaster e-Health (DEH) completed in 2019, focused on the applications of RFID and other e-health technologies to disaster management and disaster medicine. Her industrial experience, coupled with her current research in health informatics and her passion for teaching, allows her to continue to bridge the gap between academia and industry. Mandanian's research focuses on the applications of e-health technologies in healthcare, disaster management and disaster medicine which require innovative and practical solutions if they are to enhance people's quality of life.

Markus Makkonen, D.Sc. (Econ.), is a Postdoctoral Researcher (Information Systems) at the Institute for Advanced Management Systems Research (Turku, Finland). He also acts as a Visiting Researcher at the University of Jyväskylä (Finland). His research interests include technology acceptance and use, consumer behavior, and data science, especially in the contexts of electronic commerce, digital products and services, as well as sports and wellness technologies. His research has been previously published in outlets such as the Journal of Management Information Systems (JMIS), the International Journal of Information Management (IJIM), and the Communications of the Association for Information Systems (CAIS).

Anitha Mary X. completed her B.E Electronics and Instrumentation Engineeing from Karunya University, Coimbatore in the year 2001 and M.E in VLSI Design from ANNA University, Coimbatore in the year 2009. She has completed Ph.D in control system from Karunya University. she has published several international journals. Her area of interest is Embedded Systems, Control and Instrumentation, Biomedical Applications.

Ahsan Morshed commenced working in CQUniversity in May 2019 as a Lecturer in ICT. His research interests are the Machine Learning, Deep Learning, Big data, Visual Analytics, Explainable AI and Learning Analytics. Ahsan holds a PhD from the University of Trento, Italy and a Master from KTH, Sweden in the field of Computer Science. Before joining CQUniversity, he worked as a Research Fellow at Swinburne Data Science Research Institute, Swinburne University of Technology where he was actively participating in multi-disciplinary Data Science projects in collaboration with different faculties and industries. Furthermore, he worked as a senior project officer (equivalent to Data Scientist) at RMIT University and he worked as a Postdoctoral fellow at Data61, CSIRO, Australia and he worked on sensor data integration and machine learning area at CSIRO in Agriculture domain. Furthermore, he was also an information management Specialist in the OEKC division at Food and Agriculture Organization of United Nations (FAO of UN), Rome, Italy. Dr. Morshed has published over 50 peer-reviewed a book, a book chapter, journals, conference and workshop papers. Dr. Morshed is an affiliated ACM, IEEE, HISA and ACS member. Dr. Morshed has 691 citations and an h-index of 12 according to google citation.

Martinson Ofori is a PhD in Information Systems student at Dakota State University. He has worked as a Software Developer and Solutions Architect in the Banking and Telecom industries. With a specialty in decision support and analytics, Martinson's current research interests focus on two areas: designing persuasive systems to induce behavior change and the use of analytics in agriculture.Generally, however, his research covesr healthcare, agriculture, knowledge management, and project management. Martinson holds a BS and MS in Computer Science, an MBA in Fincance, and is a member of AIS and IEEE.

Shankar S. is currently working as Professor in the Department of CSE/IT at Hindusthan College of Engineering and Technology, Coimbatore. He has completed his Ph.D in Computer Science and Engineering at Anna University, Coimbatore. He has 15 years of teaching experience. He is an IBM certified DB2 professional and has obtained Brain Bench certification in various disciplines. He has presented a number of papers in various National and International conferences. Two of his papers were published in IEEE Explore. He has guided a number of research-oriented as well as application oriented projects organized by well known companies like IBM. He has to his credit 12 International journal publications with good Impact Factor. His research interests include Data Mining, Soft Computing and Database Management Systems, Big Data Analytics, Network Security and Cloud Computing.

Juergen Seitz is professor for business information systems and head of the business information systems department at Baden-Wuerttemberg Cooperative State University Heidenheim, Germany. He is co-chair of several international conferences and associated editor of several international journals. His areas of interest are digital health, digital finance, and cryptocurrencies.

Philip Smart is a Specialist Colorectal surgeon. He studied Medicine at the University of Melbourne and Royal Melbourne Hospital Clinical School, graduating in 1999. He completed surgical training at Royal Melbourne Hospital, obtaining a Fellowship in General Surgery in 2009. He completed 3 years of subspecialist training in Colon and Rectal surgery, including a Clinical Fellowship in 2013 at the Cleveland Clinic, Ohio USA, one of the leading colorectal surgery units in the world. He completed a Doctor of Medical Science degree (D.Med.Sci) at the University of Melbourne under the supervision of Professor A.Heriot and A/Prof J.Mackay. In addition, he holds a degree in Clinical Research Methods through Monash University. He completed Robotic Surgery Training at the Cleveland Clinic, Ohio, and Methodist Hospital, Texas. He is currently the Deputy Director in the Department of Surgery, Anaesthesia and Procedural Medicine at Austin Health, Head of Surgery at The Surgery Centre, Austin Health, Deputy Director of the Gastrointestinal Clinical Institute at Epworth HealthCare and Chair of the Operations Committee for the Binational Colorectal Cancer Audit (BCCA). He holds public hospital appointments at both Austin and Eastern Health.

Brita Somerkoski (phD Education) is a special researcher at the University of Turku, Department of Teacher Education. Her research interests include school and occupational safety, future technologies, injury prevention, safety promotion, multicultural issues, gender equality, student internationalization, learning outcomes and curriculum research.

Reima Suomi is a professor of Information Systems Science at University of Turku, and a part-time professor at Huazhong Normal University, Wuhan, Hubei, China, as well as a guest professor in Wuhan University of Business and Technology. He has been a professor at Turku School of Economics and Business Administration, Finland since 1994. He is a docent for the universities of Turku and Oulu, Finland. Years 1992-93 he spent as a "Vollamtlicher Dozent" in the University of St. Gallen, Switzerland, where he led a research project on business process re-engineering. Winter semester 2013-2014 he was a visiting professor at University of St. Gallen, Switzerland, and in 2013 a visiting researcher at University of Münster, Germany. Currently he concentrates on topics around management of networked activities, including issues such as management of telecommunication networks, electronic and mobile services, virtual organizations, telework and competitive advantage through telecommunication-based information systems. Different governance structures in the management of IS and are enabled by IS belong too to his research agenda, as well as application of information systems in health care.

Oleg Sytnik was born in Dneprodzerginsk, Ukraine, on May 17, 1958. He received the M.S. degree in radio engineering from the Kharkov University of Radio Electronics, Kharkov in 1980. He worked in the Design Bureau of Machine-Building Plant of Dnipropetrovsk (1980-1982), and then at the Radio Engineering Department of the Kharkov University of Radio Electronics (1982-1986). He received the Ph.D. degree in radars and navigation from the Kharkov University of Radio Electronics, Kharkov, in 1986. Since 1986 he has worked as a senior researcher at the A. Ya. Usikov Institute for Radio Physics and Electronics under the National Academy of Sciences of Ukraine in the Department of Radiophysical Introscopy and in the A.I. Kalmykov Center for Remote Sensing of the Earth under the Space Agency of Ukraine. During this time he received the Dr. Sci. degree in Radio Physics and Mathematics and Professor (2005). He has published over 163 science papers in radars theory, digital signal processing and applications. His fields of research interests are radars, digital signal and image processing, pattern recognition and stochastic non-stationary processes.

Aman Tyagi received his Ph.D. degree from Dayalbagh Educational Institute, Dayalbagh, Agra, India in 2019. He submitted his Ph.D. thesis on the topic "Healthcare Engineering: An innovative approach for better delivery of asthma care services". He was awarded Senior Research Fellowship by University Grant Commission, India. He worked as an Assistant Professor in Shri Rawatpura Sarkar Institute of Technology & Science, Datia, India and Himalayan Garhwal University, Pauri Garhwal, Uttarakhand, India. His research area of interest includes Healthcare Management and Decision Support System. He published his research work in International Journals of repute. He reviewed research papers for many International Journals.

Chinazunwa Uwaoma is a research assistant professor in the Center for Information Systems and Technology (CISAT) at Claremont Graduate University, USA. Dr. Uwaoma's research borders on the application of emerging mobile technologies and embedded systems to improve the quality of life, education, and social interaction among the underserved strata of the society. Her other research interests include communication network designs, Internet of Things, decision engineering, and healthcare. She received her PhD in computer science and MSc in digital technology from the University of the West

Indies, Jamaica. She has been involved in research projects such as design and implementation of embedded security systems, and configuring smartphones to monitor chronic health conditions, as well as other health related issues.

Saranya Vasanthamani received her B.Tech degree in Information Technology from Anna University in 2009 and M.E Software Engineering in Anna University in 2011. She is a part time research scholar in Sri Krishna College of Engineering and Technology, pursuing Ph.D in Anna University Chennai. She is currently an Assistant Professor in Department of Information Technology in Sri Krishna College of Engineering and Technology, Coimbatore. Her main research interest includes Resource Management in sensor networks and routing in self organizing networks. Have published papers in National and International Conferences and Journals on network security, resource management. She is an member in IAENG.

Cynthia Wong is a sessional lecturer at Monash University & a health statistics researcher at Swinburne University of Technology. She received her Master of Applied Econometrics degree from Monash University and she is pursuing her PhD degree in Health Sciences at Swinburne University of Technology. Cynthia is a member of the Australasian Institute of Digital Health (AIDH). Her research interests include econometric modelling, statistical analysis, health economics, health statistics, epidemiology, biostatistics, diabetes, cardiovascular disease, femur fracture surgery & digital health.

Index

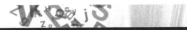
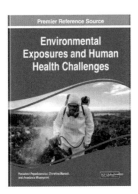
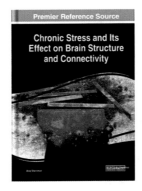
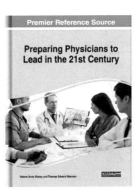
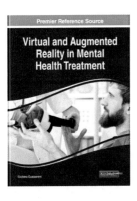
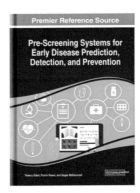
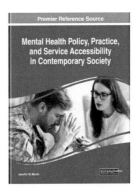
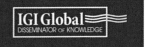

Ensure Quality Research is Introduced to the Academic Community

Become an IGI Global Reviewer for Authored Book Projects

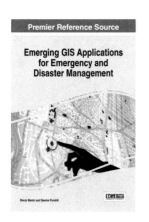
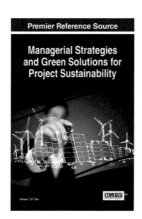
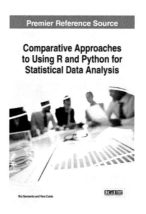
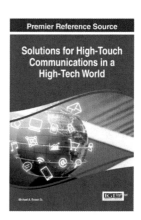

The overall success of an authored book project is dependent on quality and timely reviews.

In this competitive age of scholarly publishing, constructive and timely feedback significantly expedites the turnaround time of manuscripts from submission to acceptance, allowing the publication and discovery of forward-thinking research at a much more expeditious rate. Several IGI Global authored book projects are currently seeking highly-qualified experts in the field to fill vacancies on their respective editorial review boards:

Applications and Inquiries may be sent to:
development@igi-global.com

Applicants must have a doctorate (or an equivalent degree) as well as publishing and reviewing experience. Reviewers are asked to complete the open-ended evaluation questions with as much detail as possible in a timely, collegial, and constructive manner. All reviewers' tenures run for one-year terms on the editorial review boards and are expected to complete at least three reviews per term. Upon successful completion of this term, reviewers can be considered for an additional term.

If you have a colleague that may be interested in this opportunity,
we encourage you to share this information with them.

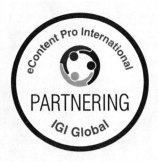

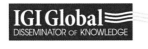

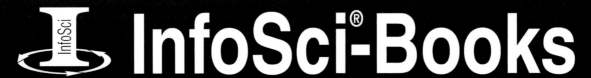
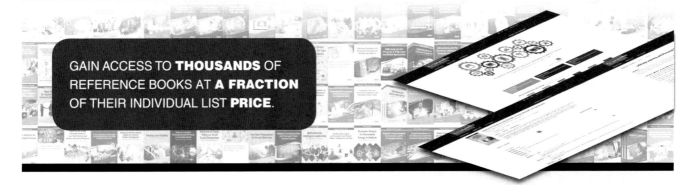

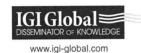
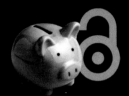
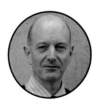

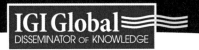
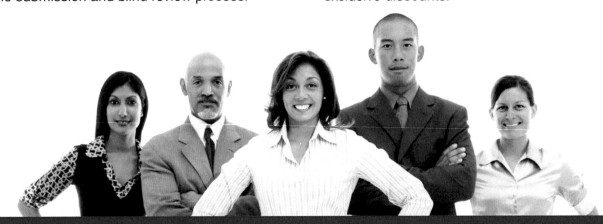

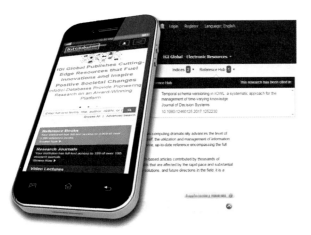
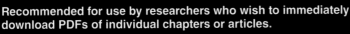
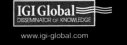

Printed in the United States
By Bookmasters